Primary Health Care

Primary Health Care

Edited by **Kelly Ward**

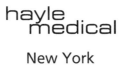

New York

Published by Hayle Medical,
30 West, 37th Street, Suite 612,
New York, NY 10018, USA
www.haylemedical.com

Primary Health Care
Edited by Kelly Ward

International Standard Book Number: 978-1-63241-324-6 (Hardback)

Contents

Preface

"In both, clinical practitioners and scientists, few find it more convenient to depend upon irrelevant clarifications, while the rest never stop looking for answers". With these astonishing words, Augusto Murri, an Italian veteran in clinical medicine, emphasizes on the fact that medical practice must be a constant journey towards knowledge and quality of care. This book is a compilation of contributions from across the globe. Distinct cultures are portrayed together, from those with developed technologies to those of indefinite spirituality, but they are all associated to each other through 5 professional characteristics, that in the 1978 the Institute of Medicine (IOM) stated as most important for practicing good Primary Care: coordination, accessibility, accountability, comprehensiveness and continuity. The content in this book is organized under two characteristics - coordination and accessibility. This would provide the reader with an international overview of hot topics and novel insights in the area.

Various studies have approached the subject by analyzing it with a single perspective, but the present book provides diverse methodologies and techniques to address this field. This book contains theories and applications needed for understanding the subject from different perspectives. The aim is to keep the readers informed about the progresses in the field; therefore, the contributions were carefully examined to compile novel researches by specialists from across the globe.

Indeed, the job of the editor is the most crucial and challenging in compiling all chapters into a single book. In the end, I would extend my sincere thanks to the chapter authors for their profound work. I am also thankful for the support provided by my family and colleagues during the compilation of this book.

Editor

Section 1

Coordination and Integration in Primary Care

Section 1

Coordination and Integration in Primary Care

Serum Ferritin and Iron Studies – Laboratory Reporting and Clinical Application in Primary Care

Catherine Ogilvie and Edward Fitzsimons
Department of Haematology, Gartnavel General Hospital, Glasgow,
UK

1. Introduction

In the primary care setting blood samples are frequently taken, following clinical assessment, in order to determine a patient's iron status. This chapter will describe the laboratory tests used to assess iron status and explain interpretation of results with respect to both iron deficiency and iron overload.

Reduced serum ferritin values confirm iron deficiency and are hugely helpful in the investigation of patients with anaemia. It has however, also been shown that elevated serum ferritin is a common finding in the primary care population (Ogilvie et al, 2010) and that General Practioners (GPs) may require more guidance from Haematologists in the management of patients with raised serum ferritin levels. This will be explained and discussed with the aim of ultimately improving the diagnosis of serious underlying conditions including Hereditary Haemochromatosis (HHC).

2. Laboratory tests

Laboratory tests assessing body iron status are performed in both the Haematology and Biochemistry departments. Serum ferritin and iron studies are most commonly requested.

2.1 Serum ferritin

In simple terms ferritin can be described as the intracellular protein which safely stores excess iron. Tiny amounts of ferritin can be detected in serum and this serum ferritin is the most frequently measured surrogate for body iron stores. The normal range for serum ferritin is generally regarded as 15-300µg/l. There is no known physiological role for serum ferritin but the results of quantitative phlebotomy studies have shown that 1µg/l of ferritin in serum is approximately equivalent to 8mg of stored reticuloendothelial system body iron. (Worwood, 1982).

Serum ferritin shows an acute phase response and can be elevated in a variety of inflammatory, metabolic, hepatic and neoplastic disorders. This can make it difficult to recognise iron deficiency in patients with inflammatory disorders as such disorders can cause serum ferritin to be elevated to levels inappropriate to the reticuloendothelial iron store.

There are however also well recognised conditions that lead to gross inappropriate elevation of serum ferritin; hepatitis, juvenile Stills disease and disseminated malignancy.

We know that total body iron content is 4g, with a daily requirement of only 1-2mg of iron. Body iron content is regulated by complex controls over iron absorption in the upper small bowel. The average Western diet provides 15-20mg of iron each day which is far in excess of the body requirement of 1-2mg iron per day. There are no regulatory pathways to eliminate iron from the body and losses occur only through shedding of cells in the GI tract, skin desquamation, pregnancy and menstrual loss.

Around 3g of total body iron is present in mature or developing red blood cells. In the developing red cells, the erythroblasts, iron (Fe^{3+}) is converted to iron (Fe^{2+}) and is then combined with protoporphyrin to form haem. Haem is then combined with 2 alpha globin and 2 beta globin chains to form haemoglobin.

The reticuloendothelial system is the main storage site of iron with approximately 0.5g of iron being found in macrophages. The reticuloendothelial system acquires its storage iron from the ingestion of effete red blood cells (lifespan 120 days) whereas other tissues accept iron from transferrin via transferrin receptors on the cell surface. Iron is found in all tissues but particularly as myoglobin in muscle, in hepatocytes and in many essential enzymes. Iron based enzymes can contain haem e.g. cytochrome P450 family, myeloperoxidase, lactoperoxidase and catalase or be non-haem iron based e.g. NADH dehydrogenase and the lipoxygenases.

2.2 Iron sudies

Iron studies in most laboratories include serum iron levels, serum transferrin or total iron binding capacity (TIBC), and transferrin saturation. Total iron binding capacity is a measurement of the maximum amount of iron that can be carried. It is therefore an indirect measurement of transferrin.

The most useful test in assessing iron supply to the tissues is transferrin saturation. Transferrin is a glycoprotein synthesised in the liver and is responsible for the transportation of iron (Fe^{3+}) in serum. This glycoprotein has 2 iron binding domains and is normally 30% saturated with iron. In iron deficiency, reduced transferrin saturation leads to iron deprivation for erythroblasts. In iron overload raised transferrin saturation leads to parenchymal iron overload.

In iron deficiency anaemia the serum iron level falls. As a result the liver is stimulated to synthesise more transferrin and the transferrin saturation falls (usually <15%). In Hereditary Haemochromatosis (HHC), a condition characterised by iron overload, iron levels rise, transferrin synthesis is reduced and transferrin saturation may reach 100%.

Serum iron concentration is a measurement of circulating iron (Fe^{3+}) bound to transferrin. Only 0.1% of total body iron is bound to transferrin at any one time. In addition, the transferrin iron pool turns over 10-20 times each day which is reflected in varying serum iron levels. Serum iron levels can fluctuate throughout the day so that measurement of serum iron concentration alone provides little useful clinical information.

Normal Iron Homeostasis

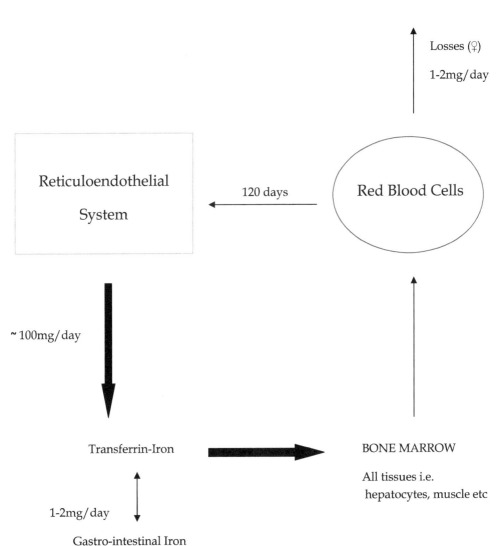

Fig. 1. Normal Iron Homeostasis

3. Iron deficiency

The majority of laboratory requests for serum ferritin and iron studies are made following a clinical suspicion of possible iron deficiency. As iron deficiency develops transferrin saturation falls to <15% and serum ferritin levels are reduced. Thereafter full blood count (FBC) parameters become abnormal, with reduced haemoglobin, low mean corpuscular haemoglobin (MCH) and low mean corpuscular volume (MCV) i.e. a hypochromic microcytic anaemia.

In the developed world IDA is most commonly seen in young women as a result of menstruation and pregnancies (each pregnancy costs the mother 500mg of iron through iron transfer to foetus and blood loss at delivery). However IDA also occurs in 2-5% of males and post-menopausal females. Blood loss from the gastro-intestinal (GI) tract is the most common cause. The British Society of Gastroenterology recommends upper and lower GI investigations and to consider screening for coeliac disease. (Goddard et al, 2011)

Specific issues are relevant in primary care. General Practioners often prescribe iron supplements and should be aware of the different elemental iron content of each preparation. For example, ferrous fumarate 210mg contains 68mg iron whereas ferrous gluconate 300mg contains 35mg iron. The amount of elemental iron often influences tolerability. Main side effects are gastrointestinal e.g. nausea and constipation. When such side effects lead to non compliance we suggest changing to a preparation containing less elemental iron. Patients who continue to have difficulty or cannot tolerate tablets may benefit from a syrup preparation. Syrups enable a smaller dose of elemental iron to be given. Parental infusions of iron should be reserved for those few patients who despite lower doses remain intolerant of oral iron. Iron infusion is also a treatment option for non compliant patients with significant anaemia. These patients should be referred and managed in secondary care.

Recurrent IDA can be difficult to manage. In a male or post menopausal female patient with normal upper and lower GI endoscopies it can be difficult to determine when repeat investigations or further procedures e.g small bowel examination are needed. In these cases however reassurance must be taken from the endoscopic exclusion of GI malignancy as the cause of IDA. Clinical assessment, severity of anaemia, speed of recurrence and response to iron supplements can be helpful. Any patients causing ongoing concern should be referred to secondary care.

4. Anaemia of Chronic Disease (ACD)

Anaemia of chronic disease (ACD) is used to describe the anaemia that develops in response to chronic illness despite normal haematinic levels (normal B12, folate and ferritin) and without blood loss. Serum iron falls but unlike IDA the transferrin level also falls (Fitzsimons et al, 2002). There are 3 main causes of ACD; inflammatory, infectious or malignant disorders. ACD can cause either a normochromic normocytic anaemia or a hypochromic microcytic anaemia. The latter may be difficult to distinguish from iron deficiency anaemia as the serum ferritin level may be elevated by the acute phase response. However, in most cases of ACD the level of storage iron remains the most important factor controlling serum ferritin concentration. Serum ferritin levels >100µg/l are thought to indicate iron replete status and the presence of storage iron in inflammatory states – so excluding iron deficiency (Witte 1991). Measurement of other acute phase proteins e.g. C-reactive protein (CRP), erythrocyte sedimentation rate (ESR) and good clinical history and examination can help to distinguish ACD from IDA. Measurement of serum soluble transferring receptor (sTfR) can reliably distinguish IDA from ACD but this assay is seldom available from UK laboratories.

In ACD treatment of the underlying condition is the most important factor in correcting the anaemia. Many inflammatory conditions are managed in secondary or tertiary care and the use of monoclonal antibody therapy to inhibit cytokine response e.g. Infliximab in rheumatoid arthritis and inflammatory bowel disease has greatly influenced the course of such diseases and their associated chronic anaemias.

General Practioners however may be required to manage chronic dysproteinaemic anaemia. This is often seen in patients with polymyalgia rheumatica (PMR) or temporal arteritis (TA). It can however be found without features of either PMR or TA. The anaemia is often hypochromic, microcytic and associated with elevated ESR >100mm/h, raised globulins without paraprotein. The anaemia is extremely sensitive to steroid although a small maintenance dose of prednisolone (ie 5mg daily) may be required longterm to maintain a normal haemoglobin. . (Fitzsimons and Brock, 2001)

5. Summary of laboratory findings

The table below summarises laboratory findings in the normal state, in iron deficiency anaemia, hereditary haemochromatosis and anaemia of chronic disease.

	Normal	Iron deficiency Anaemia	Hereditary Haemochromatosis	Anaemia of Chronic Disease
Serum Ferritin	$\leftrightarrow$ (15-300µg/l)	↓	↑	$\leftrightarrow$ / ↑
Transferrin Saturation	$\leftrightarrow$ (15-30%)	↓	↑	↓
Serum Iron	$\leftrightarrow$ (10-30µg/l)	↓	↑	↓

Table 1. Summary of Laboratory Findings

6. Hereditary Haemochromatosis

Hereditary Haemochromatosis (HHC) is a particularly important diagnosis to be considered in the further investigation of patients with unexplained elevated serum ferritin level.

6.1 Genetics of Hereditary Haemochromatosis

Hereditary Haemochromatosis is inherited as an autosomal recessive disorder and is one of the most common single gene disorders in the North European population. In the United Kingdom (UK) it is estimated that approximately 250,000 people have the genetic predisposition yet only some 5000 people have been formerly diagnosed with HHC.

The human haemochromatosis protein is named HFE – High iron (Fe). The mutation most commonly associated with HHC is the C282Y mutation. In the UK 8-12% of the population is heterozygous for C282Y (ie. carriers of HHC) and more than 90% of HHC cases are HFE homozygous for C282Y. Approximately 6% of cases are compound heterozygote for

C282Y/H63D. The cellular mechanisms by which HFE leads to increased iron gastro-intestinal iron absorption and raised serum iron levels are not understood.

6.2 Clinical features and treatment

As transferrin saturation rises to >50% tissue iron uptake increases and can lead to end organ damage; hepatic cirrhosis (and hepatocellular carcinoma), cardiomyopathy, pituitary and thyroid gland impairment, diabetes mellitus, skin pigmentation (bronze diabetes), hypogonadism and arthropathy. The presenting features can therefore be varied and diagnosis delayed until iron stores are greatly increased (20-30g) and tissue damage has occurred. Disease is seldom evident at age <30yrs. Early diagnosis and damage prevention is essential. All morbidities, once the condition is recognised, can be either prevented or lessened with simple treatment – venesection.

Phlebotomy is used to treat HHC with up to one unit of blood (500ml = 250mg iron) being venesected weekly. Serum ferritin and transferrin saturation are used to guide frequency of venesection (BCSH, 2002). The aim is to normalise iron stores - ferritin and transferrin saturation - and prevent end organ damage. Once this is achieved maintenance venesection should be tailored to maintain serum ferritin level <50µg/l and transferrin saturation <50%. It should be noted that in some patients transferrin saturations can remain >50% despite serum ferritin <50µg/l. We would suggest that these patients require more aggressive venesection programmes.

6.3 Laboratory findings

Biochemically HHC is characterised by an elevated (often grossly elevated) serum ferritin level, raised serum iron and increased transferrin saturation.

Serum ferritin is highly sensitive to iron overload in HHC (BCSH guideline 2002). A high serum ferritin level however has low specificity for HHC as the majority of patients with raised ferritin levels do not have HHC. Careful clinical history taking and examination are therefore important. Subsequent appropriate investigations and interpretation of other acute phase proteins should enable prompt diagnosis of other conditions e.g. inflammatory or neoplastic conditions. It is important to note that, even when HHC has been excluded, a serum ferritin level >1000µg/l is often indicative of serious underlying pathology e.g disseminated malignancy, liver disease of any aetiology, inflammatory arthropathy.

Serum ferritin is often elevated in hepatic cirrhosis of any aetiology. This is a major confounding factor in the use of serum ferritin in the diagnosis of HHC. The liver reticuloendothelial cells contain storage iron. The hepatocytes are a rich source of iron containing enzymes and ferritin. Any process which damages liver cells will release hepatic ferritin into the serum, causing an elevated level. It is also possible that liver impairment may interfere with the clearance of ferritin from the circulation and so further contribute to elevated levels.

The combination of a raised serum ferritin level and increased transferrin saturation however is a powerful predictor for the clinical condition of HHC. A transferrin saturation >50% together with a raised serum ferritin level is predictive of homozygosity for the C282Y mutation of the HFE gene in 90% of males and 75% of females (Gordeuk et al 2008).

6.4 Genotype versus phenotype

Assessment of body iron stores is of upmost importance in the diagnosis of HHC. Although the genetic predisposition to HHC is common, the disease penetrance is low i.e. not all people with the genetic predisposition for HHC go on to develop any evidence of iron overload or clinical disease.

Approximately 1 in 300 people in the UK are homozygous for the C282Y mutation. However, only 38-50% of C282Y homozygotes will develop laboratory evidence of iron overload and 10-33% will develop any end organ damage (Whitlock et al 2006). The other factors influencing disease penetrance are not yet clearly established. Consequently, the UK National Screening Committee does not recommend molecular screening for HFE C282Y mutation in the asymptomatic population.

We would recommend transferrin saturation as initial further investigation of elevated serum ferritin level. Clinical history and examination remain important as do other routine targeted laboratory investigations e.g liver enzymes. HFE genotyping is likely to be appropriate in patients with raised serum ferritin values when the transferrin saturation level ≥50%.

6.5 Family screening

Family screening is required for relatives of a patient with HHC.

Such screening is important primarily to identify further homozygotes and to ensure prevention of iron overload and tissue damage. Secondly, screening allows reassurance of heterozygotes and those with a normal genotype.

Laboratory screening tests should comprise assessment of iron stores (serum ferritin, serum iron and transferrin saturation) and HFE genotyping. Siblings and offspring of an affected family member should be screened. Given the high frequency of heterozygotes in the population (~10% in the UK), we would suggest that partners of known homozygous patients and heterozygous carriers should also be screened to identify the potential risk to any offspring. If both parents are heterozygous each child will have a 1 in 4 chance of being homozygous. If one parent is homozygous and the other heterozygous the risk of any child being homozygous is 1 in 2.

Family members should be counselled as to the mode of inheritance of HHC, the importance of early diagnosis and the effectiveness and ease of treatment i.e iron overload and tissue damage can be prevented by simple venesection.

The cartoon below (Figure 2) schematically demonstrates transferrin saturation; the transferrin protein (Y) combining with iron ( ). Two atoms of ferric iron bind to each transferrin molecule.

7. Elevated serum ferritin levels in primary care

Primary care physicians are often familiar with low serum ferritin values and the investigation and treatment of iron deficiency anaemia. However, a need for guidance in further investigation of elevated serum ferritin has recently been identified (Ogilvie et al, 2010).

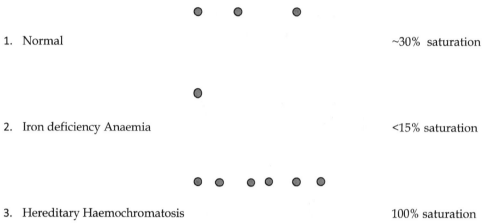

1. Normal   ~30% saturation

2. Iron deficiency Anaemia   <15% saturation

3. Hereditary Haemochromatosis   100% saturation

4. Anaemia of Chronic Disease   Reduced Tf/reduced saturation

Fig. 2. The transferrin protein and iron binding.

7.1 West of Scotland experience

Greater Glasgow and Clyde (GG&C) is located on the West coast of Scotland and is the largest single Health Board in Scotland with a population of 1.4 million. During 2009 a total of 158,495 serum ferritin measurements were performed. Approximately 50% of samples were referred from primary care and 50% of these from patients >30 years of age. We surveyed all serum ferritin results obtained in our hospital from patients aged >30yrs in primary care during a 6 month period. All requests were initiated by the General Practioner and included 3029 females (73%) and 1141 males (27%).

Only 8% of women aged 30-50 years had serum ferritin levels >100µg/l. In this age group IDA is the most frequent abnormalilty of iron metabolism reflecting the effects of menstruation and child birth. Mean serum ferritin levels rose progressively with female age. Serum ferritin levels >200µg/l were seen in 7.5% of women aged 50-59 years, 13% of women aged 60-69 years and 17% of women aged over 70 years. In contrast, irrespective of age, 17% of males over 30 years had serum ferritin levels >300µg/l. (Tables 2 and 3).

A total of 59 patients had grossly elevated serum ferritin levels >1000µg/l (30 males, 29 females). A review of the electronic individual patient case record was performed. In 27 cases the grossly elevated serum ferritin level had been noted and an explanation given. 1 patient was found to have Hereditary Haemochromatosis (HHC); 18 patients had non HHC liver disease (alcoholic liver disease, hepatitis C, hepatic steatosis). 10 of these 18 patients had HHC excluded (confirmed HFE genotype negative); 7 patients had disseminated malignancy. 1 patient had iron overload secondary to frequent packed red cell transfusion – required due to prosthetic cardiac valve haemolysis.

However, more than half of patients (n=32) with grossly elevated serum ferritin levels were neither investigated nor referred to secondary care. The investigation of patients with serum ferritin values >1000μg/l is particularly important as it has been shown that the risk of cirrhosis in HHC occurs only with serum ferritin levels >1000μg/l. HHC is an easily treatable condition once identified. Iron depletion via venesection (500mls whole blood = 250mg iron) can prevent end organ damage e.g. liver cirrhosis, diabetes. In addition, given the proportion of patients not further investigated, it is clear that more guidance to GPs on further management of these patients is needed.

Male Patients	Ferritin >100μg/l	>200μg/l	300-1000μg/l	>1000μg/l
Age 30-49yrs	153 (58%)	80 (30%)	47 (18%)	11 (4%)
50-69yrs	209 (53%)	118 (31%)	66 (17%)	9 (2%)
70yrs +	245 (50%)	130 (26%)	84 (17%)	11 (2%)

Table 2. Ferritin values in male patients >30yrs in Primary Care.

Female Patients	Ferritin >100μg/l	>200μg/l	300-1000μg/l	>1000μg/l
Age 30-49yrs	101 (8%)	40 (3%)	15 (1.5%)	3 (0.3%)
50-69yrs	215 (28%)	77 (10%)	34 (4%)	8 (1.0%)
50-59yrs	92 (22%)	31 (7.5%)	12 (3%)	5 (1.0%)
60-69yrs	123 (35%)	46 (13%)	22 (6%)	3 (1.0%)
70yrs +	452 (38%)	206 (17%)	97 (8%)	16 (1.3%)

Table 3. Ferritin values in female patients >30yrs in Primary Care

7.2 Current reporting practice

A survey of Scottish laboratories has shown that it is routine practice only to report serum ferritin levels >1000μg/l as 'grossly elevated'. No further advice is currently provided. Given the above findings it would seem appropriate for laboratory reports to recommend hospital referral for all patients with serum ferritin level >1000μg/l, unless otherwise explained. It is as yet unclear as how best to advise General Practiioners for patients with ferritin values between 300-1000μg/l. We would suggest further assessment of body iron stores with measurement of transferrin saturation. High transferrin saturation would then warrant further molecular screening for HHC. With the support of the Chief Scientist Office for Scotland we are now trying to establish an algorithm for the Scottish population based on age, sex, serum ferritin and transferrin saturation that might trigger a request for molecular screening for HHC.

8. Conclusion

We have discussed the use of laboratory tests to assess iron status in the primary care population. General Practioners frequently request serum ferritin levels and iron studies.

Often these tests are used to assess iron status when there is clinical suspicion of iron deficiency. General Practioners are familiar with the interpretation of these tests in iron deficiency (a reduced ferritin is irrefutable evidence of iron deficiency) but require more guidance when the serum ferritin level is elevated and iron overload is possible. Ferritin is an acute phase protein and can be elevated to levels inappropriately high for the degree of reticuloendothelial iron stores by infectious, neoplastic or inflammatory conditions. Even when HHC has been excluded a serum ferritin level >1000µg/l most often indicates significant underlying pathology and must be further investigated.

HHC is an autosomal recessive disorder and is one of the most common single gene disorders in the North European population. The morbidities associated are serious and preventable. Timely diagnosis is therefore important and family screening of HHC patients is essential. Molecular screening of at risk but asymptomatic population (i.e Celts) is not recommended by the UK National Screening Committee as disease penetrance is <50%. Clear guidance is required to investigate patients with unexplained raised serum ferritin values. Elevation of serum ferritin level should prompt measurement of transferrin saturation and thereafter HFE genotype if saturation exceeds 50%.

9. References

BCSH; British Committee for Standards in Haematology (2002). Dooley J and Worwood M. Guidelines for diagnosis and therapy of genetic haemochromatosis.

Fitzsimons EJ, Brock JH. (2001) The anaemia of chronic disease. *BMJ*;322:811-12.

Fitzsimons EJ, Houston T, Munro R, Sturrock RD, Speekenbrink AB, Brock LH (2002). Erythroblast iron metabolism and serum soluble transferrin receptor values in the anaemia of rheumatoid arthritis. *Arth Rh.* 15;47(2) 166-71.

Goddard AF, James MW, McIntyre AS, Scott BB on behalf of the British Society of Gastroenterology. Guidelines for the management of iron deficiency anaemia. *Gut.* 2011; 60:1309-1316.

Gordeuk VR, Reboussin DM, McLaren CE, Barton JC, Acton RT, McLaren GD, Harris EL, Reiss JA, Adams PC, Speechley M, Phatak PD, Sholinsky P, Eckfeldt JH, Chen WP, Passmore L, Dawkins FW (2008). Serum ferritin concentrations and body iron stores in a multiethnic primary care population. *American Journal of Haematology*.83;618-626.

Ogilvie C, Fitzsimons K, Fitzsimons E.(2010). Serum ferritin values in primary care: are high values overlooked. *J Clin Pathol*. 2010;63:1124-1126.

Whitlock EP, Garlitz BA, Harris EL (2006). Screening for hereditary haemochromatosis; a systematic review of the US preventive series Task Force. *Annals Int Medicine*.145;209-223.

Witte DL (1991). Can serum ferritin be effectively interpreted in the presence of the acute phase response. *Clinical Chemistry*.37;484-485.

Worwood (1982). Ferritin in human tissues and serum. *Clinics in Haematology*. 11; 275-307.

2

Cancer Diagnosis and Treatment: An Overview for the General Practitioner

Josephine Emole

University of Texas Health Center at Houston,
Houston, Texas,
USA

1. Introduction

Many cancer patients will first present to a primary care provider either in the clinic or acutely in the inpatient setting before a definite diagnosis of cancer is made. Thus, an accurate clinical evaluation - through history taking and physical examination - by a general practitioner could reveal malignant diseases at their early stages. In some instances, cancer is incidentally detected while a patient is being treated for other unrelated diseases. Plain radiographs ordered by the primary care physician for pneumonias or back pains, for instance, have been known to reveal occult lung tumors or bone metastasis.

With advances in cancer treatment, many cancer patients are living into the survivorship period and are increasingly being seen by primary care providers following active treatment. At such times, the primary care provider plays a major role in surveillance, management of cancer treatment complications and treatment of comorbid conditions. A 40 year old woman who has been treated for breast cancer, for example, will still need colorectal cancer screening as well as yearly pap smears from her primary care physician in addition to her required follow up with Breast Oncology.

Since the primary care provider plays such an invaluable role in cancer prevention, detection and control, it is imperative that the primary care provider is kept abreast of the latest advances in the ever evolving field of cancer diagnosis and therapy. While the general practitioner will likely not be responsible for cancer staging and treatment, there might be need for him or her to select the initial screening or diagnostic tests for malignant diseases prior to referral to the cancer specialist. There is therefore need for a concise literature for the generalist on the current and up-to-date approach to the diagnosis and treatment of cancers and hematological diseases.

Current classifications in surgical pathology for staging malignancies are based on anatomic features (tumor-node-metastasis) and histopathology (grade)[1]. Different modalities currently exist for the diagnosis and treatment of cancer. Most have been in use for many years whereas others have evolved as our understanding of the molecular processes that lead to carcinogenesis has increased.

2. Laboratory diagnosis of hematological and oncological diseases

2.1 Morphological methods

Morphological examinations are the easiest methods of cancer diagnosis.[2] Many sophisticated laboratory and imaging techniques have evolved in Oncology over the years but clinician still have to depend on histopathology for the definite diagnosis of many solid tumors. Only in rare occasions have imaging and appropriate biochemical assays substituted microscopic examination of a tissue sample for cancer diagnosis.

Proper pathological diagnosis begins with the referring clinician. Since certain disease processes share similar morphological and microscopic appearances, the clinical information supplied by the requesting medical provider goes a long way in helping the histopathologist to make definitive diagnoses. Proper and complete history must precede all requests for pathological evaluation.

Pertinent patient data that must accompany any tissue sample to the laboratory include the patient identity, age, gender, duration of the disease and exact location of the lesion, size and any previous treatment. With the advent of electronic medical records, the clinician should ensure that these data are in the patient's electronic records from where the pathologist can retrieve them easily as needed.

In addition to appropriate collection and reporting of clinical data to the pathologist, the referring physician must ensure that the pathological specimen is properly obtained from a well selected biopsy site and must be properly handled and transported to the laboratory.

2.2 Sampling methods for pathological exam

Incisional biopsy is easy to perform. It involves the removal of a small part of a large tumor for the purpose of laboratory diagnosis. This method is usually chosen for lesions that are easy to access. Following diagnosis, the tumor is usually completely removed surgically or treated by other modalities.

Excisional biopsy is an alternative to incisional biopsy. It enables a more complete pathological exam of the lesion and thus it is the most appropriate collection method for small tumors. It is also the best method for evaluation of lymph nodes; since pathological changes in lymph nodes may be focal and might be missed when sampled by incisional biopsy[3]. As expected, excisional biopsy might cause more local trauma than incision biopsy.

Needle aspiration allows the clinician to obtain a core of tissue from a mass for cytological examination. It is increasingly being employed for tumors in which there is a visible or readily palpable mass such as lymph nodes, breast or thyroid. Using ultrasound, computed tomography or fluoroscopy guidance, needle aspiration can also be used for deeper organs such as the liver. There is a possible complication of tumor implantation along the tract of the needle.

Cytology is a method that has been used widely in cervical cancer screening and could be employed for other suspected cancers like bladder, gastric and lung cancers. It is based on the premise that neoplastic cells are less cohesive than normal cells and are easily shed into body fluids such as urine, gastric fluid, pleural, peritoneal and bronchial fluids.[2] With improvement in accessibility of organs by endoscopy, cytological examinations are being largely replaced by direct endoscopy and biopsy of the stomach, bladder, and bronchi.[3] Cytology may still be used in follow up of patients that have been treated for cancers of the bladder or urinary tract. Routine Papanicolaou smears are still the mainstay of cervical cancer screening.

Endoscopic procedures grant access to internal organs thereby enabling biopsy of the internal organs

2.3 Specimen preparation

Following collection of tissue specimen, it undergoes preparation prior to histological exam. Specimen preparation can be permanent or frozen sections.

Permanent method involves the processes of fixation, embedding, sectioning and staining. The tissue specimen is initially fixed in formalin, and then embedded in paraffin wax to preserve its architecture and facilitate sectioning. Sectioning involves cutting the specimen into thin slices that can be examined with the microscope. The micro-sections are then finally stained prior to microscopic examination.

When the pathologist anticipates a different examination modality than histopathology, the choice of fixing and staining agents might be modified as appropriate.

Frozen section is a rapid method that quickly prepares fresh tissue for microscopic examination. It is easily used by surgeon within the operating suite to obtain an immediate pathological interpretation of the specimen and thus decide on the next therapeutic approach to pursue during surgery. It has also enabled surgeons to establish adequacy of excision margins.[3]

2.4 Molecular techniques

The diversity of genomic alterations involved in malignancy had led to the development of a variety of assays for complete tumor profiling. Thus, it is no longer adequate to know the histopathology of a cancer. The new molecular diagnostics when integrated into existing histomorphological classifications in surgical pathology provides additional stratification for a more accurate cancer prognosis.[1]

Detection of molecular markers in neoplastic tissue samples can be used to provide accurate diagnosis, prognosis and prediction of response, resistance, or toxicity to therapy. These molecular markers can be products of altered genes/DNA or abnormal pathways. Mutations in DNA can include rearrangements such as translocations, inversions, gene amplifications/deletions, point mutations and base insertions/deletions.

Cytogenetic procedures study the chromosomes in the tissue sample with the aim to identify any chromosomal changes that are peculiar to known cancer types.

FISH technique is a molecular cytogenetic technique in which probes are used to confirm presence or absence of specific DNA sequences on chromosomes. It is used in diagnosis of blood disorders or cancer which are due to specific genetic alterations on the chromosomes.

PCR is a quantitative technique that permits amplification and analysis of target DNA regions in tumor samples.

DNA microarray analysis is equipped to measure the expression levels of large number of genes concurrently.

Immunocytochemistry (IHC)is used to detect antigens or protein expression on a fixed tissue section by means of an antibody that is specific for the antigen/protein. The antibody-antigen reaction is visualized by linking the antibody to an enzyme that catalyzes a color producing reaction or to a substance that fluoresces. IHC serves as an adjunct to regular histological exam of a tissue sample and is being routinely used to detect the presence of antigens, proteins, and biomarkers in neoplastic tissue samples. It has been employed largely for the detection of estrogen and progesterone receptors on breast tissues, to detect oncogenes and tumor suppressor gene products on tumor samples as well as to characterize leukemias and lymphomas.

Flow cytometry is a technique that is used to examine and differentiate cells based on certain physical and chemical properties. A sample of blood or tissue cells in suspension is passed through the flow cytometer and the scatter emitted by the cell where it meets the light is analyzed to better characterize the cell.

Electron microscopy is used when specific cellular or intracellular structures need to be examined. Like IHC, it aids in a more accurate tumor classification.

Molecular cancer diagnostic techniques have been instrumental to identifying the brc-abl in CML, HER-2/NEU expression in breast cancer.

2.5 Biomarkers

Biomarkers are proteins which are released from cancers and whose detection or increase in the serum may screen or confirm the presence of certain cancers. Biochemical assays for tumor-associated enzymes, hormones and other markers are not being used for the definitive diagnosis of cancer[2]. Instead, cancer biomarkers complement pathological examination and thus play a role in the early detection, outcome prediction and detection of disease recurrence. In addition, in the present era of new therapeutic agents, biomarkers can help to determine which tumors will respond to which treatments.[4] Some biomarkers that are currently in clinical use are shown in **Table 1.**

The ideal biomarker should have a high specificity and sensitivity, especially if it is to be useful for staging [5]. In addition, it should be easily detected in the patient's blood or urine but not in a healthy person. Many of the current biomarkers in clinical practice lack enough sensitivity or specificity to accurately serve as the sole diagnostic tool for the diagnosis of any cancer.

It must be pointed out that despite the detection of biomarkers in a patient, a histological exam is often necessary to confirm cancer.

3. Imaging diagnosis

Histological diagnosis is still essential to establish the diagnosis of cancer. But a well-designed imaging strategy is important in the management of a patient with cancer.

Depending on circumstances, imaging can precede or follow histopathology.[6] The choice of imaging techniques are many and still evolving, and the physician must carefully select the modalities based on a good understanding of the specific neoplasm, its biological characteristics and its response to treatment.[7]

Biomarker	Type	Source	Cancer type	Clinical use
α-FP	glycoprotein	serum	nonseminomatous testicular	staging
HCG-β	glycoprotein	serum	testicular	staging
CA19-9	carbohydrate	serum	pancreatic	monitoring
CA125	glycoprotein	serum	ovarian	monitoring
CEA	protein	serum	colon	monitoring
Thyroglobulin	protein	serum	thyroid	monitoring
PSA	protein	serum	prostate	screening and monitoring
Estrogen receptor	protein	breast tumor	breast	selection for hormonal therapy
Progesterone receptor	protein	breast tumor	breast	selection for hormonal therapy
HER2/NEU	protein	breast tumor	breast	prognosis and selection of therapy
BTA	protein	urine	bladder	monitoring

Adapted from Ludwig JA, Weinstein JN. 2005. Biomarkers in cancer staging, prognosis and selection. *Nature Reviews Cancer* 5 : 845-857.

Table 1. Examples of common biomarkers in clinical use

Imaging in Oncology is used for screening, detection, diagnosis, treatment and to follow response to treatment. The choice of imaging for every type of cancer is beyond the scope of this text. Brief highlights of each of the commonly available imaging modalities will be enumerated.

Conventional radiology is widely available, and cheap. It is however largely being replaced by other techniques like CT and MRI for definition of tumor anatomy. Plain and Contrast radiography (barium or iodine) is still part of initial evaluation of GI pathology.[7] Many cancers have been discovered following radiological tests done for unrelated diseases.

Ultrasound US is relatively cheap and safe. It has become instrumental in guiding procedures such as biopsies and for assessment of fluid collections.

Mammography has become routine for breast cancer screening. This is the commonest imaging technique that is being used for mass screening for cancer.

CT plays a critical role in cancer diagnosis, staging, follow up as well as in relapse of neoplastic disease. It is increasingly being used to guide diagnostic biopsies, as part of radiotherapy simulations.

MRI is a costly imaging method. Like CT, it is useful in diagnosis, staging, therapy and follow up. It is also increasingly being used in minimally invasive procedures. CT is however more widely available.

PET makes use of labeled isotopes active which are tagged to metabolically active substances. When such substances are administered, they concentrate on certain areas of the body and yield imaging studies of metabolism. PET is useful in staging, detecting recurrences and evaluation of several cancers such as head and neck tumors, brain tumors, lymphomas, and colorectal cancers.

The last decade has seen the gradual shift to PET/CT which is an imaging modality that combines anatomy and function. It has become a powerful tool for diagnosis and staging in Oncology. PET-CT combines the functional imaging obtained by PET to the anatomical imaging of CT to a single superimposed image. The patient is therefore saved the time and costs of two separate imaging sessions. Even though this imaging technique was initially used for lung cancers, it is fast becoming a standard for most other cancers. MR and MR spectrometry are other imaging modalities that could potentially be fused with molecular PET techniques.[8]

Many other newer techniques such as magnetic resonance spectroscopy, impedance tomography, and laser optical tomography are increasingly being studied for application to cancer imaging.[6]

4. Cancer therapy

Surgery, radiation and chemotherapy are the oldest treatment modalities for malignancies. From the time cancer is first suspected or diagnosed, there is need for the different cancer disciplines to work together to formulate the best treatment plan for the patient. Since each patient and each cancer is different, treatment must be individualized. The exact treatment choice or combination of choices will depend on the patient, the disease and the stage of the disease as well as other considerations such as performance status, and comorbid conditions.

4.1 Pharmacotherapy

Cytotoxic agents still form the basis of many cancer therapy regimens. The growth pattern of individual neoplastic cells may greatly affect the overall behavior of tumors and their responses to specific types of cancer therapy.

The cell cycle gives us an insight into the kinetic behavior of dividing cells.[9] The four distinct phases of the cell cycle are: G_1, G_2 ,S and M phases. G_1 is a stage of cell increase or growth. This is followed by DNA replication or synthesis during the S (*synthesis*) phase. G_2 is another stage of cell growth. During the M (*mitosis*) stage, the cell growth is halted while active division takes place. During the G_1 and G_2 phases, the cellular constituents are synthesized. The cell cycle is well regulated with checkpoints that ensure that cells moved into the next cell cycle phase only after the proceeding phases are well completed. These checkpoints may become abnormal in cancer.

Some cytotoxics act at specific points in the cell cycle. Antimetabolites are more active against the S-phase cells while the vinca alkaloids and taxols are more M-phase specific.

Alkylating agents and platinum derivatives are cell-cycle-nonspecific agents. **Fig 1** and **Table 2** list some chemotherapeutic agents in common use and their mechanisms of action.

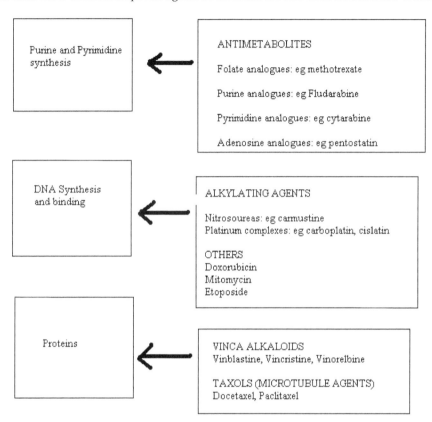

Fig. 1. Action of selected chemotherapeutic agent.

Chemotherapeutic agents are used as primary treatment for advanced disease, as neoadjucant to surgery/ radiation for localized disease or as adjuvant therapy (with surgery and/or radiation). In addition to systemic administration, anticancer agents can also be delivered regionally. Classical examples of regional delivery of chemotherapy include intrathecal administration of methothrexate in the treatment and prevention of meningeal leukemia, intraperitoneal chemotherapy in management of ovarian cancer, intravesical treatment for superficial bladder cancer, and intrahepatic arterial therapy for colon cancer metastatic to the liver.[10]

4.2 Target cancer therapies

Recent advances in genetics and molecular cellular biology has led to exponential increase in our understanding of the molecular events that either initiate or sustain cancer growth. Whereas traditional chemotherapeutic agents may not differentiate between normal and cancer cells, the newer biological agents target specific molecular pathology (pathways and aberrant genes)in cancer cells.[11] Target therapeutics can be monoclonal antibodies or small molecules. They can be used alone or in combination with other chemotherapeutics, surgery or radiation therapy.

4.3 Monoclonal antibodies

Monoclonal antibodies are antibodies that bind to antigens found specifically on cancer cells and thus induce an immune reaction against the cancer cells. These antigens are usually extra-cellular proteins or cell surface antigens that are expressed specifically by the neoplastic cells.

Many monoclonal antibodies have been produced and find use in treatment of autoimmune and oncological disorders. Their names usually end in the letters –*mab*-short for monoclonal antibodies.(**Table 3**) Some antibodies are already approved for clinical use whereas many others are still experimental and undergoing clinical trials.

4.4 Small molecules

By virtue of their size, small molecules can reach intracellular sites where they act to interact with molecular pathways and exert anti-tumor effects. **Table 4** enumerates some of the small molecules that are currently in clinical use.

4.5 Endocrine therapy

Use of hormones in Oncology is based on the recognition that some human cancers undergo changes following fluctuations in certain sex hormones. Hormone deprivation can be achieved by surgical removal of the steroid gland or by administration of inhibitors of the hormone biosynthesis. Examples of hormonal therapy for cancers include use of antiestrogens and LHRH analogues for breast cancer as well as use of antiandrogens and LHRH analogues for prostate cancer. Steroids (prednisone, dexamethasone) are used either alone or in combination with other cytotoxic agents for the treatment of leukemias, lymphomas and multiple myelomas. Steroids are also used in the management of hypercalcemia as well as for the tissue swelling that accompanied tumors of the lungs and the airway obstruction.

Alkylating agents   Bendamustine, cyclophospham, chlorambucil, ifosfamide, carmustine, lomustine, streptozocin, carboplastin, cisplatin, oxaliplatin, procarbazine, melphalan, busulphan, thiotepa   *Antimetabolites*   Methotrexate, pemetrexed, fludarabine, mercaptopurine, thioguanine, cladribine, pentostatin, capecitabine, cytarabine, floxuridinefluorouracil, gemcitabine, hydroxyurea   *Natural products*   Bleomycin, dactinomycin, daunorubicin, doxorubicin, doxil, epirubicin, idarubicin, mitomycin, etoposide, teniposide, docetaxel, paclitaxel, vinblastine, vincristine, vinorelbine, irinotecan, topotecan, asparaginase

Table 2. Chemotherapeutic agents

4.6 Radiation therapy

Radiation therapy is the administration of ionizing radiation to a cancer patient for the purpose of cure, palliation or as an adjunct to surgical treatment. Confirmation of malignancy by pathological exam, ancillary workup and staging must be completed prior to radiation therapy.

Radiation therapy is often used in conjunction with surgery for eradication of small, limited human cancers. Preoperatively, radiation therapy may be given to shrink inoperable tumors or to destroy unrecognized peripheral projections of the tumor. This method is applicable to advanced tumors of the head and neck, colorectum and bladder. On the other hand, radiation therapy can be given post operatively to eradicate residual disease or to control subclinical disease in the wound or in the lymphnodes.[12]

Radiation therapy is also used for palliation in instances like cancers of the central nervous system and pathological metastasis to the bones

4.7 Surgery

Surgery plays vital role in the prevention, diagnosis, staging, cure and palliation. Many premalignant lesions are usually surgically removed to prevent progression to cancer. Family members with familial polyposis of the colon for example, are routinely being offered colectomy to prevent eventual development of colon cancer. Mastectomy can also be done prophylactically for patients at high risk for breast cancer following the appropriate genetic counseling.

Incisional, excisional and needle biopsy techniques as well as endoscopy are surgical methods that aid cancer diagnosis.

Surgery forms the basis of therapy for early cancer in which case it is employed as local treatment for small tumors, to reduce the bulk of the disease, and for removal of metastatic tumors.

Even though late stage cancers are mainly treated by chemotherapy, surgery could offer palliation in advanced cancers. Typical examples of such instances include stenting for biliary obstruction due to advanced tumors of the biliary system or for esophageal obstruction.

4.8 Gene therapy

Cancer gene therapy is anchored on the premise that many cancers are due to genetic alterations that eventually lead to malignant changes in tissues. Gene therapy involves the transfer of genetic material into a cell to alter the cellular phenotype transiently or permanently. Gene transfer can be performed in vitro or in vivo. Different vectors exist for gene delivery into cancerous cells. Viruses (such as retroviruses) serve as a perfect tool for gene transfer. Gene therapies for cancer treatment are evolving and are largely still undergoing studies.

5. Conclusion

The general practitioner will see cancer patients at one time or the other in the course of their disease. Even though the primary care practitioner is not a medical, surgical or radio-oncologist, he is part of the interdisciplinary team that is crucial for provision of optimal care for the cancer patient or cancer survivor. Burdened with such a responsibility, the general practitioner must keep abreast of the available screening, diagnostic and therapeutic modalities that currently exist for malignant diseases. Surgery, radiation and chemotherapy still play a large role in the treatment of cancer. But with advances in molecular biology and individualized medicine, many new diagnostic and treatment options are gradually shifting towards identifying and treating cancer at the level of the genes or molecular pathways. The

Agent	Molecular target	Disease indication
Trastuzumab(Herceptin)	ERBB2	Breast cancer
Bevacizumab(Avastin)	VEGFR	Metastatic colorectal cancer
Cetuximab (Erbitux)	EGFR	Metastatic colorectal cancer
Alemtuzumab(Campath)	CD52	B-cell Chronic lymphocytic leukemia

Table 3. Examples of monoclonal antibodies

Drug	Molecular target	Uses/Disease indication
Bortezomib	26S proteosome	Multiple myeloma
Dasatinib	brc-abl,PDGFR	CML, Philadelphia positiveALL
Erlotinib	HER1/EGFR	NCSLC ,pancreas
Gefitinib	EGFR	NSCLC
Imatinib	brc-abl,PDGFR	CML,GIST
Lapatinib	EGFR,HER2	HER-2 positive metastatic breast cancer
Nilotinib	brc-abl,PDGFR	CML
Sorafenib	VEGFR,PDGFR,RAF-1	renal cell cancer
Sunitinib	VEGFR,PDGFR,RET,c-kit	renal cell cancer, GIST
Temsirolimus	mTOR	renal cell cancer

Modified from *Cancer management: A multidisciplinary approach*. 11th ed. Lawrence,Kansas: CMPMedica.

Table 4. Targeted cancer therapeutics: small molecules

primary care provider will therefore increasingly encounter patients that are being treated with these new cancer therapies. Stem cell and genetic therapies as well as some target therapies are still evolving and over the next few years will find their way into our therapeutic regimens.

6. Abbreviations

ALL	acute lymphoblastic leukemia
AML	acute myeloid leukemia
BTA	bladder tumor antigen
CML	chronic myelogenous leukemia
CT	computed tomography
BCR-ABL	oncogene fusion protein associated with the Philadelphia chromosome
EGFR	epidermal growth factor receptor
HER2-NEU	human epidermal growth factor receptor 2
DNA	deoxyribonucleic acid
FISH	fluorescence in situ hybridization
GIST	gastrointestinal stromal tumor
IHC	immunohistochemistry
MRI	magnetic resonance imaging
PET	positron emission tomography
PET-CT	positron emission tomography-computed tomography
VEGFR	vascular endothelial growth factor receptor

7. References

Bast R, Kufe D, Pollock R, Weichselbaum R, Holland J,Frei E. 2000. *Cancer medicine*. 5th ed. Ontario: BC Decker Inc.

Bernard PS, Wittwer CT. 2002. Real-time PCR technology for cancer diagnostics. *Clinical Chemistry* 48:8: 1178–1185.

Bragg DJ, Rubin P, Hricak H. 2002. *Oncologic imaging*. 2nd ed. Philadelphia: WB Saunders.

Chatterjee SK, Zetter BR. 2005. Cancer biomarkers: Knowing the present and predicting the future. *Future Oncology* 1(1) : 37-50.

Collins I, Workman P. 2006. New approaches to molecular cancer therapeutics. *Nature Chemical Biology* 2 (12).

Kumar V, Abbas AK, Fausto N, Mitchell RN. 2007. Robbins basic pathology. 8th ed., 173-222. Philadelphia: Saunders Elsevier.

Ludwig JA, Weinstein JN. 2005. Biomarkers in cancer staging, prognosis and selection. *Nature Reviews Cancer* 5 : 845-857.

Pazdur R, Wagman LD, Camphausen KA, Hoskins WJ. 2008. *Cancer management: A multidisciplinary approach*. 11th ed. Lawrence,Kansas: CMPMedica.

Regato J, Spjut HJ,Cox JD. 1985. *Cancer diagnosis, treatment and prognosis*. 6th ed. St Louis:

Schiepers C, Dahlbom M. 2011. Molecular imaging in oncology: The acceptance of PET/CT and the emergence of MR/PET imaging. *European Radiology* 21 (3) (Mar): 548-54.

Vanel D, Stark D. 1993. *Imaging strategies in oncology.* 1st ed. New York: John Wiley and Sons
        Inc.
Wang CC. 2000. *Clinical radiation oncology.* 2nd ed. Canada: John Wiley and Sons Inc.

Chronic Obstructive Pulmonary Disease in Primary Care – From Diagnosis to Therapy

Elisabetta Rovatti[1], Oreste Capelli[2,*], Maria Isabella Bonacini[3],
Imma Cacciapuoti[4] and Antonio Brambilla[2]

[1]Dept. of Pneumology – University Hospital – University of Modena and Reggio Emilia
[2]The District Primary Care, Emilia-Romagna Region, Bologna
[3]Pharmacy Department, Derriford Hospital, Plymouth NHS Trust
[4]Dpt. of Mental Health, Modena,
[1,2,4]Italy
[3]UK

1. Introduction

The Global Strategy for the Diagnosis, Management and Prevention of COPD guidelines (GOLD, 2010) and the UK National Institute of Clinical Excellence guidelines (NICE, 2010) recommend an early diagnosis of Chronic Obstructive Pulmonary Disease (COPD) in any patient over the age of 35 who has chronic cough (present intermittently or every day throughout the day), chronic sputum production, shortness of breath (dyspnoea), frequent winter 'bronchitis' or wheeze and/or a history of exposure to disease risk factors.

COPD is a progressive, but preventable and treatable disease, characterised by airflow limitation, that is not fully reversible and an abnormal inflammatory response of the lungs to noxious particles or gases; COPD is associated with significant extrapulmonary effects and comorbidities that may affect the severity (GOLD, 2010). COPD is a complex disease, a combination of emphysema and chronic bronchitis, although only one of these may be present in some people.

- Emphysema is characterized by abnormal permanent enlargement of the air spaces distal to the terminal bronchioles, accompanied by destruction of their walls, and without obvious fibrosis.
- Chronic bronchitis is characterized by chronic cough or mucous production for at least 3 months in at least 2 successive years when other causes of chronic cough have been excluded (GOLD, 2010).

The typical symptoms are cough, with large amounts of mucus, wheezing, shortness of breath, chest tightness. Cigarette smoking is the leading cause of COPD. It is estimated that over 50% of smokers will develop during the life a chronic respiratory disease (Mannino & Buist, 2007). Other than tobacco smoking, risk factors for development of COPD are being

---

* Corresponding Author

increasingly recognised (Soriano et al, 2009) and include environmental factors such as occupational exposure to dust and fumes in developed and developing countries (Blanc et al, 2009; Soriano et al, 2009) and indoor biomass fuel burning in many developing countries. Other environmental risk factors that seem unimportant for development of COPD, but that might worsen disease include outdoor pollutants and passive smoke exposure. Therefore, adequate monitoring air pollution, accompanied by appropriate strategies for cessation of cigarette smoking, are of primary importance for the care of these patients. COPD mainly affects middle-aged and older people.

The prevalence of COPD in the general population is estimated to be about 1% across all ages, rising to 8-10% or higher in individuals aged 40 years or older (Soriano et al, 2009). Actually is the fourth leading cause of death in the U.S. and is projected to be the third leading cause of death for both males and females by the year 2020. The true prevalence of this disease within the same population can vary depending on the tool used to identify COPD, such as self-reported respiratory symptoms, medical diagnosis, or lung function. The correct diagnosis and staging of the disease, based on spirometric functional assessment of the patient, are prerequisites for the implementation of rational and therapeutic measures with proven effectiveness. The prevention of complications, including through appropriate interventions vaccine, along with rehabilitation programs, is critical to positively influencing the patient's medical history (GOLD, 2010).

2. Diagnosis of COPD: From evidence to practice

In view of the increasing prevalence of the disease around the world, it is tried to create and spread worldwide guidelines and programs for the dissemination of current knowledge in order to better diagnosis and management of the disease by all health organizations (CTS, 2008; GOLD, 2010; NICE, 2010; Qaseem et al, 2011). Despite the efforts of implementation of existing guidelines COPD remains an underdiagnosed disease and it is poorly treated when diagnosed. In population studies, findings show that underdiagnosis of COPD is high and independent of overall prevalence (Buist et al, 2007; Soriano et al, 2009). Up to 80% of COPD cases remain undiagnosed until the disease is advanced and substantial end-organ damage is present (Buist et al, 2007; GOLD, 2010; Price et al, 2010). Furthermore, respiratory disease misdiagnosis is common: up to 25% of patients older than 40 years who are labelled as having asthma actually have COPD. Conversely, many patients in primary care are labelled as having COPD when they have asthma (Jones et al, 2008). It is estimated that there are twice as many patients with impaired lung function (indicative of early stage COPD) than patients with diagnosed COPD (Price et al, 2010). The symptoms of COPD may be similar to those of other respiratory conditions (Table 1) and an accurate differential diagnosis may be performed in general practice (GOLD, 2010).

2.1 Symptoms and questionnaires

The underestimation of symptoms by the patients is an important problem: despite experiencing such symptoms as dyspnoea, chronic cough, or sputum production for months or years, patients fail to recognize or report them, believing such symptoms to be a normal consequence of smoking, aging or deconditioning (Price et al, 2010; Yawn et al, 2009).

Diagnosis	Suggestive features	Recommended investigations to confirm diagnosis
COPD	Onset in midlife; symptoms slowly progressive; long history of exposure to noxious particles, typically tobacco smoking or air pollution; dyspnoea during exercise; airflow limitation that is not fully reversible	Spirometry confirms presence of airflow limitation that is not fully reversible
Asthma	Onset early in life (often childhood); variation in symptoms from day to day; symptoms at night or in early morning; other atopic conditions present (eg, allergy, rhinitis, eczema); family history of asthma	Spirometry confirms presence of largely reversible airflow limitation
Chronic heart failure	Fine basilar crackles on auscultation	CXR shows dilated heart, pulmonary edema; spirometry confirms restrictive rather than obstructive lung disease
Bronchiectasis	Large volume of purulent sputum; commonly associated with bacterial infection; coarse crackles/clubbing on auscultation	CXR or CT shows bronchial dilation, bronchial wall thickening
Tuberculosis	Onset at all ages; high local prevalence of tuberculosis	CXR shows lung infiltrate; microbiological confirmation
Obliterative bronchiolitis	Onset at younger age in nonsmokers; may have history of rheumatoid arthritis or fume exposure	CT on expiration shows hypodense areas
Diffuse pan-bronchiolitis	Most patients are men and nonsmokers; almost all have chronic sinusitis	CXR and HRCT show diffuse small centrilobular nodular opacities and hyperinflation
Carcinoma of the bronchus	Symptoms may include dyspnea, hemoptysis, coughing wheezing, pain in chest or abdomen, cachexia, fatigue and loss of appetite; history of exposure to carcinogens (such as those in tobacco smoke), ionizing radiation, or viral infection	CXR; CT; bronchoscopy

COPD = chronic obstructive pulmonary disease; CXR = Chest radiography;
CT = computed tomography; HRCT = high-resolution CT.

Table 1. Differential Diagnosis of COPD (adapted from GOLD, 2010).

A significant number of patients perceived incorrectly the severity of their disease, based on the modified Medical Research Council (MRC) dyspnoea scale (Table 2): 35.8% of subjects with the most severe breathlessness scale and 60.3% of subjects with the next most severe scale considered their condition to be mild or moderate (Rodin & Cote, 2008).

Patient questionnaires are an effective and economic instrument for discriminating between subjects with and without COPD (Barnes & Fromer, 2011; Price et al, 2011). Questions include items on age, body mass index (BMI), smoking intensity, cough, phlegm, dyspnoea on exertion and wheeze, as well as prior diagnosis consistent with asthma or COPD (Table 3) (Price et al, 2011). Examples of disease-specific instruments include the MRC dyspnoea scale (Table 2), the Clinical COPD Questionnaire (CCQ), and the COPD Assessment Test (CAT) (Jones et al, 2011).

Grade	Degree of breathlessness related to activities
1	Not troubled by breathlessness except on strenuous exercise
2	Short of breath when hurrying on the level or walking up a slight hill
3	Walks slower than most people on the level, stops after a mile or so stops after 15 minutes walking at own pace
4	Stops for breath after walking about 100 yds or after a few minutes on level ground
5	Too breathless to leave the house, or breathless when undressing

Table 2. The MRC Breathlessness Scale (from Bestall et al, 1999)

2.2 Spirometry

The diagnosis of COPD has to be confirmed by spirometry (GOLD, 2010; NICE, 2010; Qaseem et al, 2011), but in real life, only 30–50% of new cases are confirmed by this method (Barnes & Fromer, 2011; Bolton et al, 2005; Joo et al, 2008). Inadequate use of spirometry affects not only primary care but also specialised management: analysis of medical records of patients admitted to academic tertiary-care hospitals showed that only 31% of those diagnosed with COPD had spirometry, by contrast with individuals with congestive heart failure, of whom 78% had echocardiography, the golden standard examination (Soriano et al, 2009). On the contrary spirometry should not be used to screen for airflow obstruction in asymptomatic individuals (GOLD, 2010; NICE, 2010; Qaseem et al, 2011).

Spirometry is a reliable, simple, non-invasive, safe, and non-expensive procedure for the detection of airflow obstruction. Spirometry can be performed in primary care to assess lung function in terms of maximal volume of air forcibly exhaled from the point of maximal inspiration [Forced Vital Capacity (FVC)] and the volume of air exhaled during the first second of this manoeuvre [Forced Expiratory Volume in 1 s (FEV1)]. It is suggested that a postbronchodilator FEV1 < 80% of predicted, together with a FEV1/FVC ratio of < 0,7, is indicative of airflow limitation that is not fully reversible (GOLD, 2010; NICE, 2010; Qaseem et al, 2011.)

A basal spirometry, without bronchodilator, has been shown to lead to overdiagnosis of COPD by 11% in primary care (Jones et al, 2008) and by 27% in screening studies (Johannessen et al, 2005). The impairment of FEV1 in COPD is partially related to symptoms and disease severity. For this reason the main COPD guidelines define FEV1 thresholds for classifying stages of disease severity (table 4). The classifications are not all the same because the correlation between FEV1 values and clinical manifestations of COPD are not well defined. In 2012 the new GOLD guidelines will propose a new COPD severity classification, which will be based not only on spirometric evaluation but also on symptoms intensity and exacerbations frequency. However, after a medical diagnosis of COPD, guidelines (GOLD, 2010) recommend that patients should undergo a spirometry follow-up every 6 months or yearly. The assessment of sequential spirometry values in COPD is important because the Lung Health Study showed significant differences between individuals who continued to smoke (they lost 63 mL of their FEV1 per year) versus non-smokers (-30 mL of FEV1 per year) (Anthonisen et al, 2002b).

	Response choices	Points*
What is your age?	40-49 years	0
	50-59 years	5
	60-69 years	9
How many pack years of cigarettes have you smoked?	0-14 pack years	0
	15-24 pack years	3
	25-49 pack years	7
	50 + pack years	9
Have you coughed more in the last few years?	yes	0
	no	1
During the past 3 years, have you had any breathing problems that have kept you off work, indoors, at home or in bed?	Yes	0
	no	3
Have you ever been admitted to hospital with breathing problems?	yes	6
	no	0
Have you been short of breath more often in the past few years?	yes	1
	no	0
On average, how much phlegm (sputum) do you cough up most days?	None or less than 1 tablespoon (15 ml)	0
	or more per day	4
If you get a cold, does it usually go to your chest?	yes	4
	no	0
Are you taking any treatment to help your breathing?	yes	5
	no	0

***Scoring system:** Add up the total number of points based on the patient's response. 18 or fewer points suggests a diagnosis of asthma; 19 or more points suggests a diagnosis of COPD

Table 3. Differential diagnosis questionnaire to determine between COPD and asthma (adapted from Price et al, 2011)

The International Primary Care Respiratory Group (IPCRG) currently recommends a case identification spirometry in all patients over 35 years who present with respiratory symptoms and risk factors, such as prior or current smoking history (Decramer et al, 2011; Levy et al, 2006; NICE 2010). Spirometry undertaken at the primary-care level aims to exclude individuals with normal lung function and to identify those who need a complete investigation for COPD (Figure 1).

Stage	CTS 2008	NICE 2010	GOLD 2010	ACCP, ACP, ATS, ERS (Quaseem, 2011)
I - Mild	>= 80	>= 80	>= 80	> 80
II - Moderate	79,9-50	79,9-50	79,9-50	80-60 (> 50)
III - Severe	49,9-30	49,9-30	49,9-30	< 60
IV - Very severe	<30	<30	<30	

Table 4. FEV1 thresholds (% of theorical values) for classification of COPD

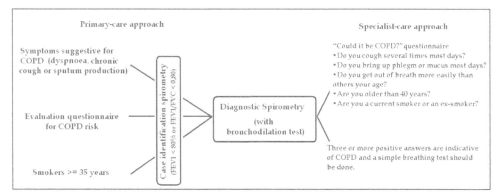

Fig. 1. Screening strategies for COPD (modified from Soriano et al, 2009)

However, spirometry is not commonly performed in primary care practice for many reasons, including limited access, lack of training, cost and time constraints (Barnes & Fromer, 2011; Perez et al, 2011). Spirometric results need a clinical interpretation, with a minimum time commitment of 2–10 min. Interpretation of one value should be assessed in conjunction with many others and by review of the shape of the best curves (ie, flow-volume loops and timing) (Soriano et al, 2009). An English survey find that most of the general practices in UK have a spirometer (82.4%) and use it (85.6%), but confidence in use and interpretation of results varied widely: 58.1% are confident in use but only 33.8% are confident in values interpretation (Bolton et al, 2005). A Swiss survey evaluated that spirometries in general practice are of acceptable quality with reproducible data in 60% of measurements (Leuppi et al, 2010). On the contrary a Dutch study (Schermer et al, 2003) assessed that the proportion of non-reproducible tests was 16% for laboratory tests and 18% for general practice tests in the first year, and 18% for both in the second year of evaluation, confirming that validity and quality of spirometric tests in general practice were as satisfactory as the procedure performed in the same group of COPD patients in a pulmonary function laboratory.

Adherence to the guidelines on the use of spirometry for diagnosis and follow-up is quite different in countries and often not comparable. A recent study (Chavez & Shokar, 2009) has estimated that only 50% of patients diagnosed with COPD performed a functional testing to confirm the presence of bronchial obstruction and only 40%, once diagnosed, received appropriate treatment. The adherence to GOLD guidelines by primary care providers have been recently evaluated (Perez et al, 2011): the study showed that less of 60% of general practitioner (GPs) complied with at least 5 to 7 key recommendations of the GLs used for evaluation. Cazzola, using an italian database in general practice, observed that a COPD population, registered in a period of 10 years, had a prevalence of chest radiograph in 67.7% while in the same period only the 31.9% of the patients had a spirometry (Cazzola et al, 2009). An important barrier to adherence is constituted by the lack of familiarity with specific recommendations due to the inadequate training in the management of COPD. In addition, medical students complain of inadequate training in the interpretation of spirometric tests (Perez et al, 2011; Soriano et al, 2009).

2.3 Radiology

There are no specific features of COPD on a plain chest radiograph. The features which are usually described are those of lung overinflation, vascular changes and bullae. However, even in patients with very appreciable disability, chest radiography results may be normal (Simon et al, 1973). The accuracy of diagnosing emphysema by plain chest radiography increases with the severity of the disease and it has been reported as being 50–80% accurate in patients with moderate-to-severe disease (Remy-Jardin et al, 1993). Modern imaging techniques, particularly with the advent of CT and, more recently, high resolution CT (HRCT), have provided a more sensitive means of diagnosing macroscopic emphysema during life (Gevenois & Yernault, 1995; Klein et al, 1992).

3. Treatments for stable COPD

The pharmacological treatment of COPD is based on the severity of the disease, defined by functional impairment and frequency of exacerbations (CTS, 2008; NICE, 2010; GOLD, 2010;

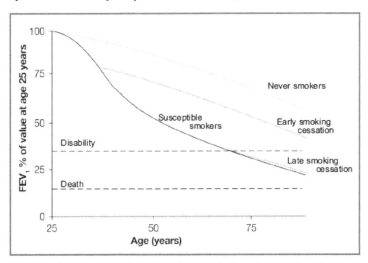

Fig. 2. Effects of smoking and smoking cessation on decline in lung function among adults with COPD (modified from Jones & Østrem, 2011).

Qaseem et al, 2011). It is currently under definition an algorithm that takes into account the intensity of symptoms, assessed with different scales (MRC and CAT). Smoking cessation is the first therapeutic measure, and perhaps most important in changing the natural history of disease. As it has been well demonstrated (Anthonisen et al, 2002a; Fletcher & Peto, 1977; Jones & Østrem, 2011) smoking cessation significantly improves survival, including the reduction of the pulmonary function decay. The relationship between long-term cigarette smoking, decline in lung function (FEV1 reduction) and life expectancy was demonstrated by Fletcher & Peto in 1977, but recently Jones & Østrem (2011) have redrawn the curves (Figure 2) to take into account data from recent studies.

3.1 Treatment strategies with inhaled drugs and COPD severity

The therapeutic approach to stable COPD is progressive, in steps, in relation to the 4 levels of severity defined by all guidelines (GLs) (CTS 2008; NICE, 2010; GOLD, 2010; Qaseem et al, 2011). As an example, the treatment schedule proposed by GOLD GLs (2010) is reported in figure 3.

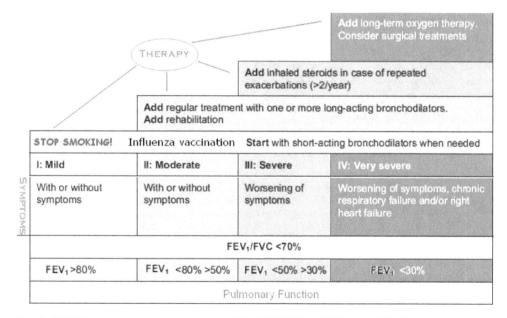

Fig. 3. COPD treatment strategies proposed by GOLD GLs (2010 – modified)

- **Stage 1 (mild COPD):** Initially, the drug treatments are based on the use to need of short-acting bronchodilators (in particular beta2-agonists with short duration of action - SABA). Some GLs (NICE, 2010; GOLD, 2010) suggest starting to use a long-acting bronchodilator (LABA or tiotropium) if symptoms (including cough and dyspnoea) are not well controlled with SABA.
- **Stage 2 (moderate COPD):** All recent GLs (CTS, 2008; NICE, 2010; GOLD, 2010; Qaseem et al, 2011) agree in recommending the use of a long-acting bronchodilator alone (LABA

or tiotropium) as first choice. If the symptoms persist or in the presence of frequent exacerbations (2 or more in the previous year) it is recommended to combine LABA and tiotropium and sometimes even an inhaled corticosteroid (ICS).

- **Stage 3 (severe COPD):** All recent GLs (CTS, 2008; NICE, 2010; GOLD, 2010; Qaseem et al, 2011) agree in recommending the use, as first choice, of a long-acting bronchodilator alone (LABA or tiotropium) and, in case of ineffectiveness, of associating LABA and tiotropium. The introduction of an ICS, usually associated with a LABA in a fixed combination, should be reserved for patients who have frequent exacerbations (at least 2 or more in the previous year).
- **Stage 4 (very severe COPD):** Treatment strategy is the same as Stage 3, although the introduction of an ICS, or the simultaneous use of LABA + ICS + tiotropium (Triple association) is from an early diagnostic findings (Karner & Cates 2011).

3.2 Efficacy of Inhaled treatments for COPD

In recent years the inhalation therapy of COPD has been shown to be effective in reducing symptoms, the frequency and severity of exacerbations, improve health status and exercise tolerance (NICE, 2010; GOLD, 2010; Spencer et al, 2011). In severe cases the only fixed combination of LABA and ICS, given twice a day and for several years, has also been shown to reduce mortality compared to placebo (Baker et al, 2009; Kliber et al, 2010; Nannini et al, 2007a; Wilt et al, 2007). However, the benefit is very modest, so that combination therapy (LABA + ICS, with or without tiotropium) does not appear to significantly improve clinically important outcomes (such as mortality, hospitalizations, severe exacerbations) than treatment with single products (Baker et al, 2009; Kliber et al, 2010; Nannini et al, 2007b; Puhan et al, 2009; Rodrigo et al, 2009; Welsh et al, 2010; Wilt et al, 2007). The association between LABA and tiotropium does not demonstrate advantages when compared with tiotropium alone (Wang et al, 2011).

The choice of the drug to start with, and any subsequent associations has to be customized, since the relationship between the severity of symptoms and the severity of airflow obstruction is influenced by other factors, such as the frequency and severity of exacerbations, presence of one or more complications, respiratory failure, comorbidities (cardiovascular disease, sleep disorders, etc.) and general health.

Fundamental to the effectiveness of prescribed treatments is that the patient has been properly taught on how to use various devices inhalers (Al-Showair et al, 2007; Dolovich et al, 2011). Patients with COPD may have problems in coordination and find it difficult to use a metered-dose inhaler (MDI) or, in cases of severe emphysema, fail to produce the inspiratory depression (Peak Inspiratory Flow - PIF) required to inhale the powder of a device DPI (Dry Powder Inhaler). The inhaler technique should be checked at each visit (see Table 5).

Many drugs are available for nebulising to be used in patients who have very low inspiratory flow (PIF), i.e. for severe hyperinflation. However, there are few randomized studies on their benefits compared to many other devices, and the use of nebulizers often depends on personal preferences, the availability and price. The nebulizer treatment should be continued only if patients report a clear benefit on symptoms.

Metered dose inhalers (MDI)	Dry powder inhalers (DPI)
	Load the dispenser
Exhale away from device	Exhale away from device
Put mouthpiece in your mouth	Put mouthpiece in your mouth
Take a slow, deep breath at the same time you press down on the medication canister.	Take a deep breath and breath in quickly.
Continue inhaling slowly for 4-5 seconds	Hold your breath for 10 second or as long as possible.
	Do not exhale through the mouthpiece to avoid wetting the chamber.
At the end of inhalation always rinse the mouth.	

Table 5. Patient information for optimal use of inhaled devices
(adapted from Dolovich et al, 2011)

3.3 Safety of Inhaled treatments for COPD

β2-agonists. The β2-adrenergic receptors stimulation can give sinus tachycardia at rest and induce changes in heart rate in patients highly susceptible. A recent review of the literature has also ruled out that prolonged treatment with LABAs increase the risk of cardiovascular death (Rodrigo et al, 2008). In older patients treated with high doses of β2-agonists can occur over a tremor that creates problems, regardless of the administration route, thus limiting the tolerated dose. Other metabolic effects, subject to tachyphylaxis, are hypokalaemia, especially when the beta2-agonist therapy is associated with a thiazide diuretic (Lipworth et al, 1990), and the increase of oxygen consumption at rest (Uren et al, 1993).

Anticholinergics. Inhaled anticholinergic drugs are poorly absorbed, which limits the occurrence of important systemic adverse effects (AEs), that are atropine-like (Tashkin, 2010). The most common AE is dry mouth. Some patients using ipratropium report a bitter and metallic taste. It has rarely been reported prostate (dysuria, urinary retention) and ocular (worsening of acute glaucoma) disorders. A slight increase in cardiovascular events compared with placebo, was observed in COPD patients regularly treated with ipratropium (Anthonisen et al, 2002b; Michele et al, 2010) or tiotropium used with Respimat MDI device, (a death in every 124 patients treated per year) (Singh et al, 2011).

Inhaled corticosteroids. Inhaled steroids in COPD are used almost exclusively associated with LABAs and at doses lower than those used in the treatment of asthma in adults. There are adverse events (AEs) both local and systemic:

- **Topic AEs** (oral candidiasis, dysphonia and pharyngitis): affect 8-10% of patients and the frequency increases by increasing the administered dose (Rachelefsky et al, 2007). Typically there is a lower incidence of AEs using DPI formulations compared to MDI formulations. The risk of such AEs can be reduced by rinsing the mouth after inhalation.
- **Systemic AEs**: the most important are the increased frequency of pneumonia and fractures. An increased frequency of pneumonia and severe pneumonia (respectively +2.7% and +2.1%), without increasing total mortality, has been documented with ICS treatment, alone or in combination with LABAs (Singh et al, 2009). The risk of pneumonia increases especially in patients with more severe COPD (FEV1 <40%). A

modest increase (+0.3%) in the risk of bone fractures related to the dose of ICS has been recently documented in a systematic review of 16 randomized controlled trials with 17,513 patients affected with moderate to severe COPD (Loke et al, 2011). In prolonged treatments with high doses of ICS were also reported cases of adrenal cortical insufficiency, cataracts, glaucoma and dermal dystrophy (thinning skin, easy bruising). (Tashkin et al, 2004).

3.4 Oral treatments for COPD

Methylxanthines (theophylline). The most commonly used methylxanthine is theophylline, whose clearance decreases with age. Low-dose theophylline reduces exacerbations, but do not improve post-bronchodilator lung function (Zhou et al, 2006). The evidence supporting the use of theophylline in stable COPD, limited because of its side effects, is insufficient. The toxicity of theophylline is dose-dependent, the therapeutic index is low and most of the benefits appear only with the administration of doses close to those toxic (Ram, 2006b). The AEs include the development of atrial and ventricular arrhythmias (which can be fatal), grand mal seizures (which may occur regardless of a previous history of epilepsy). Other AEs include headache, insomnia, nausea and epigastralgia, which can also occur within the therapeutic range of theophylline. Methylxanthines also have significant interactions with commonly used medications, such as digitalis, warfarin, etc..

Phosphodiesterase-4 inhibitors (roflumilast). The main activity of the inhibitors of phosphodiesterase-4 (PDE4 inhibitors) is to reduce inflammation by inhibiting intracellular cyclic AMP degradation (Rabe, 2011). The use of roflumilast is not worldwide approved. This drug is administered orally once a day, without direct bronchodilator activity, although it has been shown to improve FEV1 in patients treated with tiotropium or salmeterol (Calverley et al, 2009; Fabbri et al, 2009). In patients with severe to very severe COPD and a history of exacerbations, the roflumilast is able to reduce moderate and severe exacerbations (Calverley et al 2009; Rabe, 2011). There is a lack of evidence for comparing roflumilast vs or added to inhaled corticosteroids. The PDE4 inhibitors cause more AEs than inhaled medications for COPD (Calverley et al, 2009; Fabbri et al, 2009; Rabe, 2011). The most frequent AEs are nausea, decreased appetite, abdominal pain, diarrhoea, headache and sleep disorders; these AEs seem to occur early during treatment, are reversible and reduced over time during continued treatment. Since in registrative clinical trials was seen a decline in average weight of 2 kg in patients treated with roflumilast, the drug is not recommended in patients underweight. Roflumilast should be used with caution in patients with depression, too. The roflumilast and theophylline should not be administered concurrently.

3.5 Oxygen therapy

The long-term oxygen therapy (LTOT) is usually administered in patients with stable COPD who have:

- PaO_2 equal to or less than 7.3 kPa (55 mmHg) or SaO_2 equal to or less than 88%, with or without hypercapnia or
- PaO_2 between 7.3 kPa (55 mmHg) and 8.0 kPa (60 mmHg), or $SaO_2 > 88\%$, if there is pulmonary hypertension, peripheral edema suggesting congestive heart failure, or polycythemia (hematocrit > 55%).

LTOT has been shown to increase survival in patients with chronic respiratory failure and severe hypoxemia at rest only if practiced over 15 hours a day (Stoller et al, 2010).

Oxygen therapy can be administered in three ways (ATS, 1995; Celli & McNee, 2004):

- Long-term continuous therapy,
- during physical exertion and
- to relieve acute dyspnoea.

The main goal of oxygen therapy is to increase the baseline PaO_2 to a minimum of 8.0 kPa (60 mmHg) at sea level and at rest, and / or produce an O_2 saturation of at least 90%. Oxygen is usually released through face masks, with adequate flow concentrations, ranging from 24 to 35%. The facemask get an accurate titration of oxygen; however, many patients prefer the oxygen released by nasal cannula. The release of oxygen by this route requires additional monitoring of blood gases to ensure a satisfactory oxygenation, and may require individual titration. Additional oxygen at home is usually the most expensive part of the therapy of patients with COPD (Petty & O'Donohue, 1994). The oxygen concentrators can be cheaper than the systems of delivery of liquid or gaseous oxygen (Heaney et al, 1999).

3.6 Non-pharmacologic treatments for stable COPD

Vaccinations. The annual flu vaccination has been shown to reduce both hospitalizations and mortality in patients with COPD (Nichol et al, 1999a; Poole et al, 2006). Pneumococcal vaccination has been shown to produce important benefits, such as the reduction of hospitalizations and total mortality, particularly in patients with severe COPD (Nichol et al, 1999b).

Pulmonary Rehabilitation The main goals of pulmonary rehabilitation are to reduce symptoms, improve quality of life and increased physical and emotional participation in everyday activities (Nici et al, 2006; Ries et al, 2007).

The minimum length of an effective rehabilitation period is 6 weeks, but better results are obtained with activities even longer. However, no effective program has been developed so far to maintain the effects over time (Ries et al, 2007). Although the benefits have not been studied, it is reasonable to suggest to COPD patients, who can not follow a structured rehabilitation program, to exercise on their own (such as walking for 20 minutes a day). In any case, patients with more severe dyspnea (stage MRC 4 - see table 2) may not have the benefit of rehabilitation (Wedzicha et al, 1998)

The components of pulmonary rehabilitation programs are:

- **Physical training.** The exercise tolerance can be assessed with various tests, the simplest of which is the 6-minute walking test, measuring the distance traveled. The duration of physical training generally ranges from 4 to 10 weeks, resulting in greater effects for longer than the shorter lengths (Lacasse et al, 1996). The patient should be encouraged to move until it has been completed a walking period of 20 minutes. In patients severely disabled, the use of a simple walker with wheels improves walking distance and decreases the sensation of dyspnoea. The addition of upper limb exercises or other aerobic training is effective in improving the muscular strenght, but does not improve the quality of life or exercise tolerance (Bernard et al, 1999).

- **Smoking cessation.** Smoking cessation has the greatest impact on the natural history of COPD (figure 2). The evaluation of smoking cessation in a multicenter, long-term study (Anthonisen et al, 1994) indicates that, if effective resources and time are devoted to smoking cessation, can be maintained long-term quit rate of 25%.
- **Nutritional counselling.** Nutritional status is an important part of certain symptoms, disability and prognosis of COPD. Both overweight and underweight can be a problem (Nici et al, 2006). Approximately 25% of patients with COPD shows a reduction in body mass index, especially against the lean mass, which turns out to be an independent risk factor for mortality (Schols et al, 1998). The current evidence suggests that the nutritional supplement alone may not be sufficient if a strategy is not associated with exercise. In patients with COPD, nutritional supplements (eg creatine) do not substantially increase the training effect of a multidisciplinary pulmonary rehabilitation program (Deacon et al, 2008). Anabolic steroids in COPD patients with weight loss increase body weight and lean body mass, but have little or no effect on exercise ability (Weisberg et al, 2002).
- **Education.** Most pulmonary rehabilitation program includes an educational component, but the specific contributions of education to the improvements obtained after pulmonary rehabilitation are still not clear. Patient education alone does not improve exercise performance or lung function, but may play a role in improving the skills, the ability to cope with the disease and health status (Celli, 1995).

Table 6 summarizes the benefits of pulmonary rehabilitation in descending order with respect to the robustness of available evidences (from A to C grading system).

Grading*	
A	Improves the ability to exercise
A	Reduces the intensity of the perceived sense of breathlessness
A	Improves the quality of life related to health
A	Reduces the number and days of hospitalisation
A	Reduces anxiety and depression associated with COPD
B	Strength and endurance training of the upper limbs improves the function of the arms.
B	The benefits extend beyond the immediate period of training
B	Improves survival
B	Increases the effect of long-acting bronchodilators
B	Improves recovery after hospitalisation for an exacerbation
C	Training of respiratory muscles is useful, especially when combined with physical training
C	Psychosocial intervention is helpful

*The grading system express the robustness of scientific evidence: an A recommendation is sustained by a strong scientific proofs, while a D evidence is mainly based on expert-opinion. Grade B and C express intermediate levels of evidence.

Table 6. Benefits of pulmonary rehabilitation in patient with COPD (modified from GOLD GLs, 2010)

4. COPD and comorbidity

COPD often coexists with other diseases that have a significant impact on prognosis (Barnes & Celli, 2009; Mannino et al, 2008; Soriano et al, 2005; Sin et al, 2006). Some of these more often coexist and may be correlated, both for shared risk factors that impact on the mutual development (Fabbri et al, 2008), although the risk of comorbidity may also be the result of consequences of COPD, for example, reduced physical activity.

Cardiovascular disease is probably the main comorbidity in COPD (Fabbri et al, 2008; Soriano et al, 2005). Heart Failure (HF) is common in COPD: about 30% of patients with stable COPD have some degree of HF (Rutten et al, 2005). Worsening of HF is a significant differential diagnosis to an acute exacerbation of COPD. About 30% of patients in a cardiologic clinic is diagnosed with COPD (Hawkins et al, 2009) which will often be the cause of hospitalization for acute HF, with significant implications on prognosis (Iversen et al, 2010). In the treatment of HF with concomitant COPD is preferable to use a β-selective blocker (β-1 selective) compared to a non-selective β-blocker (Jabbour et al, 2010). Patients with COPD also have an increased incidence of Atrial Fibrillation (AF) (Buch et al, 2003). There are no reliable data on the use of drugs in COPD patients with AF and these patients were often excluded from clinical trials. In cardiac patients, however, it seems reasonable to avoid particularly high doses of β-agonists.

Other diseases commonly associated with COPD are osteoporosis (often under-diagnosed and at risk of deterioration with the use of systemic corticosteroids) and depression (associated with poor prognosis, but can favorably affected by exercise rehabilitation - Knubben et al, 2007). Lung cancer is often observed in patients with COPD and was found to be the most frequent cause of death in patients with mild COPD (Anthonisen et al, 2002a).

5. Management of acute exacerbations of COPD (AECOPD)

An authoritative definition of acute exacerbation of COPD (AECOPD) is the American Thoracic Society (ATS)/European Respiratory Society (ERS) consensus statement one: "an exacerbation of COPD is an event in the natural course of the disease characterised by a change in the patient's baseline dyspnoea, cough and/or sputum beyond day-to-day reliability sufficient to warrant a change in management" (Celli & McNee, 2004).

On average, COPD patients have one to four AECOPD per year, of various intensity/severity (Hagedorn, 1992). Patients who have frequent exacerbations (more than 3 per year) have a more rapid decline in lung function than patients who relapsed less frequently (-40 mL FEV1/year vs. -32 mL FEV1/year) (Donaldson et al, 2002). The economic burden of this common condition is extremely high, taking into consideration that during an AECOPD there is an intensification of treatment and often the need for hospitalisation, or even use of the intensive care unit (ICU). Hospital mortality for AECOPD is about 10% per year (Siafakas & Wedzicha, 2006) and the long-term outcome is rather poor: 3 years after hospitalization mortality from all causes rises up to 49% (Gunen et al, 2005; Wouters, 2003).

5.1 Diagnosis of AECOPD

The diagnosis of COPD exacerbation is clinical and does not depend on the results of ad hoc surveys, however, such investigations may help to define an optimal strategy of treatment.

The presence of greenish phlegm is a good indicator of high bacterial load and the potential success of antibiotic therapy; patients with light-colored phlegm do not derive additional benefit from antibiotic treatment (Stockley et al, 2000). Pulse oximetry may be useful in assessing the severity of an exacerbation and to identify patients who may benefit from oxygen (Bach et al, 2001). Chest radiographs are useful in the differential diagnosis, distinguishing pneumonia, congestive heart failure, pneumothorax, pleural effusion , etc. (Emerman & Cydulka 1993; Sherman et al, 1989; Tsai et al, 1993). During an exacerbation, lung function changes are usually limited , then spirometry takes little diagnostic significance (Bach et al, 2001).

5.2 Causes of AECOPD

For adequate management of the patient it is of paramount importance to identify the causes of AECOPD (Celli & McNee, 2004; GOLD, 2010) (Figure 4); however, in approximately one-third of the cases, this is not feasible. In more than half of the episodes, the cause of an exacerbation is a viral infection. Bronchoscopic studies have shown that at least 50% of patients have bacteria in high concentrations in their lower airways during exacerbations of COPD (Pela et al, 1998), but a significant proportion of these patients have bacteria in their lower airways in the stable phase of the disease, too (Sethi & Murphy, 2008). Conditions that may mimic the symptoms of an COPD exacerbation in a patient with COPD include pneumonia, congestive heart failure and/or arrhythmias, pulmonary embolism, pneumothorax, pleural effusion, metabolic diseases, inappropriate use of drugs (hypnotics) or end-stage disease (Siafakas & Wedzicha, 2006).

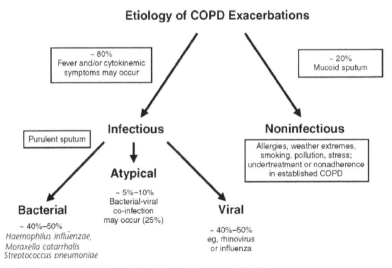

Etiology of COPD Exacerbations

Fig. 4. **Etiology of AECOPD** (modified from Anzueto, 2010)

5.3 Home management of AECOPD

Proper decision about the management of an AECOPD requires information on the previous condition of the patient in the stable state and a precise assessment of the severity of the present episode (Celli & McNee, 2004; GOLD 2010). In table 7 the factors to consider to decide whether to manage an AECOPD at home or in hospital are reported (NICE, 2010).

	Treat at home?	Treat in hospital?
Able to cope at home	Yes	No
Breathlessness	Mild	Severe
General condition	Good	Poor/deteriorating
Level of activity	Good	Poor/confined to bed
Cyanosis	No	Yes
Worsening peripheral oedema	No	Yes
Level of consciousness	Normal	Impaired
Already receiving LTOT	No	Yes
Social circumstances	Good	Living alone/not coping
Acute confusion	No	Yes
Rapid rate of onset	No	Yes
Significant comorbidity (particularly cardiac disease and insulin-dependent diabetes)	No	Yes
$SaO_2 < 90\%$	No	Yes

Table 7. Patient's factors to consider when deciding where to manage an AECOPD (modified from NICE, 2010)

A review shows that, when the patient does not require intensive hospital care and can be adequately cared at home, the home management of exacerbations is effective as the hospital management (mortality and hospital readmissions are similar) (Ram et al, 2004) and is most appreciated by patients and carers. The objectives of outpatient or home management are (Hurst & Wedzicha, 2004; Ram et al, 2004):

- educate patients and families on the signs of deterioration and the actions to be taken (with written instructions);
- increase maximum airflow;
- remove excess bronchial secretions;
- treat infection, if present;
- improve respiratory muscle strength and, thus, facilitate cough;
- avoid or monitor adverse events of treatment.

A decisional algorithm to facilitate decisions in treating at home a mild to moderate AECOPD exacerbation is reported in figure 5 (modified from Siafakas & Wedzicha, 2006).

Education: it was shown that education can reduce utilisation of health services and result in better survival rates after an AECOPD (Nici et al, 2006; Tougaard et al, 1992). Educational intervention (better with written instructions) should underline the following features:

- The patient, but just as importantly the family, should be instructed on the signs and symptoms that indicate a worsening of the patient's condition and the actions that should be taken, e.g. contact a physician or go to the hospital.

- Self-clearance of sputum by frequent coughing and/or by performing forced expiratory manoeuvres from middle lung volume. An effective cough consists of a slow, deep inspiration, a few seconds of breath holding followed by a cascade of two to three voluntary cough efforts.
- If the patient is on LTOT, advise him/her not to change the dose by him/herselve;
- Adequate training in usage of treatment to ensure maximum compliance to prescribed treatment.
- Usual nutrition may need to be modified (i.e. small and frequent meals with low carbohydrate content) and fluid intake increased.
- Advise the patient or his/hers family to avoid sedatives and hypnotics, as well as cough mixtures that contain such agents.

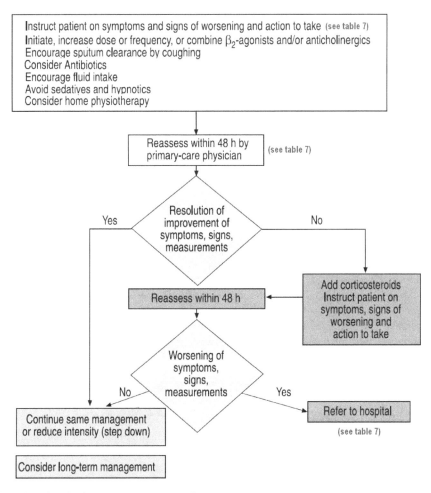

Fig. 5. Algorithm for the home management of an AECOPD
(Modified from Siafakas & Wedzicha, 2006)

Bronchodilators (short acting and long acting): increasing doses of beta 2 agonists "short acting" (isoprenaline, salbutamol, terbutaline) may effectively counteract the increased dyspnoea; standard pressurized inhalers (MDI) and nebulizers are equally effective dose inhalers to administer bronchodilators; doses to be administered and the patients' conditions may influence the choice of method of administration (see table 5). There is no evidence on the effectiveness of LABAs in the treatment of exacerbations. The use of ipratropium or tiotropium (alone or in combination) does not appear justified in the first instance (McCrory & Brown, 2003).

Inhaled and Oral Corticosteroids: Initiating or increasing the dose of inhaled corticosteroids (ICS) is the first step-up when steroid treatment is required. If a spacer is used and an adequate dose is given, this mode of administration (inhaled) is efficient in most cases. However, oral corticosteroids may be needed in more severe cases, often with beneficial results (Thompson et al, 1996; Siafakas & Wedzicha, 2006). A daily dose of 30–40 mg of prednisolone for 10–14 days may be required. Systemic corticosteroids shorten the length of hospital stay, improve lung function (FEV_1) and arterial hypoxemia (PaO_2) (Davies et al, 1999, Maltais et al, 2002; Thompson et al, 1996); they also reduce the risk of early recurrence and treatment failure (Aaron et al, 2003; Davies et al, 1999).

Antibiotics: although only half of AECOPD are due to infections, and a large part of these are viral (Wedzicha, 2004), it is common practice to administer a course of antibiotics for 7–14 days. A systematic review of the few placebo-controlled studies available has shown that antibiotics reduce the risk of short-term mortality by 77%, by 53% of the treatment failure and sputum purulence by 44%. This review supports antibiotics for patients with moderate or severe AECOPD, with increased cough and sputum purulence (Quon et al, 2008; Ram et al, 2006a). The benefits of antibiotics are still more pronounced in patients with more severe exacerbations (Bach et al, 2001).

The local bacterial resistance should be taken into account when empirical treatment is given (Celli & McNee, 2004). Broad-spectrum antibiotics, such as amoxicillin, with or without clavulanic acid, tetracyclines, erythomycin or oral cephalosporin are recommended (Siafakas et al, 2005). In particular conditions (patients with frequent episodes of exacerbation, recent antibiotic treatments or hospitalizations, stays at facilities for the elderly) is likely the selection of multiresistant (bacterial strains especially Pseudomonas or Staphylococcus aureus). In these cases, when the targeted therapy is not possible, you should choose between fluoroquinolones or cephalosporins (Woodhead al, 2005).

Mucolytic agents: recent guidelines conclude that: "there is no evidence to support prescription of mucolytics in acute exacerbation". However, these agents can be beneficial in a few cases with copious and tenacious sputum (Celli & McNee, 2004; GOLD, 2010).

Oxygen therapy: Initiation of oxygen therapy at home during an exacerbation of COPD may lead to serious complications and should be avoided. If the patient is on long-term oxygen therapy (LTOT), a thorough inspection of the apparatus and dosage of oxygen administered is recommended (see paragraph 3.5). In addition, a clinical evaluation of adequate oxygenation is required. However, when the evaluation is in doubt, the assessment should take place in the hospital with emogasanalysis. (Siafakas & Wedzicha, 2006; NICE 2010).

5.4 Hospital discharge and follow-up

The following features were found to be predictive of re-hospitalization (Bahadori & Fitzgerald, 2007): a previous hospitalization, use of oral corticosteroids or long-term oxygen, the poor quality of life associated with reduced physical activity. Regular home visits by a community nurse may permit earlier discharge of patients hospitalized for AECOPD without increasing re-hospitalizations (Celli & McNee, 2004; Hermiz et al, 2002; Hughes et al, 2000; Siafakas et al, 2005). However, the exact criteria for this approach remain uncertain and vary depending on the scope rated health (Hermiz et al, 2002). The use of a written action plan increased therapeutic interventions appropriate for an acute exacerbation, an effect that does not diminish, however, the use of health resources (Wood-Baker et al, 2006). For patients who are hypoxemic during the AECOPD, blood gases and / or pulse oximetry should be reevaluated before hospital discharge and if the patient remains hypoxemic, it may be necessary to add an additional long-term oxygen therapy.

5.5 Prevention of AECOPD

Smoking cessation, anti-flu and anti-pneumococcal vaccines, knowledge of current treatment, including inhaler technique, the constant treatment with inhaled bronchodilators in long duration of action, with or without inhaled corticosteroids, significantly reduces the number of exacerbation and hospitalization (Calverley et al, 2007; Nannini et al, 2007a; Nannini et al, 2007b; Tashkin et al, 2008). Early outpatient pulmonary rehabilitation after hospitalization is safe (see paragraph 3.6) and leads to significant clinical improvements in terms of exercise capacity and health status at 3 months (Man et al, 2004). If the patient has a significant persisting disability should be evaluated in social welfare issues, identifying the main caregivers with whom agree the treatment plan.

6. Conclusions

COPD is a chronic disease whose prevalence is increasing, and the diagnosis and management is primarily the task of general practitioners. Screening for COPD is not recommended in asymptomatic smokers, but running an office spirometry in heavy smokers older than 35 years and with symptoms can be an initial framework for early detection of COPD and provide effective interventions to reduce mortality. Smoking cessation has been shown to improve the prognosis of patients with COPD, especially if applied early. Treatments with combined inhaled LABA and ICS have also been shown to reduce mortality in patients with more severe COPD, while the use of long-acting bronchodilators (LABAs or/and tiotropium) reduces only the number of exacerbations and hospitalizations. Pulmonary rehabilitation is a key to improving treatment outcomes (important for patients with COPD), but is rarely used, especially in home management of COPD. Able to prevent or control the AECOPD at home is a very important goal of the GP, for which it is necessary to apply the recommendations of the best guidelines and obtain the cooperation of patients and their families.

7. References

Aaron SD, Vandemheen KL, Hebert P, Dales R, Stiell IG, Ahuja J, Dickinson G, Brison R, Rowe BH, Dreyer J, Yetisir E, Cass D, Wells G. (2003) Outpatient oral prednisone after emergency treatment of chronic obstructive pulmonary disease. *N Engl J Med* 348: 2618-2625.

Al-Showair RA, Tarsin WY, Assi KH, Pearson SB, Chrystyn H. (2007) Can all patients with COPD use the correct inhalation flow with all inhalers and does training help? *Respir Med* 101: 2395-2401.

American Thoracic Society (1995) Standards for the diagnosis and care of patients with chronic obstructive pulmonary disease. *Am J Respir Crit Care Med* 152: S77–S120.

Anthonisen NR, Connett JE, Kiley JP, Altose MD, Bailey WC, Buist AS, Conway WA Jr, Enright PL, Kanner RE, O'Hara P, et al.. (1994) Effects of smoking intervention and the use of an inhaled anticholinergic bronchodilator on the rate of decline of FEV1. The Lung Health Study. *JAMA* 272: 1497-1505.

Anthonisen NR, Connett JE, Enright PL, Manfreda J. (2002 a) Hospitalizations and mortality in the Lung Health Study. *Am J Respir Crit Care Med* 166: 333-339.

Anthonisen NR, Connett JE, Murray RP. (2002 b) Smoking and lung function of Lung Health Study participants after 11 years. *Am J Respir Crit Care Med* 166: 675-679.

Anzueto A. (2010) Primary Care Management of Chronic Obstructive Pulmonary Disease to reduce Exacerbations and Their Consequences. *Am J Med Sci* 340 (4): 309–318.

Bach PB, Brown C, Gelfand SE, McCrory DC. (2001) Management of Acute Exacerbations of Chronic Obstructive Pulmonary Disease: A Summary and Appraisal of Published Evidence. *Ann Intern Med* 134: 600-620.

Bahadori K, FitzGerald JM. (2007) Risk factors of hospitalization and readmission of patients with COPD exacerbation--systematic review. *Int J Chron Obstruct Pulmon Dis* 2: 241-251.

Baker WL, Baker EL, Coleman CI. (2009) Pharmacologic treatments for chronic obstructive pulmonary disease: a mixed-treatment comparison meta-analysis. *Pharmacotherapy* 29(8): 891-905.

Barnes PJ, Celli BR. (2009) Systemic manifestations and comorbidities of COPD. *Eur Respir J* 33: 1165-1185.

Barnes TA, Fromer L. (2011) Spirometry use: detection of chronic obstructive pulmonary disease in the primary care setting *Clinical Interventions in Aging* 6: 47–52

Bernard S, Whittom F, Leblanc P, Jobin J, Belleau R, Bérubé C, Carrier G, Maltais F. (1999) Aerobic and strength training in patients with chronic obstructive pulmonary disease. *Am J Respir Crit Care Med* 159: 896-901.

Bestall JC, Paul EA, Garrod R, Garnham R, Jones PW, Wedzicha JA. (1999) Usefulness of the Medical Research Council (MRC) dyspnoea scale as a measure of disability in patients with chronic obstructive pulmonary disease. *Thorax* 54: 581–586.

Blanc PD, Menezes AM, Plana E, Mannino DM, Hallal PC, Toren K, Eisner MD, Zock JP. (2009) Occupational exposures and COPD: an ecological analysis of international data. *Eur Respir J* 33: 298 – 304.

Bolton CE, Ionescu AA, Edwards PH, Faulkner TA, Edwards SM, Shale DJ. (2005) Attaining a correct diagnosis of COPD in general practice. *Respir Med* 99: 493 – 500.

Buch P, Friberg J, Scharling H, Lange P, Prescott E. (2003) Reduced lung function and risk of atrial fibrillation in the Copenhagen City Heart Study. *Eur Respir J* 21: 1012-1016.

Buist AS, McBurnie MA, Vollmer WM, Gillespie S, Burney P, Mannino DM, Menezes AM, Sullivan SD, Lee TA, Weiss KB, Jensen RL, Marks GB, Gulsvik A, Nizankowska-Mogilnicka E. BOLD Collaborative Research Group. (2007) International variation in the prevalence of COPD (The BOLD Study): a population-based prevalence study. *Lancet* 370: 741 – 750.

Calverley PM, Anderson JA, Celli B, Ferguson GT, Jenkins C, Jones PW, Yates JC, Vestbo J. TORCH investigators. (2007) Salmeterol and fluticasone propionate and survival in chronic obstructive pulmonary disease. *N Engl J Med* 356: 775-789.

Calverley PM, Rabe KF, Goehring UM, Kristiansen S, Fabbri LM, Martinez FJ. (2009) Roflumilast in symptomatic chronic obstructive pulmonary disease: two randomised clinical trials. *Lancet* 374: 685-694.

Cazzola M, Bettoncelli G, Sessa E, Cricelli C. (2009) Primary care of the patient with chronic obstructive pulmonary disease in Italy. *Respiratory Medicine* 103: 582-588.

Celli BR. (1995) Pulmonary rehabilitation in patients with COPD. *Am J Respir Crit Care Med* 152: 861-864.

Celli BR, MacNee W. (2004) Standards for the diagnosis and treatment of patients with COPD: a summary of the ATS/ERS position paper. *Eur Respir J* 23: 932-946.

Chavez PC, Shokar NK. (2009) Diagnosis and management of chronic obstructive pulmonary disease (COPD) in a primary care clinic. *COPD* 6 (6): 446-451.

CTS (2008) Canadian Thoracic Society recommendations for management of chronic obstructive pulmonary disease – 2008 update - highlights for primary care. O'Donnell DE, Hernandez P, Kaplan A, Aaron S, Bourbeau J, Marciniuk D, Balter M, Ford G, Gervais A, Lacasse Y, Maltais F, Road J, Rocker G, Sin D. *Can Respir J* 15 Suppl A:1A-8A. www.lung.ca/cts-sct/guidelines-lignes_e.php

Davies L, Angus RM, Calverley PM. (1999) Oral corticosteroids in patients admitted to hospital with exacerbations of chronic obstructive pulmonary disease: a prospective randomised controlled trial. *Lancet* 354: 456-460.

Deacon SJ, Vincent EE, Greenhaff PL, Fox J, Steiner MC, Singh SJ, Morgan MD. (2008) Randomized controlled trial of dietary creatine as an adjunct therapy to physical training in chronic obstructive pulmonary disease. *Am J Respir Crit Care Med* 178: 233-239.

Decramer M, Miravitlles M, Price D, Roman-Rodrìguez M, Llor C, Welte T, Buhl R, Dusser D, Samara K, Siafakas N. (2011) New horizons in early stage COPD - Improving knowledge, detection and treatment. *Respiratory Medicine* 105: 1576-1587

Dolovich M, Dhand R. (2011) Aerosol drug delivery: developments in device design and clinical use. *Lancet* 377: 1032-1045

Donaldson GC, Seemungal TA, Bhowmik A, Wedzicha JA. (2002) Relationship between exacerbation frequency and lung function decline in chronic obstructive pulmonary disease. *Thorax* 57: 847-852.

Emerman CL, Cydulka RK. (1993) Evaluation of high-yield criteria for chest radiography in acute exacerbation of chronic obstructive pulmonary disease. *Ann Emerg Med* 22: 680–684.

Fabbri LM, Calverley PM, Izquierdo-Alonso JL, Bundschuh DS, Brose M, Martinez FJ, Rabe KF. M2-127 and M2-128 study groups. (2009) Roflumilast in moderate-to-severe chronic obstructive pulmonary disease treated with long-acting bronchodilators: two randomised clinical trials. *Lancet* 374: 695-703.

Fabbri LM, Luppi F, Beghé B, Rabe KF. (2008) Complex chronic comorbidities of COPD. *Eur Respir J* 31: 204-212.

Fletcher C, Peto R. (1977) The natural history of chronic airflow obstruction. *BMJ* 1: 1645-1648.

Gevenois PA, Yernault JC. (1995) Can computed tomography quantify pulmonary emphysema? *Eur Respir J* 8: 843–848.

GOLD (2010) Global Strategy for the Diagnosis; Management and Prevention of COPD, update 2010. www.goldcopd.org

Gunen H, Hacievliyagil SS, Kosar F, Mutlu LC, Gulbas G, Pehlivan E, Sahin I, Kizkin O. (2005) Factors affecting survival of hospitalised patients with COPD. *Eur Respir J* 26: 234-241.

Hagedorn SD (1992) Acute exacerbations of COPD. How to evaluate severity and treat the underlying cause. *Postgrad Med* 91: 105–112.

Hawkins NM, Huang Z, Pieper KS et al. (2009) Chronic obstructive pulmonary disease is an independent predictor of death but not atherosclerotic events in patients with myocardial infarction: analysis of the Valsartan in Acute Myocardial Infarction Trial (VALIANT) *Eur J Heart Fail* 11: 292-298.

Heaney LG, McAllister D, MacMahon J. (1999) Cost minimisation analysis of provision of oxygen at home: are the drug tariff guidelines cost effective? *BMJ* 319: 19-23.

Hermiz O, Comino E, Marks G, Daffurn K, Wilson S, Harris M. (2002) Randomised controlled trial of home based care of patients with chronic obstructive pulmonary disease. *BMJ* 325: 938-942.

Hughes SL, Weaver FM, Giobbie-Hurder A, Manheim L, Henderson W, Kubal JD, Ulasevich A, Cummings J. Department of Veterans Affairs Cooperative Study Group on Home-Based Primary Care. (2000) Effectiveness of team-managed home-based primary care: a randomized multicenter trial. *JAMA* 284: 2877-2885.

Hurst JR, Wedzicha JA. (2004) Chronic obstructive pulmonary disease: the clinical management of an acute exacerbation. *Postgrad Med* 80: 497–505.

Iversen KK, Kjaergaard J, Akkan D, Kober L, Torp-Pedersen C, Hassager C, Vestbo J, Kjoller E; ECHOS Lung Function Study Group. (2010) The prognostic importance of lung function in patients admitted with heart failure. *Eur J Heart Fail* 12: 685-691.

Jabbour A, Macdonald PS, Keogh AM, Kotlyar E, Mellemkjaer S, Coleman CF, Elsik M, Krum H, Hayward CS. (2010) Differences between beta-blockers in patients with chronic heart failure and chronic obstructive pulmonary disease: a randomized crossover trial. *J Am Coll Cardiol* 55: 1780-1787.

Johannessen A, Omenaas ER, Bakke PS, Gulsvik A. (2005) Implications of reversibility testing on prevalence and risk factors for chronic obstructive pulmonary disease: a community study. *Thorax* 60 (10): 842-847.

Jones RC, Dickson-Spillmann M, Mather MJ, Marks D, Shackell BS. (2008) Accuracy of diagnostic registers and management of chronic obstructive pulmonary disease: the Devon primary care audit. *Respir Res* 9: 62.

Jones PW, Price D, van der Molen T. (2011) Role of clinical questionnaires in optimizing everyday care of chronic obstructive pulmonary disease. *International Journal of COPD* 6: 289–296

Jones R, Østrem A. (2011) Optimising pharmacological maintenance treatment for COPD in primary care. *Primary Care Respiratory Journal* 20(1): 33-45

Joo MJ, Lee TA, Weiss KB. (2008) Geographic variation of spirometry use in newly diagnosed COPD. *Chest* 134: 38 – 45.

Karner C, Cates CJ. (2011) Combination inhaled steroid and long-acting beta2-agonist in addition to tiotropium versus tiotropium or combination alone for chronic obstructive pulmonary disease. *Cochrane Database of Systematic Reviews*, Issue 3. Art. No.: CD008532. DOI: 10.1002/14651858.CD008532.pub2.

Klein JS, Gamsu G, Webb WR, Golden JA, Muller NL. (1992) High-resolution CT diagnosis of emphysema in symptomatic patients with normal chest radiographs and isolated low diffusing capacity. *Radiology* 182: 817–821.

Kliber A, Lynd LD, Sin DD (2010) The effects of long-acting bronchodilators on total mortality in patients with stable chronic obstructive pulmonary disease *Respiratory Res* 11: 56-70

Knubben K, Reischies FM, Adli M, Schlattmann P, Bauer M, Dimeo F (2007) A randomised, controlled study on the effects of a short-term endurance training programme in patients with major depression. *Br J Sports Med* 41: 29-33.

Lacasse Y, Wong E, Guyatt GH, King D, Cook DJ, Goldstein RS. (1996) Meta-analysis of respiratory rehabilitation in chronic obstructive pulmonary disease. *Lancet* 348: 1115-1119.

Leuppi JD, Miedinger D, Chhajed PN, Buess C, Schafroth S, Bucher HC Tamm M. (2010) Quality of Spirometry in Primary Care for Case Finding of Airway Obstruction in Smokers. *Respiration* 79: 469–474

Levy ML, Fletcher M, Price DB, Hausen T, Halbert RJ, Yawn BP. (2006) International Primary Care Respiratory Group guidelines: diagnosis of respiratory diseases in primary care. *Prim Care Respir J* 15 (1): 20-34.

Lipworth BJ, McDevitt DG, Struthers AD. (1990) Hypokalemic and ECG sequelae of combined beta-agonist/diuretic therapy. Protection by conventional doses of spironolactone but not triamterene. *Chest* 98: 811-815.

Loke YK, Cavallazzi R, Singh S. (2011) Risk of fractures with inhaled corticosteroids in COPD: systematic review and meta-analysis of randomized controlled trials and observational studies. *Thorax* 66: 699-708

Maltais F, Ostinelli J, Bourbeau J, Tonnel AB, Jacquemet N, Haddon J, Rouleau M, Boukhana M, Martinot JB, Duroux P. (2002) Comparison of nebulized budesonide and oral prednisolone with placebo in the treatment of acute exacerbations of chronic obstructive pulmonary disease: a randomized controlled trial. *Am J Respir Crit Care Med* 165: 698-703.

Man WD, Polkey MI, Donaldson N, Gray BJ, Moxham J. (2004) Community pulmonary rehabilitation after hospitalisation for acute exacerbations of chronic obstructive pulmonary disease: randomised controlled study. *BMJ* 329: 1209-1211.

Mannino DM, Buist AS. (2007) Global burden of COPD: risk factors, prevalence, and future trends. *Lancet* 370: 765–773.

Mannino DM, Thorn D, Swensen A, Holguin F. (2008) Prevalence and outcomes of diabetes, hypertension and cardiovascular disease in COPD. *Eur Respir J* 32: 962-969.

McCrory DC, Brown CD. (2003) Anticholinergic bronchodilators versus beta2-sympathomimetic agents for acute exacerbations of chronic obstructive pulmonary disease. *Cochrane Database of Systematic Reviews* Issue 1. Art. No.: CD003900. DOI: 10.1002/14651858.CD003900.

Michele TM, Pinheiro S, Iyasu S. The safety of tiotropium-the FDA's conclusions. (2010) *N Engl J Med* 363: 1097-1099.

Nannini LJ, Cates CJ, Lasserson TJ, Poole P. (2007a) Combined corticosteroid and long-acting beta-agonist in one inhaler versus placebo for chronic obstructive pulmonary disease. *Cochrane Database of Systematic Reviews*, Issue 4. Art. No.: CD003794. DOI:10.1002/14651858.CD003794.pub3.

Nannini LJ, Cates CJ, Lasserson TJ, Poole P. (2007b) Combined corticosteroid and long-acting beta-agonist in one inhaler versus long-acting beta-agonists for chronic obstructive pulmonary disease. *Cochrane Database of Systematic Reviews*, Issue 4. Art. No.: CD006829. DOI: 10.1002/14651858.CD006829.

NICE (2010) Management of Chronic Obstructive Pulmonary Disease in Adults in Primary and Secondary Care. Update NICE Clinical Guideline 12 - www.nice.org.uk/cg101

Nichol KL, Baken L, Nelson A. (1999a) Relation between influenza vaccination and outpatient visits, hospitalization, and mortality in elderly persons with chronic lung disease. *Ann Intern Med* 130(5): 397-403.

Nichol KL, Baken L, Wuorenma J, Nelson A. (1999b) The health and economic benefits associated with pneumococcal vaccination of elderly persons with chronic lung disease. *Arch Intern Med* 159(20): 2437-2442.

Nici L, Donner C, Wouters E, Zuwallack R, Ambrosino N, Bourbeau J, Carone M, Celli B, Engelen M, Fahy B, Garvey C, Goldstein R, Gosselink R, Lareau S, MacIntyre N, Maltais F, Morgan M, O'Donnell D, Prefault C, Reardon J, Rochester C, Schols A, Singh S, (2006) American Thoracic Society/European Respiratory Society statement on pulmonary rehabilitation. *Am J Respir Crit Care Med* 173: 1390-1413.

Pela R, Marchesani F, Agostinelli C, Staccioli D, Cecarini L, Bassotti C, Sanguinetti CM. (1998) Airways microbial flora in COPD patients in stable clinical conditions and during exacerbations: a bronchoscopic investigation. *Monaldi Arch Chest Dis* 53: 262-267.

Perez X, Wisnivesky JP, Lurslurchachai L, Kleinman LC, Kronish IM. (2011) Barriers to adherence to COPD guidelines among primary care providers. *Respiratory Medicine* xx, 1-8 (in press)

Petty TL, O'Donohue WJ, Jr. (1994) Further recommendations for prescribing, reimbursement, technology development, and research in long-term oxygen therapy. Summary of the Fourth Oxygen Consensus Conference, Washington, D.C., October 15-16, 1993. *Am J Respir Crit Care Med* 150: 875-877.

Poole P, Chacko EE, Wood-Baker R, Cates CJ. (2006) Influenza vaccine for patients with chronic obstructive pulmonary disease. *Cochrane Database of Systematic Reviews*, Issue 1. Art. No.: CD002733. DOI: 10.1002/14651858.CD002733.pub2.

Price D, Chir MBB, Yawn BP, Jones RCM. (2010) Improving the Differential Diagnosis of Chronic Obstructive Pulmonary Disease in Primary Care. *Mayo Clin Proc* 85(12): 1122-1129.

Price D, Freeman D, Cleland J, Kaplan A, Cerasoli F. (2011) Earlier diagnosis and earlier treatment of COPD in primary care. *Primary Care Respiratory Journal* 20 (1): 15-22.

Puhan MA, Bachmann LM, Kleijnen J, Ter RG, Kessels AG. (2009) Inhaled drugs to reduce exacerbations in patients with chronic obstructive pulmonary disease: a network meta-analysis. *BMC Med* 7: 2 doi:10.1186/1741-7015-7-2

Qaseem A, Wilt TJ, Weinberger SE, Hanania NA, Criner G, van der Molen T Marciniuk DD, Denberg T, Schunemann H, Wedzicha W, MacDonald R, and Shekelle P (2011) Diagnosis and Management of Stable Chronic Obstructive Pulmonary Disease: A Clinical Practice Guideline Update from the American College of Physicians, American College of Chest Physicians, American Thoracic Society, and European Respiratory Society *Ann Intern Med* 155: 179-191.

Quon BS, Gan WQ, Sin DD. (2008) Contemporary management of acute exacerbations of COPD: a systematic review and metaanalysis. *Chest* 133: 756-766.

Rabe KF. (2011) Update on roflumilast, a phosphodiesterase 4 inhibitor for the treatment of chronic obstructive pulmonary disease. *Br J Pharmacol* 163: 53-67.

Rachelefsky SG, Liao Y, Faruqi R. (2007) Impact of inhaled corticosteroid-induced oropharyngeal adverse events: results from a meta-analysis. *Ann Allergy Asthma Immunol* 98: 225-238

Ram FS, Wedzicha JA, Wright J, Greenstone M. (2004) Hospital at home for patients with acute exacerbations of chronic obstructive pulmonary disease: systematic review of evidence. *BMJ* 329: 315. doi:10.1136/bmj.38159.650347.55

Ram FS, Rodriguez-Roisin R, Granados-Navarrete A, Garcia-Aymerich J, Barnes NC. (2006a) Antibiotics for exacerbations of chronic obstructive pulmonary disease. *Cochrane Database of Systematic Reviews*, Issue 2. Art. No.: CD004403. DOI:10.1002/14651858.CD004403.pub2.

Ram FS. (2006b) Use of theophylline in chronic obstructive pulmonary disease: examining the evidence. *Current opinion in pulmonary medicine* 12: 132-139.

Remy-Jardin M, Remy J, Gosselin B, Becette V, Edme JL. (1993) Lung parenchymal changes secondary to cigarette smoking: pathologic–CT correlations. *Radiology* 86: 643–651.

Ries AL, Bauldoff GS, Carlin BW et al. (2007) Pulmonary Rehabilitation: Joint ACCP/AACVPR Evidence-Based Clinical Practice Guidelines. *Chest* 131: 4S-42S.

Rodin A, Cote C. (2008) Primary care of the patient with chronic obstructive pulmonary disease–part 1: frontline prevention and early diagnosis. *Am J Med* 121 (7 suppl): S3-S12.

Rodrigo GJ, Nannini LJ, Rodriguez-Roisin R. (2008) Safety of long-acting beta-agonists in stable COPD: a systematic review. *Chest* 133(5): 1079-1087.

Rodrigo GJ, Castro-Rodriguez JA, Plaza V. (2009) Safety and Efficacy of Combined Long-Acting β-Agonists and Inhaled Corticosteroids vs Long-Acting β-Agonists Monotherapy for Stable COPD. *Chest* 136: 1029–1038.

Rutten FH, Cramer MJ, Grobbee DE, Sachs AP, Kirkels JH, Lammers JW, Hoes AW. (2005) Unrecognized heart failure in elderly patients with stable chronic obstructive pulmonary disease. *Eur Heart J* 26: 1887-1894.

Schermer TR, Jacobs JE, Chavannes NH, Hartman J, Folgering HT, Bottema BJ, van Weel C. (2003) Validity of spirometric testing in a general practice population of patients with chronic obstructive pulmonary disease (COPD). *Thorax* 58: 861–866 .

Schols AM, Slangen J, Volovics L, Wouters EF. (1998) Weight loss is a reversible factor in the prognosis of chronic obstructive pulmonary disease. *Am J Respir Crit Care Med* 157: 1791-1797.

Sethi S, Murphy TF. (2008) Infection in the pathogenesis and course of chronic obstructive pulmonary disease. *N Engl J Med* 359: 2355-2365.

Sherman S, Stoney JA, Ravikrishnan KP. (1989) Routine chest radiographs in exacerbations of chronic obstructive pulmonary disease. Diagnostic value. *Arch Intern Med* 149: 2493–2496.

Siafakas NM, Tzortzaki E, Tsoumakidou M. Antibiotics in COPD. (2005) In: *Long-Term Intervention in Chronic Obstructive Pulmonary Disease*. Pauwels RA, Postma DS, Weiss S, eds. New York, Marcel Dekker Inc., pp. 423–443.

Siafakas NM, Wedzicha JA (2006) Chapter 24. Management of acute exacerbation of chronic obstructive pulmonary disease. *European Respiratory Society Monograph* n. 38 (Management of Chronic Obstructive Pulmonary Disease): 387-400; DOI: 10.1183/1025448x.00038024

Simon G, Pride NB, Jones NL, Raimondi AC. (1973) Relation between abnormalities in the chest radiograph and changes in pulmonary function in chronic bronchitis and emphysema. *Thorax* 28: 15–23.

Sin DD, Anthonisen NR, Soriano JB, Agusti AG (2006) Mortality in COPD: Role of comorbidities. *Eur Respir J* 28: 1245-1257.

Singh S, Amin AV, Loke YK. (2009) Long-term use of inhaled corticosteroids and the risk of pneumonia in chronic obstructive pulmonary disease: A Meta-analysis. *Arch Intern Med* 169: 219-229

Singh S, Loke YK, Enright PL, Furberg CD. (2011) Mortality associated with tiotropium mist inhaler in patients with chronic obstructive pulmonary disease: systematic review and meta-analysis of randomised controlled trials. *BMJ* 342: d3215

Soriano JB, Visick GT, Muellerova H, Payvandi N, Hansell AL. (2005) Patterns of comorbidities in newly diagnosed COPD and asthma in primary care. *Chest* 128: 2099-2107.

Soriano JB, Zielinski J, Price D. (2009) Screening for and early detection of chronic obstructive pulmonary disease. *Lancet* 374: 721–732.

Spencer S, Karner C, Cates CJ, Evans DJ. (2011) Inhaled corticosteroids versus long-acting beta2-agonists for chronic obstructive pulmonary disease. *Cochrane Database of Systematic Reviews*, Issue 12. Art. No.: CD007033. DOI:10.1002/14651858. CD007033.pub3.

Stockley RA, O'Brien C, Pye A, Hill SL. (2000) Relationship of sputum color to nature and outpatient management of acute exacerbations of COPD. *Chest* 117: 1638-1645.

Stoller JK, Panos RJ, Krachman S, Doherty DE, Make B. (2010) Oxygen therapy for patients with COPD: current evidence and the long-term oxygen treatment trial. *Chest* 138: 179-187.

Tashkin DP, Murray HE, Skeans M, Murray RP. (2004) Skin manifestations of inhaled corticosteroids in COPD patients: results from Lung Health Study II. *Chest* 126: 1123-1133

Tashkin DP, Celli B, Senn S, Burkhart D, Kesten S, Menjoge S, Decramer M. UPLIFT Study Investigators. (2008) A 4-year trial of tiotropium in chronic obstructive pulmonary disease. *N Engl J Med* 359: 1543-1554.

Tashkin DP. (2010) Long-acting anticholinergic use in chronic obstructive pulmonary disease: efficacy and safety. *Current opinion in pulmonary medicine* 16: 97-105.

Thompson WH, Nielson CP, Carvalho P, Charan NB, Crowley JJ. (1996) Controlled trial of oral prednisone in outpatients with acute COPD exacerbation. *Am J Crit Care Med* 154: 407–412.

Tougaard L, Krone T, Sorknaes A, Ellegaard H. (1992) Economic benefits of teaching patients with chronic obstructive pulmonary disease about their illness. *Lancet* 339: 1517–1520.

Tsai RW, Gallager EJ, Lombarti G, Gennis P, Carter W. (1993) Guidelines for the selective ordering of admission chest radiography in adult obstructive airway disease. *Ann Emerg Med* 22: 1854–1858.

Uren NG, Davies SW, Jordan SL, Lipkin DP. (1993) Inhaled bronchodilators increase maximum oxygen consumption in chronic left ventricular failure. *Eur Heart J* 14: 744-750.

Wang J, Jin D, Zuo P, Wang T, Xu Y , Xiong W (2011) Comparison of tiotropium plus formoterol to tiotropium alone in stable chronic obstructive pulmonary disease: A meta-analysis. *Respirology* 16: 350–358

Wedzicha JA, Bestall JC, Garrod R, Garnham R, Paul EA, Jones PW. (1998) Randomized controlled trial of pulmonary rehabilitation in severe chronic obstructive pulmonary disease patients, stratified with the MRC dyspnoea scale. *Eur Respir J* 12: 363-369.

Wedzicha JA. (2004) Role of viruses in exacerbations of chronic obstructive pulmonary disease. *Proc Am Thoracic Soc* 1: 115–120.

Weisberg J, Wanger J, Olson J, Streit B, Fogarty C, Martin T, Casaburi R. (2002) Megestrol acetate stimulates weight gain and ventilation in underweight COPD patients. *Chest* 121: 1070-1078.

Welsh EJ, Cates CJ, Poole P. (2010) Combination inhaled steroid and long-acting beta2-agonist versus tiotropium for chronic obstructive pulmonary disease. *Cochrane Database of Systematic Reviews*, Issue 5. Art. No.: CD007891. DOI: 10.1002/14651858. CD007891.pub2.

Wilt TJ, Niewoehner D, MacDonald R, Kane RL. (2007) Management of stable chronic obstructive pulmonary disease: a systematic review for a clinical practice guideline. *Ann Intern Med* 147(9): 639-653.

Wood-Baker R, McGlone S, Venn A, Walters EH. (2006) Written action plans in chronic obstructive pulmonary disease increase appropriate treatment for acute exacerbations. *Respirology* 11: 619-626.

Woodhead M, Blasi F, Ewig S et al. (2005) Guidelines for the management of adult lower respiratory tract infections. *Eur Respir J* 26: 1138-1180.

Wouters EF. (2003) The burden of COPD in The Netherlands: results from the Confronting COPD survey. *Respir Med* 97 Suppl C: S51-59.

Yawn BP. (2009) Differential assessment and management of asthma vs chronic obstructive pulmonary disease. *Medscape J Med* 11 (1): 20.

Zhou Y, Wang X, Zeng X, Qiu R, Xie J, Liu S, Zheng J, Zhong N, Ran P. (2006) Positive benefits of theophylline in a randomized, double-blind, parallel-group, placebo-controlled study of low-dose, slow-release theophylline in the treatment of COPD for 1 year. *Respirology* 11: 603-610.

4

Diagnosis of Chronic Obstructive Pulmonary Disease with Special Reference to Over- and Underdiagnosis Using Spirometry

Peter Montnemey and Sölve Elmståhl
Lund University
Sweden

1. Introduction

Chronic Obstructive Pulmonary Disease (COPD) is increasingly recognized as a major public health problem. In the western world it is the 4th -5th most common cause of death and the only one that is rising among the top ten causes (Murray & Lopez, 1997). The disease is estimated to become the third leading cause of death worldwide by 2020 (Chapman et al., 2006). However, depending on the criteria used and the population studied, the estimated prevalence rates may vary. Historically, COPD has been defined symptomatically as chronic bronchitis, anatomically as emphysema. The current definition is physiologically based on airway obstruction as measured by a spirometer.

By searching PubMed for population based prevalence studies extending back to mid-1962 Halbert et al. identified 32 studies that had a satisfactory methodology to be included in the interpretation (Halbert et al., 2003). The methodology included spirometry with or without clinical examination, the presence of respiratory symptoms, self reported disease and expert opinion (WHO). In all, the prevalence rates of COPD were ranging from 2%-22% depending on the criteria used for definition. Eleven studies used spirometry either in combination with clinical examination or alone to estimate the prevalence rates of COPD. In the spirometry studies the prevalence rates of COPD also varied but most of them were between 4% and 10 %. Recently Chapman et al. (Chapman et al., 2006) and Mannino & Buist have reported that COPD affects 5-15% of all adults in industrialized countries (Mannino & Buist, 2007). A growing number of women are affected.

However, since COPD is such a common disease and new treatments have been introduced, it is important that it can be diagnosed accurately. According to the current definition of COPD, the diagnosis requires a spirometry examination.

2. History

The ancient Egyptians described a condition similar to asthma more than 3000 years ago. Hippocrates (460-370 BC) is supposed to be the first European to describe asthma. The knowledge concerning COPD and its manifestations emphysema, chronic bronchitis and asthmatic bronchitis goes back to Badham 1814 (Badham, 1814), who described the bronchiolitis and chronic cough and mucus hypersecretion that are the cardinal symptoms of COPD.

Emphysema and its symptoms has been described by Laënnec, the inventor of the stethoscope, in 1827. The CIBA Guest Symposium in 1959 (CIBA Guest Symposium, 1959) and the American Thoracic Society Committee on Diagnostic Standards in 1962 defined the components of COPD that are the foundation for the present definitions (Committtee on Diagnostic Standards for Nontuberculous Respiratory Diseases, American Thoracic Society, 1962). William Briscoe is supposed to be the first person to use the term COPD in 1965 (Briscoe & Nash, 1965).

3. Definitions

There is a lack of a generally accepted definition of COPD. American Thoracic Society (ATS) and European Respiratory Society (ERS) define COPD as: " A preventable and treatable disease state characterized by airflow limitation that is not fully reversible. The airflow limitation is usually progressive and associated with an abnormal inflammatory response of the lungs to noxious particles or gases, primarily caused by cigarette smoking. Although COPD affects the lungs, it also produces significant systemic consequences." (Celli & MacNee, 2004).

Global Initiative for Chronic Obstructive Lung Disease (Global Initiative for Chronic Obstructive Lung Disease GOLD, 2010) define COPD as: "A preventable and treatable disease with some significant extra-pulmonary effects that may contribute to the severity in individual patients. Its pulmonary component is characterized by airflow limitation that is not fully reversible. The airflow limitation is usually progressive and associated with an abnormal inflammatory response of the lung to noxious particles or gases".

A simple spirometric definition and classification of disease severity into four stages has been recommended by GOLD. The classification has recently been updated (GOLD, 2010). GOLD recommends that a post-bronchodilator Forced Expiratory Volume in one second (FEV1)/Forced Vital Capacity (FVC) < 0.7 confirms the diagnosis of COPD. FEV1 provides a way to stage the severity of the disease.

Stages of COPD according to GOLD

Stage I: Mild COPD Mild airflow limitation (FEV1/FVC<0.7; FEV1 ≥80% predicted) and sometimes, but not always, chronic cough and sputum production.
At this stage, the individual may not be aware that his or her lung function is abnormal.

Stage II: Moderate COPD Worsening airflow limitation (FEV1/FVC < 0.7; 50%≤FEV1<80% predicted), with shortness of breath typically developing on exertion.
This is the stage at which patients typically seek medical attention because of chronic respiratory symptoms or an exacerbation of their disease.

Stage II: Severe COPD Further worsening of airflow limitation (FEV1/FVC < 0.7; 30%≤FEV1<50% predicted), greater shortness of breath, reduced exercise capacity, and repeated exacerbations which have an impact on patients´ quality of life.

Stage IV: Very Severe COPD Severe airflow limitation (FEV1/FVC < 0.7; FEV1<30% predicted or FEV1<70% predicted plus chronic respiratory failure. Patients may have Very Severe (Stage IV) COPD even if the FEV1 is >30% predicted, whenever this complication is present.
At this stage, quality of life is very appreciably impaired and exacerbations may be life-threatening.

However, the usage of a fixed Quotient FEV1/FVC to define pulmonary obstruction or COPD has been questioned. Considering that the FEV1/(F)VC ratio falls with age (Hedenstrom et al., 1985; Hedenstrom et al., 1986; Quanjer et al., 1993), the use of a fixed cut-off point for defining COPD overestimates the prevalence in the elderly and underestimates the prevalence in younger patients (Cerveri et al., 2008). The diagnosis and possible overestimation of COPD among elderly has previously been reported (Hansen et al., 2007; Lundbäck et al., 2003; Swanney et al., 2008; Vollmer et al., 2009).

While the current definitions of obstructive pulmonary disease are founded on spirometry measurements, the applied spirometric reference values and the applied guidelines are crucial. Several spirometric reference values are in use. In Europe the prediction equations by the European Coal and Steel Community (ECSC) are widely used for adults although the data were derived from lung function measurements over a long time period (1954-1980) and from different European countries. (Quanjer et al., 1993)

Globally several other spirometry reference values are in use or have been proposed, e.g. the prediction equations for Caucasian adult males and females derived from the Third US National Health and Nutrition Examination Survey (NHANES-III) (Hankinson et al., 1999) Brändli et al have published reference values of a Swiss population (Brädli et al., 1996; Brädli et al., 2000). In 2001 Langhammer et al. published forced spirometry reference values for Norwegian adults (Langhammer et al., 2001)

Recently Kuster et al published another set of reference equations for lung function of never smoking Swiss adults aged 18-80 years (Kuster et al., 2008). Falaschetti et al. have published reference values predicted for an English adult population using data from the 1995/1996 Health Survey for England (Falaschetti et al., 2004). Pistelli et al. have published spirometry reference equations from a general population sample aged 8-74 years in central Italy (P Pistelli et al., 2007). Recently reference equations have been published for Brazilian adults (Pereira et al., 2007), Polish adults (Ostrowoski et al., 2005), Chinese adults (Ip et al., 2006) and Kazakh adolescents (Facchini et al., 2007).

For ethnic populations of north-western Europe (Iceland, Norway, Denmark, Finland and Sweden), the almost 40-year-old Swedish reference material of Berglund et al has been used. The subjects were not randomly selected and included smokers as well as occupational exposures to dust. (Berglund et al., 1963).

In 1985 and 1986 Hedenström et al have published spirometric reference equations for Swedish females and males, which are widely used in Sweden. A total of 186 females, 100 never smokers and 86 smokers, and 270 males, 124 never smokers and 146 smokers respectively were investigated. The subjects were aged 20-70 years and divided in five age decades. Only subjectively healthy subjects with normal chest radiograms and who had had no significant occupational exposure to noxious dusts or fumes were included (Hedenstrom et al., 1985; Hedenstrom et al., 1986).

4. Risk factors

4.1 Smoking

Smoking is the major cause of COPD (Anto et al., 2001), and 85-90% of all patients with COPD are current or ex-smokers. In the literature it has been proposed that approximately

20% of smokers develop a clinically significant COPD (American Thoracic Society 1995; Fletcher et al.,1976; Rijcken et al., 1998). Lundbäck et al. have reported that as much as 50% of smokers who continue to smoke develop COPD (Lundbäck et al., 2003). Their results were based on the British Thoracic Society criteria (British Thoracic Society [BTS], 1997) and the GOLD criteria (GOLD, 2001) by the using the Swedish reference values published by Berglund et al. in 1963 (Berglund et al., 1963). Rennard et al have also proposed that far more than 15% of smokers get COPD: in fact, most develop some amount of pulmonary impairment. (Rennard & Vestbo, 2006).

4.2 Occupational and environmental exposure

Other factors are thought to modulate the risk of developing COPD. Occupational exposure to dust and fumes are important risk factors (Trupin et al., 2003). Bakke et al have examined a Norwegian general population aged 18-73 years. The authors concluded that exposure to specific agents and work processes may be independent risk factors for COPD when adjusted for gender, age and smoking. (Bakke et al., 1991). Urban air pollution may affect lung function. In a cross sectional study by Lindgren et al., living within 100 m of a road with >10 cars per minute was associated with prevalence of COPD diagnosis (OR = 1.64, 95%CI=1.11- 2.40) as well as chronic bronchitis symptoms as increased cough and sputum production compared with having no heavy road within this distance (Lindgren et al., 2009). Exposure to biomass fuels is also an important risk factor (Perez-Padilla, 1996; Varkey, 2004). It can be supposed that genetic and environmental factors interact to cause COPD. α_1 - antitrypsin deficiency has been recognized as one major genetic factor (Laurell & Eriksson , 1963).

4.3 Nasal features

In addition, a recent epidemiological study suggests that certain nasal features may be associated with COPD (Hurst, 2010; Montnemery et al., 2008).

4.4 Socio-economic status

Several previous studies have shown a relation between COPD and socioeconomic status as well as a recent study by Kanervisto et al. (Kanervisto, 2011) that measured low socioeconomic status by educational and income levels as risk factors using age, gender smoking and body mass index as possible confounders.

4.5 Alcohol

Alcohol intake has been proposed to be a risk factor, but the results are inconsistent. Garshick et al. found that lifetime alcohol consumption was a predictor of lower levels of FEV1 in a model that included age and pack years (Garshick et al., 1989). Lange et al found that consumption of 350 g of alcohol per week had an effect on FEV1 comparable to the effect of 15 g tobacco per day (Lange et al., 1988). Schunemann et al. did not find any correlation between total alcohol intake and lung function when adjusting for smoking, education and nutritional factors but a positive effect for wine intake, especially white wine (Schunemann et al., 2002). Tabak et al. found a beneficial effect of low alcohol consumption (1-30 g per day). The FEV 1 was higher and the prevalence of COPD symptoms lower than in non-drinkers (Tabak et al., 2001).

4.6 Co-morbidity

Some data suggest that co-morbidity of coronary heart disease (CHD), chronic congestive heart failure (CHF) and COPD are common. van Manen et al. found that comorbidity was more common among COPD patients seventy three percent and sixty three percent respectively (van Manen et al., 2001). Comorbidity and COPD has also been emphasized by Siebeling et al. (Siebeling et al., 2011).

Left ventricular dysfunction has been found in 32% of patients with COPD (Render et al., 1995). In a prospective cohort study including >60 years old patients with echocardiographically confirmed CHF (n=201) and clinical spirometry confirmed COPD (n=218), the prevalence of airway obstruction among CHF patients was 37.3% and the prevalence of ventricular dysfunction among COPD patients was 17 %. (Macchia et al., 2011).

4.7 Gender

The role of gender is unclear. Previous studies have shown a greater prevalence in men related to a more frequent smoking compared to females. (Foreman et al., 2011; Silverman et al., 2000). Results from the worldwide BOLD study indicate that not only smoking is a risk factor for COPD but also female gender (Buist et al., 2007). There might be a higher susceptibility for tobacco-induced COPD among different population groups.

Recently Kikpatrick and Dransfield have suggested that women and African-Americans are particularly susceptible to tobacco smoke. (Kikpatrick & Dransfield, 2009). The underlying physiological mechanisms for females to be at an increased risk have been considered to involve either hormonal homeostasis or structural development of lungs. The racial disparities in a higher susceptibility for COPD among African Americans have also been emphasized by Garcia-Aymerich (Garcia-Aymerich , 2011).

5. Normal ageing of the lung

Maximal lung function is reached at approximately the age of 20 years for females and 20 years for males. Thereafter, ageing is associated with a decrease of lung function. The most important physiologic lung changes with normal ageing are characterized by significant reduction in the elastic recoil of the lung, greater chest wall rigidity, and loss of respiratory muscle strength. (Knudson et al., 1977; Turner et al., 1968). However, in contrast to COPD, the morphologic changes consist of alveolar enlargement but without destructive wall changes of the alveoli (Fukuchi, 2009). As a result of the ageing process residual volume increases (air trapping) by approximately 50% between 20 and 70 years of age (Janssens et al., 1999). These changes are responsible for the lowered FEV1/FVC quotient observed in the elderly (Hedenstrom et al., 1985; Hedenstrom et al., 1986; Quanjer et al., 1993)., Thus, there is a risk of an over diagnosis of COPD when the disease is defined by a fixed ratio of FEV1/FVC (Swanney et al., 2008).

6. Pathology and pathogenesis of COPD

6.1 Pathology

The chronic airflow limitation characteristic of COPD is caused by inflammatory processes of the airways and lung tissue as a result of exposure to inhaled irritants. The airflow limitation is caused by a mixture of small airway disease (obstructive bronchiolitis) and parenchymal destruction (emphysema). The relative contributions vary from person to person. The inflammation causes structural changes and narrowing of the small airways and airway remodeling. Destruction of the lung parenchyma leads to loss of alveolar attachments to the small airways and decreases lung elastic recoil. These changes diminish the ability of the airways to remain open during expiration. (GOLD, 2010 ; Snider, 2000). The inflammation also leads to excess mucus production due to hypertrophy of the goblet cells and mucous glands of the airways. There is also a reduction of mucociliary clearance.

6.2 Pathogenesis

There are two major views of the pathogenesis of COPD.

6.2.1 The British hypothesis

The British hypothesis says that recurrent bronchial infections are the reason that some smokers develop airway obstruction. COPD (Anthonisen, 2004). The British hypothesis emphasizes that repeated chest infections and air pollution contribute to the development of the disease (Anthonisen, 2004).

6.2.2 The Dutch hypothesis

The Dutch hypothesis suggests that allergy and airway hyperresponsiveness interacting with genetic and environmental factors are important in the development both of asthma and COPD. (Dirjke et al., 2004; Vestbo & Prescott, 1998).

British hypothesis emphasizes exogenous factors but the Dutch hypothesis emphasizes endogenous factors. Both hypotheses are probably correct. Both bronchial hyperreactivity and recurrent pulmonary infections interacting with exposure to air irritants such as cigarette smoke or air pollution contribute to the development of and COPD and chronic bronchitis (Petty, 2006)

7. The natural history of COPD

The natural history of COPD begins with cellular and biochemical changes in the small airways and alveoli due to a chronic inflammation caused by the long term inhalation of noxious gases and particles such as cigarette smoke. COPD is characterized by a reduced FEV1 and an accelerated decline of FEV1 compared to healthy subjects. The airflow limitation measured by reduced FEV1 progresses over a long time, most often over several decades without any symptoms (Huib et al., 1997). In non-smokers without respiratory disease, FEV1 declines by 20-30 ml per year beginning at an age of about 35 years (Burrows et al., 1983; Huib et al., 1997). The rate of decline in smokers is steeper and the heavier the smoking, the steeper the rate of decline (Anthonisen et al., 1994; George, 1999). This indicates some dose – response relationship in the deterioration. In addition there are individuals who are unusually susceptible to the effects of tobacco smoke and in whom FEV1 declines at even at greater rates. Burrows et al. have described that a low FEV1/FVC ratio on entry of a spirometric study was associated with a high rate of decline in FEV1 at least among male smokers. This phenomena is called the horse racing effect (Burrows et al., 1987).

7.1 Smoking cessation

Almost every study on the effect of smoking cessation has shown that it has clinical and physiological benefits. Indeed it is the only measure that so far has been proven to stop the decline of FEV1 . In 1961 Fletcher and Peto started to investigate 792 working males aged 30 to 59 with spirometry, of whom 103 were non-smokers (Fletcher & Peto, 1977).

All the men were seen regularly over the next eight years. The decline of FEV1 in ex-smokers was slower than that in smokers, 37 and 62 mL/year respectively. After, smoking cessation the abnormal rate in FEV1 decline in ex-smokers gradually becomes similar to that found in non-smokers (Fletcher & Peto, 1977).

Their findings of reduced decline of FEV1 after quitting smoking have been confirmed by several other investigators as reviewed by Willemse et al. and Lee & Fry (Lee and Frey, 2010; Willemse et al., 2004). After having reviewed 47 studies, Lee and Fry concluded that never smokers had a decline of FEV1 10.8 mL/year less than continuing smokers and for quitters 8.5 mL/year less. Some but not all studies showed that the annual decline of FEV1 was greater in those with reduced lung function, particularly in those who continued smoking.

8. Spirometry

Hutchinson invented the spirometer in 1846.

The diagnosis of COPD is confirmed by spirometry, a test that measures the forced expiratory volume in one second (FEV1), which is the greatest volume of air that can be breathed out in the first second of a large breath. Spirometry also measures the forced vital capacity (FVC), which is the greatest volume of air that can be breathed out in a whole large breath. Normally at least 70% of the FVC comes out in the first second (FEV1/FVC ratio >0.7). Spirometric diagnosis and severity classification of COPD are based on post bronchodilator values after the administration of an adequate dose of an inhaled bronchodilator. (e.g. 400 µg salbutamol or 1000 µg terbutalin). Most investigators perform the spirometry according to the ATS guidelines (American Thoracic Society, 1995).

Fig. 1 shows a normal spirogram of a 57 years old female. The FVC and FEV1 values are normal. The FEV1/FVC ratio is normal. There was no increase of the lung volumes after a bronchodilator (400 µg salbutamol) was given.

Fig. 2. shows an abnormal spirogram (COPD) of a 62 years old female with a life long smoking history with about 44 pack years. One pack year is defined as 20 cigarettes a day for one year.

9. Over and under-diagnosis of COPD

COPD is one of the leading causes of morbidity and mortality among the adult population worldwide (GOLD, 2010). However, differences in the definition of COPD make it difficult to quantify the morbidity. Spirometry is the golden standard for diagnosing COPD but there are also different recommendations in the guidelines concerning how to perform spirometry (Nathell et al., 2007). Most guidelines define airway obstruction by a FEV1/FVC ratio less than 0.7. It is well known that the FEV1/FVC ratio declines with

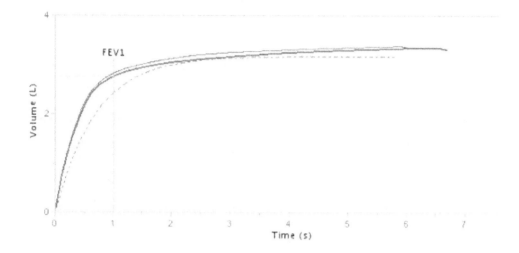

Fig. 1. Normal spirogram. Female 57 years old, height 162 cm. Predicted values according to Hedenström et al., 1985.

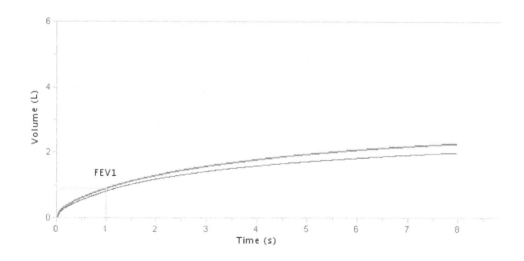

Fig. 2. Severe COPD according to the GOLD criteria. Female 62 years old, height 175 cm. Predicted values according to Hedenström et al., 1985.

Normal spirogram Fig.1.

	Pre-bronchodilator values (grey line)	Post-bronchodilator values (green line)	Percent (%) of predicted values. Post bronchodilator	Predicted values
FVC	3.4	3.4	97%	3.5
FEV1	2.8	2.8	104%	2.7
FEV1/FVC	0.82	0.82	106%	0.77

Abnormal spirogram (COPD) Fig.2.

	Pre-bronchodilator values (grey line)	Post-bronchodilator values (green Line)	Percent (%) of predicted values. Post bronchodilator	Predicted values
FVC	2.3	2.5	61%	4.1
FEV1	0.8	0.9	31%	2.9
FEV1/FVC	0.35	0.36	51%	0.71

increasing age, even in healthy non-smokers (Falaschetti et al., 2004; Quanjer et al., 1993; Stanojevic et al., 2010). Thus, there is a risk of an over-diagnosis of COPD in the elderly patient but a risk of under-diagnosis in younger individuals when the disease is defined by a fixed ratio of FEV1/FVC (Swanney et al., 2008). By using four prediction equations derived from large European studies, Schermer et al. have illustrated the decline of the FEV1/FVC ratio by age (Schermer et al., 2007) They concluded that the fixed 0.70 ratio leads to false negative results in younger adults and to false positive test results in older adults. Using the large NHANES III database (Hankinson et al., 1999) it has been demonstrated that above the age of 50 years, about 50% of subjects regarded to be obstructive were false positives (Schermer et al., 2007).

Celli et al. have also used the NHANES III database to evaluate the impact of different definitions of airway disease by different criteria: 1) self-reported disease, 2) the GOLD criteria FEV1/FVC<0.7 and FEV1<80% predicted, 3) FEV1/FVC < LLN, FEV1/FVC <88% predicted in males and <89% predicted in females and FEV1/FVC<0.7. They concluded that prevalence rates can vary by >200% depending on which definition was used (Celli et al., 2003). Vollmer et al. have analyzed data from the large international Burden of Obstructive Lung Disease (BOLD) study including data from 10,001 individuals aged ≥ 40 years recruited from 14 sites (Vollmer et al., 2009). They concluded that using FEV1/FVC<LLN criterion instead of the fixed FEV1/FVC criterion should minimize known age biases and better reflect clinically significant irreversible airflow limitation (Vollmer et al., 2009). Miller et al. determined the discrepancy rates in pulmonary function test interpretation between the GOLD guidelines of FEV1/FVC<0.7 for detecting airway obstruction and an FEV1 of 80% predicted for detecting and classifying the severity of COPD (Miller et al., 2011). They investigated 11,413 patients with pre bronchodilator lung function tests and concluded that using 80% predicted and fixed thresholds can lead to substantial misclassification of disease that affects >20% of patients compared to using LLN in diagnosing pulmonary obstruction. Shirtcliffe et al. investigated 749 people by post bronchodilator spirometric tests (Shirtcliffe et al., 2007). For adults ≥ 40 years, 14.2% were obstructive according to the GOLD definition and 9.0% according to obstruction defined using LLN.

In an editorial published in the European Respiratory Journal in 2007, Mannino argued for the fixed FEV1/FVC quotient to define pulmonary obstruction in favor of simplicity and that it is more sensitive to identify patients at risk of death and COPD related hospitalization (Mannino et al., 2003).

The latter position was also argued by Firdaus et al (Firdaus et al., 2011). However, the prediction of death and hospitalization has nothing to do with defining the diagnosis of the disease (Pellegrino et al. 2008). Spirometry software and hardware have changed and there is no longer a need for manual calculations of predicted spirometric values.

In a recent Swedish study, a random sample of 518 men and women in nine age cohorts 60, 66, 72, 78, 81, 84, 87, 90 and 93 years were drawn from the municipality registers and were investigated with spirometry using different guidelines and reference values (Szanto, et al., 2010). In the whole population, the prevalence of airway obstruction was 22.5% using FEV1/(F)VC <0.7 and 10.1% using the FEV1/(F)VC<expected for age and gender to define obstruction by using the Swedish spirometric reference values by Hedenström et al. Smoking habits had a great impact on the prevalence figures. Among current smokers the prevalence of pulmonary obstruction was 41.7%, among ex-smokers 22.7% and 15.5% among never-smokers using FEV1/(F)VC <0.7 to define obstruction. The corresponding figures using FEV1/(F)VC<expected for age and gender to define obstruction were 25.0%, 9.7% and 4.9% respectively. Using the FEV1/(F)VC<expected for age and gender definition yielded lower prevalence rates in all age groups and in both genders. The highest prevalence, 76.9%, was seen among current male smokers in the age cohort 72-81 years when airway obstruction was defined as FEV1/(F)VC <0.7. Using the FEV1/(F)VC< expected for age and gender definition yielded a prevalence of 46.2% in the same group. It is notable that 23.9% of never-smokers in the age cohort 84-93 years were classified as obstructive using FEV1/(F)VC <0.7 to define obstruction but 10.1% using the age and gender adjusted ratio (Table1).

Age cohorts	60-94			60-71			72-82			83-94		
Gender	All	M	F	All	M	F	All	M	F	All	M	F
	(n=565)	(n=223)	(n=342)	(n=200)	(n=90)	(n=110)	(n=208)	(n=83)	(n=125)	(n=157)	(n=50)	(n=107)
Current-smokers												
FEV1/(F)VC)<0.7	41.7	50.0	35.7	35.2	33.3	36.7	57.7	76.9	38.5	37.5	66.7	30.8
FEV1/(F)VC<LLN	25.0	30.0	21.4	22.2	20.8	23.3	34.6	46.2	23.1	18.8	33.3	15.4
Ex-smokers												
FEV1/(F)VC)<0.7	22.7	19.8	27.0	14.9	7.3	24.2	25.3	27.7	21.9	34.4	26.1	55.6
FEV1/(F)VC<LLN	9.7	9.0	10.8	9.5	2.4	18.2	8.9	12.8	3.1	12.5	13.0	11.1
Never-smokers												
FEV1/(F)VC)<0.7	15.5	18.1	14.6	6.9	8.0	6.4	12.6	13.0	12.5	23.9	33.3	21.2
FEV1/(F)VC<LLN	4.9	6.9	4.2	1.4	0	2.1	1.9	0	2.5	10.1	20.8	7.1

Table 1. Variation in prevalence of airway obstruction defined FEV1/(F)VC<0.7 and Lower Limit of Normal (FEV1/(F)VC<expected for age and gender) in the study population (n=565) related to smoking habits. Hedenstrom et al. normal spirometric values. No smoking data in 9 subjects. M= males, F= females. Figures in percent.

In an open letter by Philip Quanjer, Paul Enright, Martin Miller, Janet Stocks, Gregg Ruppel, Maureeen Swanney, Robert Crapo, Ole Pedersen, Emanuel Falaschetti, Jan Schouten and Robert Jensen to the members of the GOLD committee, the group appealed to change the method by which mild airway obstruction is defined by the GOLD guidelines in order to abandon the fixed ratio in favor of the lower limit of normal (Quanjer et al., 2010).

10. Conclusions

A diagnosis of COPD should be considered in any smoker, especially in smokers who have breathing symptoms characterized by dyspnea, chronic cough or sputum production and who are aged 40 years or more. For the diagnosis and assessment of COPD, spirometry is the golden standard.

However, the diagnosis of pulmonary obstruction depends very much on the criteria used for definition of airway obstruction and on which spirometric normal values are applied. Normal values derived from the population investigated should be used.

Defining and diagnosing pulmonary obstruction using a fixed FEV1/(F)VC quotient <0.7 is simple to use in clinical practice but might result in an under-diagnosis in younger subjects and a substantial over-diagnosis in older subjects. Using an age-adjusted FEV1/(F)VC quotient to define pulmonary obstruction can be suggested to reduce the risk of over-diagnosis among elderly and under-diagnosis in younger subjects.

COPD is usually a progressive disease and lung-function can be expected to degrade over time. Therefore spirometry should be repeated over time, E.g. once a year.

Earlier diagnosis will allow earlier, and more aggressive efforts to make the patients quit smoking, the most important and effective therapy.

11. Appendix

11.1 Reference equations

The range of spirometric values obtained from a healthy population is assumed to represent normal. There are an overwhelming number of published reference equations.

11.2 Abbreviations

NA = Not Available
VC = Vital Capacaty
FVC = Forced Vital Capacaty
FEV1 = Forced Expiratory Volume in one second
FEV6 = Forced Expiratory Volume in six seconds
H = Height (cm or m)
A = Age (yrs)
pr = Predicted

LLN = Lower Limit of Normal (The lower fifth percentile of the reference population. Can be calculated by subtracting 1.64 times the standard deviation from the mean, i.e. the expected value (Firdaus et al., 2011).

11.3 Equations

Swedish participants. Between 7 to 70 years of age. Smokers and non smokers. (Berglund et al., 1963).

Male subjects:

FVC Berglund= $(4.81 \times H) - (0,020 \times A) - 2.81$
FEV1Berglund = $(3.44 \times H) - (0,033 \times A) - 1.00$

Female subjects:

FVC Berglund = $(4.04 \times H) - (0,022 \times A) - 2.35$
FEV1 Berglund = $(2.67 \times H) - (0,027 \times A) - 0.54$

Swedish participants. Between 20 to 70 years of age. Smokers and non smokers. (Hedenström et al., 1985; Hedenström et al.,1986)

Male subjects:

VC Hedenstrom = $(7.52 \times H) + (0.0471 \times A) - (0.000686 \times A^2) - 8,56$
FVC Hedenstrom = $(7.44 \times H + (0.0467 \times A) - (0.000705 \times A^2) - 8,44$
FEV1 Hedenstrom = $(5.09 \times H) + (0.0145 \times A) - (0.000406 \times A^2) - 4.67$

Female subjects:

VC Hedenstrom = $(5.52 \times H) - (0.0119 \times A) - (0.000145 \times A^2) - 4.329$
FVC Hedenstrom = $(5.45 \times H) - (0.0143 \times A) - (0.000118 \times A^2) - 4.205$
FEV1 Hedenstrom = $(2.58 \times H) - (0.0281 \times A) + 0.13$ (A^2 this term is not included)

The European Community of Coal and Steel (ECCS) European Participants. Between 18 to 70 years of age. Smokers and non smokers. (Quanjer et al., 1993)

Male subjects:

VC ECCS NA
FVC ECCS = $(5.76 \times H) - (0.0260 \times A) - 4.340$
FEV1 ECCS = $(4.30 \times H) - (0.0290 \times A) - 2.49$

Female subjects:

NA NA
FVC ECCS = $(4.43 \times H) - (0.0260 \times A) - 2.89$
FEV1 ECCS = $(3.95 \times H) - (0.0250 \times A) - 2.60$

Lifelong asymptomatic non-smoking Caucasian US subjects as part of NHANS III. Between 20 to 80 years of age. (Hankinson et al., 1999).

Male subjects:

FVC pr Hankinson = $(0.00018642 \times H^2) + (0.00064 \times A) - (0.000269 \times A^2) - 0.1933$
FVC $_{LLN}$ = $(0.00015695 \times H^2) + (0.00064 \times A) - (0.000269 \times A^2) - 0.1933$
FEV1pr = $(0.00014098 \times H^2) - (0.01303 \times A) - (0.000172 \times A^2) + 0.5536$
FEV1 $_{LLN}$ = $(0.00011067 \times H^2) - (0.01303 \times A) - (0.000172 \times A^2) + 0.5536$
FEV6 pr = $(0.00018188 \times H^2) - (0.00842 \times A) - (0.000223 \times A^2) + 0.1102$

$FEV6_{LLN} = (0.00015323 \times H^2) - (0.00842 \times A) - (0.000223 \times A^2) + 0.1102$

Female subjects:

$FVC\ pr = (0.00014815 \times H^2) + (0.01870 \times A) - (0.000382 \times A^2) - 0.3560$
$FVC_{LLN} = (0.00012198 \times H^2) + (0.01870 \times A) - (0.000382 \times A^2) - 0.3560$
$FEV1pr = (0.00011496 \times H^2) - (0.00361 \times A) - (0.000194 \times A^2) + 0.4333$
$FEV1_{LLN} = (0.00009283 \times H^2) - (0.00361 \times A) - (0.000194 \times A^2) + 0.4333$
$FEV6\ pr = (0.00014395 \times H^2) + (0.01317 \times A) - (0.000352 \times A^2) - 0.1373$
$FEV6_{LLN} = (0.00011827 \times H^2) + (0.01317 \times A) - (0.000352 \times A^2) - 0.1373$

H=height in cm!

Asymptomatic never smoking adults in Norway. Between 20 to 80 years of age. (Langhammar et al., 2001)

Male subjects:

$FVC\ Langhammar = e^{(-12.396 + 2.7333 \times lnH - 0.0000592 \times AA)}$
$FEV1\ Langhammar = e^{(-10.556 + 2..342 \times lnH - 0.0000685 \times AA)}$

Female subjects:

$FVC\ Langhammar = e^{(-9.851 + 2.189 \times lnH - 0.000143 \times AA + 0.006439 \times A)}$
$FEV1\ Langhammar = e^{(-9.091 + 2.004 \times lnH - 0.000163 \times AA + 0.007237 \times A)}$
H=height in cm!

12. References

American Thoracic Society. Standardization of spirometry, 1994 update. Am J Respir Crit Care Med, 152, 1107- 1136.

American Thoracic Society. Standards for the diagnosis and care of patients with chronic obstructive pulmonary disease. (1995) *Am J Respir Crit Care Med*, 152, 77s-120s.

Anthonisen, N.R., Connett, J.E., Kiley, J.P., Altose, M.D. & Bailey, W.C. (1994) Effects of smoking intervention and the use of inhaled anticholinergic bronchodilator on the rate of decline of FEV1. The lung health study. *JAMA*, 272(19), 1497-14505.

Anthonison, N.R. (2005) The British hypothesis revisted. *Eur Respir J*, 23, 657-658.

Antó, J.M., Vermiere, P., Vestbo, J., & Dunyer, J. (2001) Epidemiology of chronic obstructive pulmonary disease. *Eur Respir J*, 17(5), 982-984.

Badham C, (1814) An essay on bronchitis: with a supplement containing remarks on simple pulmonary abscess. 2nd ed. London: J Callow

Bakke, P.S., Baste, V., Hanoa, R., & Gulsvik, A. (1991) Prevalence of obstructive lung disease in a general population: telation to occupational title and exposure to some airbone agents. *Thorax*, 46(12), 863-870.

Berglund, E., Birath, G., Grimsby, G., Kjellmer, I., Sandqvist, L., & Söderholm, B. (1963) Spirometric studies in normal subjects. Forced expirograms in subjects between 7 and 70 years of age. *Acta Med Scand* 173, 185- 192.

Briscoe W.A., Nash E.S. (1965) The slow space in chronic obstructive pulmonary disease Ann *NY Acad Sci*, 121, 706-722.

Brändli,O., Schindler,C., Künzli,N,.Keller,R., & Perruchoud,A.P. (1996) Lung function in healthy never smoking adults: reference values and lower limits of normal of a Swiss population. *Thorax*, 51(3), 277-283.

Brändli,O., Schindler,C., Leuenberger,P.H., Baur,X., Degens,P., et al. (2000) Re-estimated equations for 5th percentiles of lung function variables. *Thorax*, 55(2), 173-174.

Buist, A.S., McBurnie, M.A., Vollmer, W.M., Gillespie, S., Burney, P., et al. (2007) International variation in the prevalence of COPD (The Bold Study): a population-based prevalence study. *Lancet*, 370, 741-750.

Burrows, B., Cline, M.G., Knudson, R.J., Taussig, L.M., & Lebowitz, M.D. (1983) A descriptive analysis of the growth and decline of the FVC and FEV1. *Chest*, 83(5), 717-724.

Burrows, B., Knudson,. R.J., Camilli., A.E., Lyle, S.K., & Lebowitz, M.D. (1986) The "Horse-Racing Effect" and predicting decline in forced expiratory volume in one second from screening spirometry. *Am Rev Respir Dis*, 135, 788-793.

Celli, B.R., Halbert, R.J., Isonaka, S., & Schau, B. (2003) Population impact of differen definitions of airway obstruction. *Eur Respir J*, 22, 268-273.

Celli B.R. & MacNee W. (2004) Standards for diagnosis and treatment of patients with COPD: a summary of the ATS/ERS position paper. *Eur Respir J*, 23(6), 932-946.

Cerveri,I., Corsico,A.G., Accordini,S., Ansaldo, E., Anto, J.M., et al. (2008) Underestimation of airflow obstruction among young adults using FEV1/FVC<70% as a fixed cut-off: a longitudinal evaluation of clinical and functional outcomes. *Thorax*, 63(12), 1040-1045.

Chapman, K.R., Mannino D.M., Soriano J.B., Vermiere P.A., et al. (2006) Series "The Global Burden of Chronic Obstructive Pulmonary Disease. *Eur Respir J*, 27, 188-207.

Ciba Guest Symposium 1959. Terminology, definition, and classificationof chronic pulmonary emphysema and related conditions. *Thorax*, 14, 286-299

Committee on Diagnostic Standards for Nontuberculous Respiratory Diseases, American Thoracic Society. Definitions and classification of chronic bronchitis, asthma, and pulmonary emphysema. (1962) *Am Rev Respir Dis*, 85, 762-769

Facchini, F., Flori, G., Bedogni, G,. Galetti, L., Ismagulov, O., et al. (2007) Spirometric reference values for children and adolescents from Kazakhstan. *Ann hum Biol*, 34(5), 519-534.

Falaschetti, E., Laiho, J., Primatesta, P., & Purdon, S. (2004) Prediction equations for normal and low lung function from the Health Survey for England. *Eur Respir J*, 23, 456-463.

Firdaus, A.A., Hoesein, M., Zanen., & Lammers, J-W.J (2011) Lower limit of normal or FEV1/FVC < 0.70 in diagnosing COPD: An evidence-based review. *Respir Med*, 105, 907-915.

Fletcher, C., Peteo., R., Tinker, R., & Speitzer, F.E. (1976) The natural History of Chronic Bronchitis and Emphysema. Oxford University Press.

Fletcher, C., & Peto., R. (1977) The natural history of chronic airflow obstruction. *Br Med J*, 1, 1645-1648.

Foreman, M.G., Zhang, L., Murphy, J., Hansel., Make, B., et al. (2011) Early-onset Chronic Obstructive Pulmonary Disease is associated with female sex, material factors and African American race in COPDGene study. Am J *Respir Crit Care Med*, 184(4), 414-420.

Fukuchi., Y. (2009) The aging lung and chronic obstructive pulmonary disease. *Proc Am Thorac Soc*, 6(7), 570-572.

Garcia-Aymerich, J., (2011) Are we ready to say that sex and race are key risk factors for COPD. *Am J Respir Crit Care Med*, 184, 388-390.

Garshick, E., Segal, M.R., Worobec, T.G., Salekin, CM., & Miller, M.J. (1989) Alcohol consumption and chronic obstructive pulmonary disease. *Am Rev Respir Dis*, 140, 373-378.

George, R.B. (1999) Course and prognosis of chronic obstructive pulmonary disease. *Am J Med Sci*, 318(2), 103-106.

Global Initiative for Chronic Obstructive Lung Disease [GOLD] Updated 2010 http://www.goldcopd.org/guidelines-resources.html

Halbert R.J., Isonaka S., George D., Iqbal. (2003) Interpreting COPD Prevalence Esimates. What is the True Burden of the Disease? *Chest*, 123(5), 1684-1692

Hankinson ,J.L., Odencrantz,J.R., & Feden,K.B. (1999) Spirometric reference values from a sample of the general U.S. population. *Am J Respir Crit Care Med*, 159(1), 179-187.

Hansen,J.E., Sun,X.G, &Wasserman,K. (2007) Spirometric criteria for airways obstruction:Use percentage of FEV1/FVC ratio below the fifth percentile, not<70%. *Chest*, 131,349-355.

Hedenstrom, H., Malmberg, P., & Agarwal K. (1985) Reference values for lung function tests in females. Regression equations with smoking variables. *Bull Eur Physiopathol Respir*, 21,551-557

Hedenstrom, H., Malmberg, P., & Fridriksson, H.V. (1986) Reference values for pulmonary function tests in men. Regression equations which include tobacco smoking variable. *Uppsala J Med Sci*, 91,299-310.

Hurst, J.R. (2010) Upper airway.3: Sinonasal involvement in chronic obstructive pulmonary disease. *Thorax*, 65(1), 85-90.

Ip, M.S., Ko, F.W., Lau, A.C., Tang, K.S. & Choo, K., et al. (2006) Updated spirometric reference values for adult Chinese in Hong Kong and implications on clinical utilization. *Chest*, 129(2), 384-392.

Janssens, J.P., Pache,. J.C., & Nicod,. L.P. (1999) Physiological changes in respiratory function associated with ageing. *Eur Respir J*, 13, 197-205,

Kanervisto, M., Vasankari, T., Laitinen, T., Heliövaara, M., Jousilathi, S., et al. (2011) Low socioeconomic status is associated with chronic obstructive diseases. *Respire Med*, 105(8), 1140-1146.

Kerstjens, H.A.M., Rijcken, B., Schouten, J.P., & Postma, D.S. (1997) Decline of FEV1 by age and smoking status : facts, figures, and fallacies. *Thorax*, 52, 820-827.

Kirkpatrick, P., & Dransfield, M.T. (2009) Racial and sex differences in chronic obstructive pulmonary disease susceptibility, diagnosis, and treatment. *Curr Opin Pulm Med*, 15(2), 100-104.

Knudson, R.J., Clark, D.F., Kennedy, T.C., & Knudson, D.E. (1977) Effect of ageing alone on mechanical properties of the normal adult human lung. *J Appl Physiol*, 43, 1054-1062.

Kuster, S.P., Kuster, D., Schindler, C., Rochat, M.K., Braun, J., et al. (2008) Reference equations for lung function screening of healthy never-smoking adults 18-80 years. *Eur Respir J*, 31, 860-868.

Lange, P., Groth, S., Mortensen, J., Appleyard, M., Nyboe,J., et al. (1998) Pulmonary function is influenced by heavy alcohol consumption. *Am Rev Respir Dis*, 137, 1119-1123.

Langhammer, A., Johnsen, R., Gulsvik, A., Holmen, T.R., & Bjermer, L. (2001) Forced spirometri reference values for Norwegian adults: the Bronchial Obstruction in Nord-Trøndelag Study. *Eur Respir J*, 18(5), 770-779.

Laurell, C.B., Eriksson. S, (1963). The electrophoretic alpha 1-globulin pattern of serum in alpha 1-antitrypsin deficiency. *Scand J Clin Lab Invest*, 15 (2), 132–140.

Lee, P.N., & Fry, J.S. (2010) Systematic review of the evidence relating FEV1 decline to giving up smoking. BMC Med, 8 (84).

Lindgren, A., Stroh, E., Montnémery, P., Nihlén, U., Jakobsson, K., & Axmon A. (2009) Traffic-related air pollution associated with the prevalence of asthma and COPD/chronic bronchitis. A cross-sectional study in Southern Sweden. *Int J Health Geogr*, 8:2.

Lundbäck,B., Lindberg,A., Lindström,M., Rönnmark,E., Jonsson,A.C. et al. (2003) Not 15 but 50% of smokers develop COPD? Report from the Obstructive Lung Disease in Northern Sweden Studies. *Respir Med*, 97(2),115-122.

Macchia, A., Moncalvo, J.J., Kleinert, M., Comignani, P.D., Gimeneo, G., et al. (2011) Unrecognized ventricular dysfunction in chronic obstructive pulmonary disease. *Eur Respir J* Jun 23. [Epub ahead of print]

van Manen, J.G., Bindels, P.J., Jzermans, C.J., van der Zee, J.S., Bottema, B.J., et al. (2001) Prevalence of comorbidity in patienets with a chronic airway obstruction and controls over the age of 40. *J Clin Epidemiol*, 54(3), 287-293.

Mannino, D.M., Buist, A., Petty, T., Enright, P., & Redd, S. (2003) Lung function and mortality in the United States: data from the First National Health and Nutrition Examination Survey follow up study. *Thorax*, 58(5), 388-393.

Mannino D.M., & Buist A.S. (2007) Global burden of COPD: risk factors, prevalence, and future trends. *Lancet*, 370(9589), 765-773.

Mannino, D.M. (2007) Defining chronic obstructive pulmonary disease... and the elephant in the room. *Eur Respir J*, 30, 189-190.

Miller, M.R., Quanjer, P.H., Swanney, M.P., Ruppel, G., & Enright, P.L. (2011) Interpreting lung function data using 80% predicted and fixed thresholds misclassifies more than 20% of patients. *Chest*, 139(1), 52-59.

Murray, C.J., & Lopez A.D. (2007) Global mortality, disability, and the contribution of risk factors: Global Burden of Disease study. *Lancet*, 349(9063), 1436-1442

Nathell, L., Nathell, M., Malmberg., & Larsson, K. (2007) COPD diagnosis related to different guidelines and spirometry techniques. *Respir Res*, 8(89)

Nihlén, U., Montnémery, P., Andersson, M., Persson, C.G., Nyberg, P., et al. (2008) Specific nasal symptoms and symptom-provoking factors may predict increased risk of developing COPD. *Clin Physiol Funct Imaging*, 28(4), 240-250.

Ostrowski, S., Grzywa-Celinska,A., Mieczkowska,J., Rychlik,M., Lachowska-Kotowska,P., et al. (2005) Pulmonary function between 40 and 80 years of age. *J Physiol Pharmacol*, 56, Suppl 4, 137-133.

Pellegrino, P., Brusasco, V., Viegi, R.O., Crapo., Burgos, F., et al. (2008) Definition of COPD: based on evidence or opinion? *Eur Respir J*, 31, 681-690.

Pereira, C.A., Sato,T., & Rodriques, S.C. (2007) New reference values for forced spirometry in white adults in Brazil. *J Bras Pneumol*, 33(4), 397-406.

Pérez-Padilla, R., Regalado, J., Vedal, S., Paré, P. Chapela, R., et al. (1996) Exposure to biomass smoke and chronic airway disease in Mexican women. A case-control study. *Am J Respir Crit Care Med*, 154(3 Pt 1), 701-706.

Petty,T.L. (2006) The history of COPD. *Int J Chron Obstruct Pulmon Dis*, 1(1), 3-14.

Pistelli, F., Bottai, M., Carrozzi, L., Baldacci, S., Simoni, M., et al. (2007) Reference equations for spirometry from a general population in central Italy. *Respir Med*, 101(4), 814-824.

Postma, D.S., & Boezen, H.M. (2004) Rationale for the Dutch hypothesis. Allergy and airway hyperresponsiveness as genetic factors and their interaction with environment in the development of asthma and COPD. *Chest*, 126(2 Suppl), 96S-104S.

Quanjer, P.H., Tammeling, G.J., Cotes, J.E., Pedersen, O.F., Peslin, R., & Yernault,J.C. (1993) Lung volumes and forced ventilatory flows. Report Working Party Standardization of Lung Function Tests. European Community for steel and Coal. Official Statement of the European Respiratory Society. *Eur Respir J*, 6(Suppl. 16) 5s-40s.

Quanjer, P., Enright, P., Miller, M., Stocks., Ruppel, G., et al. (2010) Open letter to the members of the GOLD committee.
http://www.spirxpert.com/controversies/Open_Letter.pdf

Render, M.L., Weinstein, A.S., & Blaustein, A.S. (1995) Left ventricular dysfunction in deteriorating patients with chronic obstructive pulmonary disease. *Chest*, 107, 162-168.

Rennard, S.I., & Vestbo, J. (2006) COPD: the dangerous underestimate of 15%. Lancet, 367(9518), 1216-1219.

Rijcken, B., & Britton, J. (1998) Epidemiology of chronic obstructive pulmonary disease. *Eur Respir Mon*, 7, 41-73.

Schermer, T.R.J., & Quanjer, P.H. (2007) COPD screening in primary care: who is sick? *Prim Care Respi J*, 16(1), 49-52.

Schuneman, H.J., Grant, B.J., Frudenheim, J.L., Muti, P., McCann, S.E., et al. (2002) Evidence for a positive association between pulmonary function and wine intake in a population-based study. *Sleep Breath*, 6, 161- 173.

Shirtcliffe, P., Weatherall, M., Marsh, S., Travers, J., & Hansell, A. (2007) COPD prevalence in a random population survey: a matter of definition. *Eur Respir J*, 30(2), 232-239.

Siebling, L., Puhan, M.A., Muggensturm, P., Zoller, M., & ter Riet, G. (2011) Characteristics of Dutch and Swiss primary care COPD patients – baseline data of the ICE COLD ERIC study. *Clinical Epidemiology*, 3, 273-283.

Silverman, E.K., Weiss, S.T., Drazen, J.M., Chapman, H.A., Carey, V., et al. (2000) Gender-Related Differences in Severe, Early-onset Chronic Obstructive Pulmonary Disease. *Am J Respir Crit Care Med*, 162(6), 2152-2158.

Snider, G.L. (2000) Clinical relevance summary: Collagene vs elastin in pathogenesis of emphysema; cellular origin of elastases; bronchiolitis vs emphysema as a cause of airflow obstruction. *Chest*, 117, 244S-246S.

Stanojevic, S., Wade, A., & Stocks, J. (2010) Reference values for lung function: past present and future. *Eur Respir J*, 36, 12-19.

Swanney,M.P., Ruppel,G., Enright,P.L., Pedersen, O.F., Crapo,R.O., et al. (2008) Using the lower limit of normal for the FEV1/FVC ratio reduces the misclassification of airways obstruction. *Thorax*, 63,1046-1051.

Szanto, O., Montnemery., & Elmstahl., S. (2010) Prevalence of airway obstruction in the elderly: results from a cross-sectional spirometric study of nine age cohorts between the ages of 60 and 93 years. *Prim Care Respi J*, 19(3), 231-236.

Tabak,C., Smit, H.A., Rasanen, L., Fidanza, F., Menotti, A., et al. (2001) Alcohol consumption in relation to 20-year COPD mortality and pulmonary function in middle-aged men from three European countries. *Epidemiology*, 12, 239-245.

Trupin, L., Earnest, G., San Pedro, M., Balmes, J.R., & Eisner. (2003) The occupational burden of chronic obstructive pulmonary disease. *Eur Respir J*, 22(3), 462-469.

Turner, J.M., Mead, J., & Wohl, M.E. (1968) Elasticity of human lungs in relation to age. *Appl Physiol*, 25, 664-671. Varkey, A.B. (2004) Chronic obstructive pulmonary disease in women: exploring gender differences. *Curr Opin Pulm Med*, 10(2), 98-103.

Vestbo, J., & Prescott, E. (1998) Update on the "Dutch hypothesis" for chronic respiratory disease. *Thorax*, 53(Suppl 2), 15S-19S.

Vollmer,W., Gislason,P., Burney,P., Enright,P., Gulsvik,A. et al. (2009) Comparison of spirometric criteria for the diagnosis of COPD: results from the BOLD study. *Eur Respir J*, 34,588-597.

Willemse, B.W.M., Postma, D.S., Timens, W, & ten Hacken, N.H.T. (2004) The impact of smoking cessation on respiratory symptoms, lung function, airway hyperresponsiveness and inflammation. *Eur Respir J*, 23, 464- 476.

5

The Management of Peripheral Arterial Disease (PAD) in Primary Care

Andrew P. Coveney

Department of Vascular Surgery, Cork University Hospital, Cork,
Ireland

1. Introduction

Peripheral arterial disease (PAD) encompasses a range of non-coronary arterial syndromes that are caused by the altered structure and function of the arteries that supply the brain, visceral organs, and the limbs. Numerous pathophysiological processes can contribute to the creation of stenoses or aneurysms of the non-coronary arterial circulation, but atherosclerosis remains the most common disease process affecting the aorta and its branch arteries. (Hirsch et al., 2006) While "peripheral arterial disease" encompasses disorders affecting arterial beds exclusive of the coronary arteries, this chapter is limited to a review of disease of the lower extremity arteries as these can be easily assessed in the primary care setting.

Vascular disease is the leading cause of death globally (Murray and Lopez, 1997). With an aging global population, this is expected to continue and the burden on healthcare systems from cardiovascular disease is expected to rise. Vascular disease in one arterial territory predicts the presence of disease in other territories (Rothwell, 2000). The risk of a myocardial infarction or death increases significantly after a transient ischemic attack or stroke (Touze et al., 2005). The presence of PAD significantly increases your risk of a vascular event also (Banerjee et al., 2010). Of particular importance is the fact that asymptomatic PAD is a significant predictor of cardiovascular morbidity and mortality (Hooi et al., 2004). These findings demonstrate the systemic nature of cardiovascular disease and the underlying pathophysiology of atherosclerosis. Patients who present with symptoms of single territory arterial disease need to be screened and treated for multiterritory vascular disease.

In a recent observational study, 62% of patients presenting to a vascular outpatient service had symptoms of PAD and more than half of these patients had been managed solely by their primary care physcian (Coveney et al., 2011). This demonstrates the importance for primary care physcians to identify high risk cardiovascular patients and commence appropriate secondary preventative measures. Primary care physicians are best placed to identify and screen high risk vascular patients and to initate and monitor long term secondary preventative measures in these patients.

This book chapter focuses on the importance and significance of screening for PAD in the primary care setting and aims to review existing guidelines for optimising the secondary management of patients with peripheral arterial disease.

A pubmed search to identify recent reviews and articles on the epidemiology, assessment and treatment of peripheral arterial disease using the terms "intermittent claudication", peripheral arterial disease" and "peripheral vascular disease" was performed and existing international guidelines on the management of peripheral arterial disease (Hirsch et al., 2006, Norgren et al., 2007) provide the evidence on which this chapter is based and referenced.

The chapter is divided into different sections which include,

Epidemiology of PAD.
Risk factors for PAD
Diagnosis and assessment of PAD,
Screening for PAD in appropriate patients,
Treatment of PAD
When to refer to a vascular surgeon,
Vascular surgical interventions for PAD.

A summary of the important factors to consider when managing patients with PAD in the primary care setting will be given along with up to date evidence based guidelines.

2. Epidemiology of Peripheral Arterial Disease

Lower extremity PAD affects approximately 8 million men and women in the United States and is associated with significant morbidity and mortality (Hirsch et al., 2001). PAD prevalence increases dramatically with age and disproportionately affects the black ethnic population (Selvin and Erlinger, 2004). As people survive longer with chronic illness, PAD is likely to become increasingly more prevalent. In the general population, only 11% of patients with PAD have the classic symptoms of intermittent claudication (Hirsch et al., 2001). The term claudication is derived from the latin verb claudicare, meaning to limp. Interestingly, the Roman emperor Claudius (AD 41-54) was so named as he limped, most likely due to a birth defect. Classical intermittent claudication describes aching, crampy leg pain brought on by exercise and relieved by rest and is a symptom of leg muscle ischemia due to PAD. Up to 40% of patients with PAD are asymptomatic, while the remaining 50% of patients describe a variety of leg symptoms different from intermittent claudication (McDermott et al., 2001). Non-invasive testing in populations indicates that the true prevalence of PAD is at least five times higher than would be expected based on the reported prevalence of intermittent claudication (Criqui et al., 1997). The Edinburgh artery study (Fowkes et al., 1991), showed that one in five of the middle aged (65-75 years) population of the United Kingdom have evidence of peripheral arterial disease on clinical examination, although only a quarter of them had symptoms. The Rotterdam study (Meijer et al., 1998), demonstrated a 19.1% prevalence of PAD among 7,715 dutch members of the public over 55yrs of age, using the non-invasive ankle-brachial index (ABI), with <0.9 taken as the cut off for diagnosis. A recent french study demonstrated a PAD prevalence of 27.8% when non-invasive ABI screening was performed on 5,679 primary care patients over 55-years old considered at risk (Cacoub et al., 2009).

Patients with PAD have impaired function and quality of life. This is true even for people who do not report leg symptoms. Furthermore, PAD patients, including those who are asymptomatic, experience significant decline in lower extremity functioning over time (McDermott et al., 2002).

Despite the high prevalence of peripheral arterial disease, the number of people requiring a major amputation is small. A recent german study reported a major amputation rate of only 25.1 per 100,000 population in 2008, down from 27 in 2005. The same study reported an increase in the minor amputation rate due to vascular disease from 47.4 to 53.7 per 100,000 population over the same period from 2005 to 2008 (Moysidis et al., 2011). Among patients with intermittent claudication, there is a 1.0 to 3.3% risk of major amputation over 5 years which increases significantly in diabetic patients (Norgren et al., 2007).

3. Risk factors for PAD

The risk factors for PAD are similar to those for coronary artery disease. Although diabetes and cigarette smoking are particularly strong risk factors for PAD (Criqui et al., 1997), additional risk factors include age and male sex, hypercholesterolemia, hypertension, chronic kidney disease, hyperhomocystinemia, elevated fibrinogen levels, family history of athersclerosis and being of a non-white ethnic background (Norgren et al., 2007).

3.1 Smoking

Smoking is an exceptionally powerful etiologic risk factor for lower extremity PAD (Criqui et al., 1997). Cigarette smoking is a stronger risk factor for PAD than for coronary artery disease (Price et al., 1999). An interesting case-control study (Cole et al., 1993) estimated, using logistic regression analysis to adjust for confounding variables, that 76% of PAD is attributable to smoking. The same study reported the relative risk for PAD in ex-smokers as 7 and in current smokers as 16 when compared to men who had never smoked and the relative risk increased directly with the lifetime number of cigarettes smoked. Among smokers, the risk of developing PAD increases with plasma concentration levels of cotinine, which is a more accurate marker of tobacco exposure, as it takes into account the degree of inhalation per cigarette as well as the amount of cigarettes smoked (Powell et al., 1997).

3.2 Diabetes

Diabetes mellitus increases the risk of lower extremity PAD by 2- to 4-fold (Criqui et al., 1997) and is present in 12% to 20% of people with lower limb PAD (Hiatt et al., 1995, Beks et al., 1995, Coveney et al., 2011). The risk of developing PAD is proportional to the duration and severity of diabetes (Beks et al., 1995, Katsilambros et al., 1996). In the Framingham Heart Study, diabetes increased the risk of intermittent claudication by 3.5-fold in men and 8.6-fold in women (Kannel and McGee, 1985). The risk of developing critical limb ischemia is also greater in diabetic patients than in non-diabetic patients (Bowers et al., 1993, McDaniel and Cronenwett, 1989). Diabetic patients with lower extremity PAD are 7- to 15-fold more likely to undergo a major amputation than non-diabetics with lower extremity PAD (Dormandy and Murray, 1991, McDaniel and Cronenwett, 1989, Most and Sinnock, 1983).

3.3 Dyslipideamia

As seen with coronary artery disease, lipid abnormalities that are associated with lower extremity PAD include elevated total and low-density lipoprotein (LDL) cholestrol, decreased high-density lipoprotein (HDL) cholestrol, and hypertriglyceridemia (Fowkes et al., 1992, Kannel and Shurtleff, 1973, Murabito et al., 2002, Hiatt et al., 1995). In the Framingham study, a fasting cholestrol level greater than 7 mmol/L (270mg/dL) was associated with a doubling of the incidence of intermittent claudication, but the ratio of total to HDL cholesterol was the best predictor of occurrence of PAD. The risk of developing lower extremity PAD increases by approximately 5% to 10% for each 10 mg/dL rise in total cholestrol (Newman et al., 1993, Ingolfsson et al., 1994, Murabito et al., 1997). It has also been suggested that cigarette smoking may synergistically enhance the effects of hypercholestroleamia.

3.4 Hypertension

Hypertension which has a longstanding association with coronary artery disease and cerebrovascular disease, is also associated with PAD but to a weaker extent (Criqui et al., 1997, Murabito et al., 1997, Novo et al., 1992, Hooi et al., 1998). In some, but not all epidemiological studies, hypertension increased the risk of developing PAD (Fowkes et al., 1992, Smith et al., 1990, Murabito et al., 1997, Reunanen et al., 1982). In the Framingham Heart Study, hypertension increased the risk of intermittent claudication 2.5-fold in men and 4-fold in women, and the risk was proportional to the severity of the hypertension. (Murabito et al., 1997)

3.5 Hyperhomocysteineamia

Elevated levels of homocysteine are associated with a 2- to 3-fold increased risk for developing atherosclerotic arterial disease (Boushey et al., 1995, Graham et al., 1997). Approximately 30% to 40% of patients with lower extremity PAD have high levels of homocysteine (Taylor et al., 1991). Hyperhomocysteineamia is prevalent in both the elderly and younger patients with lower extremity PAD and appears to increase the risk of progression of their PAD. Approximately 25% of patients with intermittent claudication have plasma homocysteine levels exceeding the 95th percentile (Molgaard et al., 1992).

Homocysteine metabolism is influenced by nutritional factors. Supplementation with B-vitamins, especially folate, reduces plasma homocysteine levels. Multiple trials based on the hypothesis that folate supplementation would reduce homocysteine levels and lead to a reduction in cardiovascular risk have failed to show any beneficial results (Lonn, 2008, Toole et al., 2004, Song et al., 2009). Therefore, B-vitamin supplementation cannot currently be recommended for the prevention of CVD events and there is no role for the routine screening for elevated homocysteine levels.

Despite the convincing epidemiological evidence linking high homocysteine levels with atherothrombotic disease, it is possible that hyperhomocysteineamia is not a common primary cause of the atherothrombotic disorder in the general population, but rather a marker of systemic or endothelial oxidant stress that is a major mediator of these disorders (Hoffman, 2011).

4. The presentation of Peripheral Arterial Disease

Clinically PAD has been recognised since as early as 1831 and the disease spectrum varies from asymptomatic PAD to gangrene and critical limb ischemia requiring amputation. Two separate classification systems based on symptoms and clinical measures are commonly used to classify the severity of PAD. These are the Fontaine classification system and the more recently developed Rutherford classification system (Norgren et al., 2007). (Tables 1&2).

Fontaine Stages

Stage	Symptoms
I	Asymptomatic
II	Intermittent claudication
IIa	Pain-free, claudication walking >200m
IIb	Pain-free, claudication walking <200m
III	Rest / Nocturnal pain
IV	Necrosis / Gangrene

Table 1. Fontaine stages of peripheral arterial disease (adapted from TASC II guidelines)

Rutherford Classification

Grade	Category	Clinical Description
0	0	Asymptomatic
I	1	Mild claudication
	2	Moderate claudication
	3	Severe claudication
II	4	Ischemic rest pain
	5	Minor tissue loss; nonhealing ulcer, focal gangrene with diffuse pedal oedema
III	6	Major tissue loss extending above transmetatarsal level; foot no longer salvageable

Table 2. Rutherford classification of peripheral arterial disease (adapted from TASC II guidelines)

4.1 Intermittent claudication

The majority of patients with PAD have limited exercise performance and walking ability. As a consequence, PAD is associated with reduced physical functioning which impacts on quality of life. While a large proportion of patients are asymptomatic from their PAD, (emphasising the importance of screening for the disease, discussed below), the most common symptom among patients is intermittent claudication. The classical symptom of intermittent claudication is muscle discomfort in the lower limb reproducibly brought on by exercise and relieved by rest within 10 minutes. Patients may describe a cramping muscle pain, ache or muscle fatigue brought on by exertion, most commonly localised to the calf, that is relieved by rest. Symptoms may also affect the thigh or buttock when the arterial lesion is more proximal, such as in iliac disease. Patients with intermittent claudication have normal blood flow at rest and therefore have no limb symptoms. However, on exercising the oxygen demand of the leg muscles increases, necessitating increased blood flow. Occlusive lesions in the arterial supply of the leg muscles limits this increase in blood flow, resulting in a mismatch between oxygen supply and muscle metabolic demand that leads to the symptoms of claudication.

When the prevalence of PAD in population based studies diagnosed using an ABI <0.9 is compared to the prevalence of intermittent claudication using questionnaires, it becomes apparent that only about 25% of patients with PAD complain of intermittent claudication. Of further relevance is the fact that between 10% and 50% of patients with intermittent claudication have never consulted a doctor about their symptoms, considering it a normal part of the aging process (Norgren et al., 2007). This highlights further the need for primary care physicians to actively seek out patients that would benefit from secondary preventative treatment.

Peripheral arterial disease patients without typical claudication symptoms commonly have walking limitations that may be associated with atypical or no limb symptoms (McDermott et al., 2001). It should also be noted that patients with PAD commonly have multiple co-morbidities that may restrict their exercise capacity (musculoskeletal disease, pulmonary disease, congestive heart failure) and prevent sufficient activity to produce limb symptoms. So patients with severe PAD might not necessarily complain of intermittent claudication. Equally patients who complain of apparent symptoms of intermittent claudication may not have PAD, as some conditions can mimic the symptoms of intermittent claudication such as nerve root compression, compartment syndrome, arthritis, spinal stenosis and venous claudication.

4.2 Rest pain

As seen from tables 1&2, as PAD progresses clinically, patients start to develop rest pain. Classically, patients describe being woken at night by severe pain in their leg, which forces them to sit up and hang the leg out over the edge of the bed for relief. The pain is similar to intermittent claudication, except the arterial disease has progressed to a stage where exercise is no longer required to precipitate a lack of sufficient blood supply to the leg muscles. Increased ambient heat while in bed, diverts available blood away from muscles to superficial skin in order to maintain normal body temperature. Lying horizontal in bed also reduces the orthostatic pressure that contributes to the intra arterial pressure in the blood vessels of the leg, reducing leg perfusion further. Hanging the legs out of the warm bed, cools them down and makes them more dependent, resulting in increased blood flow to the muscles and some relief from the symptoms.

4.3 Tissue loss and impaired healing.

Occasionally patients present with a chronic leg ulcer or wounds that simply refuse to heal as a consequence of poor peripheral blood supply secondary to PAD. Diabetic patients are particularly at risk, due to their increased risk of infection and impaired healing due to known immunological dysfunction and the presence of peripheral neuropathy contributing to foot trauma. Prevention of foot trauma is an essential part of diabetic management and the use of appropriate footwear and access to podiatry services are important elements of the secondary prevention of amputation in diabetics. Trauma to a diabetic foot such as that seen in figure 1B, can lead to a cascade of events resulting ultimately in a below knee amputation.

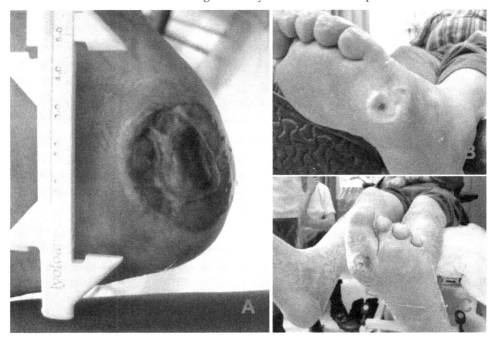

Fig. 1. A. Chronic arterial ulcer on heal, B. Trauma to a diabetic foot, C. Chronic arterial ulcer on patient with previous 2nd toe amputation.

Recognition of PAD in patients with chronic tissue loss is essential so as to expedite appropriate referral to teritary centres for potential revascularisation procedures. Often the aim of revascularisation procedures is to ensure adequate healing after an inevidable amputation.

5. Diagnosis and assessment of peripheral arterial disease

As with any clinical condition or disease, a full history and thorough physical examination is the cornerstone of making the correct diagnosis. Patients with risk factors for PAD, limb symptoms on exertion or reduced limb function should undergo a vascular history to evaluate for symptoms of claudication or other limb symptoms that limit walking ability. They should also undergo a vascular examination evaluating their peripheral pulses.

A comprehensive physical examination in a suspected PAD patient should assess the circulatory system as a whole. Key components of the general examine include blood pressure measurement in both arms, assessment of cardiac rate and rhythm, assessment for cardiac murmurs and palpation of abdomen for an abdominal aortic aneurysm (although non-palpation of one does not exclude an anuerysm). Close inspection of the feet should be performed examining closely for signs of PAD, which might include, non-healing ulcers, muscle atrophy, hair loss, hypertrophied slow growing nails, reduced temperature, pallor or reactive hypereamia. A peripheral vascular examination also requires palpation of the radial, ulnar, brachial, carotid, femoral, popliteal, dorsalis pedis and posterior tibial artery pulses. A small number of healthy adults will have an absent doralis pedis due to anatomical variation. An especially prominent pulse at the femoral or popliteal artery should raise suspicion for an aneursym. It is important to compare the pulses of both legs and correlate any abnormalities with leg symptoms to determine lateralisation of disease. Absent pedal pulses tends to over-diagnose PAD, whereas using the symptom of classical intermittent claudication for diagnosing patients tends to underdiagnose PAD (Criqui et al., 1985). Palpable pedal pulses on examination have a negative predictive value of over 90% that may rule out the diagnosis of PAD in many cases.

Patients with a history or examination suggestive of PAD should proceed to objective testing including ankle-brachial index (ABI) measurement. The ABI which is the ratio of systolic blood pressure at the ankle to the arm, is used in the diagnosis of peripheral arterial disease. A low ABI is associated with concomitant coronary and cerebrovascular disease. The lower the ABI, the greater the increase in cardiovascular risk; however, even those with modest, asymptomatic reductions in the ABI (0.8 to 1.0) appear to be at increased risk of cardiovascular disease (Newman et al., 1993). A meta-analysis of 16 cohort studies of healthy individuals, demonstrated a 10-year risk of a major coronary event in men with an ABI < 0.90 or less to be 27% compared to 9% in those with a normal range 1.11 to 1.40 (Fowkes et al., 2008). This highlights the main benefit of diagnosing PAD is not to treat the symptoms of PAD , but is instead to initiate the secondary preventative measures against systemic arterial disease and prolong patient survival. The ABI can also be used to assess the progression of existing PAD.

The gold standard method of diagnosing PAD is angiography. While this has the benefit of also offering the possibilty of intervention in the form of angioplasty, it is an invasive test not without risk. It also requires significant expertise and resources. Patients with PAD should be on an antiplatelet as disccused later and are therefore at increased risk of bleeding from their arterial puncture site. Vascular surgeons are not uncommonly asked to repair iatrogenic trauma of the common femoral artery after angiography. A metaanalysis of over 30 randomised control trials looking at the efficacy of vascular closure devices found a 0.7% rate of vascular surgical intervention after diagnostic angiography, with no significant difference in vascular complications found between patients treated with vascular closure devices and manual compression (Biancari et al., 2010). Bleeding, heamatoma formation, pseudoaneurysm formation, arterial stenosis and embolic complications are all potential complications of angiography that my require vascular surgical intervention. Advances in the quality of CT scanners have made CT angiography a reasonable alternative to formal diagnostic angiograms, thus eliminating the complications of arterial access but the potential side effects of intravenous contrast, including allergy and nephrotoxicity remain.

Some patients with PAD will have non-compressible arteries due to calcified atherosclerotic vessels resulting in falsely high ankle blood pressures. This is particularly prevalent in diabetic patients. Caution should be taken in interpreting ABI measurements in such patients, which may have an ABI > 1.4. Alternative non-invasive objective tests should be used to assess these patients. Transcutaneous oxygen saturation levels is one alternative non-invasive method for assessing PAD. Others include toe systolic pressures, pulse volume recordings or duplex ultrasound. Unfortunately, these tests generally require referral to a specialised vascular laboratory.

A proportion of patients diagnosed with PAD will have underlying undiagnosed diabetes. It is therefore important to screen newly diagnosed PAD patients for diabetes. PAD is more aggressive in diabetic patients compared to non-diabetics, with the need for amputation five- to ten-times higher. This is contributed to by sensory neuropathy and decreased resistance to infection. Based on these observations, the American Diabetes Association recommends PAD screening with an ABI every 5 years in all diabetic patients(2003).

6. Screening for PAD

The principles of health screening were well documented by the World health Organisation (WHO) in a document published in 1968 (Wilson and Jungner, 1968). The document outlined ten important principles when initiating screening for disease which remain as relevant today as in 1968 and are summarised below in table 3. The adherence of screening for PAD to each of these ten principles requires further elaboration.

Health Screening Principles

1. The condition sought should be an important health problem.
2. There should be an accepted treatment for patients with recognized disease.
3. Facilities for diagnosis and treatment should be available.
4. There should be a recognizable latent or early symptomatic stage.
5. There should be a suitable test or examination.
6. The test should be acceptable to the population.
7. The natural history of the condition, including development from latent to declared disease, should be adequately understood.
8. There should be an agreed policy on whom to treat as patients.
9. The cost of case-finding (including diagnosis and treatment of patients diagnosed) should be economically balanced in relation to possible expenditure on medical care as a whole.
10. Case-finding should be a continuing process and not a "once and for all" project.

Table 3. Health Screening Principles (Wilson and Jungner, 1968)

Regarding the first principle that "the condition sought should be an important health problem", is evident from epidemiological studies already discussed which estimate a prevalence of PAD to be around 20% in the over 55 at risk population. The risk of a person with claudication progressing to critical limb ischemia and requiring major amputation is low (1%-3.3% over 5 years). However the risk of death in patients diagnosed with PAD is high (5-10% a year) mainly from coronary and cerebrovascular events, representing 3-4 times the risk to an age and sex matched population without PAD. So while the symptoms of PAD may not represent a major health problem on their own, the fact that PAD is an indirect measurement of a patient's cardiovascular disease which is the greatest killer in the world today, makes PAD a very important health problem.

Patients diagnosed with PAD, can be initated on secondary preventative treatment for their cardiovascular disease. There are multiple accepted treatments for patients identified as being at increased cardiovascular risk, which have been shown to improve surival and reduce morbidity. These treatments include life-style, medical and surgical interventions which will be discussed later in the chapter. By initiating secondary preventative measures earlier in these increased risk cardiovascular patients, their overall survival is lengthened and their cardiovascular morbidity reduced.

The ankle-brachial index measurement is a non-invasive accurate test that can be performed in an office setting, by a family physican, general practitioner or trained nurse practitioner. The accepted threshold for the diagnosis of PAD on ABI is 0.90. (Hirsch et al., 2006, Norgren et al., 2007). Studies comparing the ABI threshold of 0.90 to invasive angiography have demonstrated a sensitivity of 89-95% and a specificity of 99-100% in diagnosing PAD (Fowkes, 1988, Feigelson et al., 1994). The mean time required among 1,219 french general practioners performing 5,679 ABI measurements in their own practices was 11.5 minutes (Cacoub et al., 2009). This represents a very acceptable time demand for both the patient and physician for a non-invasive test that is harmless and costs nothing (excluding the intial capital cost of the hand held doppler), yet can yield accurate diagnostic results that impact significantly on patient management.

Recommendations for
ankle-brachial index (ABI) screening

An ABI should be measured in :

1. All patients with exertional leg symptoms.
2. All patients aged 50-69 and have a cardiovascular risk factor (particularly diabetes or smoking).
3. All patients age ≥ 70 years, regardless of risk factors status.
4. All patients with a Framingham risk score 10%-20%

Table 4. At risk patients who should undergo ABI screening (TASC II guidelines, 2007).

A large proportion of patients with PAD confirmed by an ABI< 0.9 are asymptomatic from their disease, however they have a significantly increased risk of cardiovascular morbidity and mortality (Hooi et al., 2004) as seen in symptomatic patients. The use of questionnaires as used in some screening programs in the past rely on patients having symptoms and would be of little use in identifying PAD in asymptomatic patients. It is these asymptomatic patients who stand to benefit most from screening with ABI measurement and general practioners are best placed to perform this screening for several reasons. Firstly, due to their indepth knowledge of their patients, they are able to appropriately select at risk patients for screening, which should include those listed in table 4 below. Evidence from the recent eurpoean PANDORA study looking at the prevalence of asymptomatic PAD using ABI<0.9, found that many PAD diagnosed patients failed to meet the screening requirements for ABI testing, which may lead to a broadening of the screening criteria to include more patients (Sanna et al., 2011).

Patients may benefit from opportunistic screening performed on patients who present for other reasons to their general practitioner. Those patients found to have PAD are best managed initially by their doctor in the community, who can monitor their progress in relation to lifestyle interventions and medication side effects. Finally, screening by their general practitioner is more convenient and cost effective for the patient and also reserves secondary and teritary referral centres for the more symptomatic and complex vascular cases.

7. Treatment for peripheral arterial disease

The treatment of peripheral arterial disease has two goals. The first, is to improve the patient's function and reduce their local symptoms, by minimising progression of their disease towards critical limb ischemia and reduce the need for amputation. The second goal is to reduce their overall increased risk of cardiovascular death or morbidity, most commonly due to a coronary or cerebrovascular event. Initial management of patients diagnosed with PAD should consist of modification of vascular risk factors and implementation of best medical treatment with the expectation that this will prolong life, reduce morbidity and improve functional status. A sufficient time should elapse before assessing the success of initial medical treatment before referring for endovascular or surgical intervention. Most patients' symptoms improve sufficiently that further invasive treatment is no longer needed (Leng et al., 1996). In those that do require surgical or endovascular intervention, the success and durability of their intervention is improved if best medical treatment has already been initiated and adherred to (Whyman et al., 1997).

7.1 Smoking cessation

Smoking is the single most important modifiable risk factor in PAD. Complete and permanent cessation of smoking is by far the single most important factor determining the outcome of patients with PAD. While this sounds like an easy intervention, it is very difficult to achieve, as most patients with PAD are life-long smokers and have failed on many occasions in the past to quit.

In middle aged smokers with reduced pulmonary function, physician advice to stop smoking, coupled with a formal cessation program and nicotine replacement was associated with a 22% cessation rate at 5 years, compared with only 5% cessation in the usual care group (Anthonisen et al., 2005). The same study showed a significant survival advantage for the interventional group after 14 years follow up. Nicotine replacement can be delivered via multiple methods, including gum, patches, and inhaler devices.

The use of the antidepressant bupropion in patients with cardiovascular disease to improve the cessation rate of smoking has been supported in a number of randomised trials, with one study demonstrating 3-, 6- and 12-month abstinence rates of 34%, 27% and 22%, respectively, compared with 15%, 11% and 9% respectively, with placebo treatment (Tonstad et al., 2003). Nicotine replacement therapy in combination with bupropion has been shown to be more effective than either treatment alone. There is also some evidence that group therapy increases the rate of smoking cessation and is comparable to intensive individual therapy, which is often impractical due to limited resources (Stead and Lancaster, 2000).

The practical approach as advocated in the TASC II guidelines is to encourage physician advice at every patient visit, combined with behaviour modification, nicotine replacement and bupropion treatment in order to achieve the best cessation rates. These are summarised in table 5 below.

Recommendations for smoking cessation

1. All patients who smoke should be strongly and repeatedly advised to stop smoking.
2. All patients who smoke should receive a program of physician advice, group counseling sessions, and nicotine replacement.
3. Cessation rates can be enhanced by addition of antidepressant drug therapy (bupropion) and nicotine replacement.

Table 5. Smoking cessation recommendations (TASC II guidelines).

Smoking cessation does not necessarily improve the symptoms of intermittent claudication, with improved walking distance seen in only some patients. However, smoking cessation is associated with a reduced risk of cardiovascular events and a reduced risk of amputation. Those patients that do undergo bypass surgery have a three-fold increased risk of graft failure with continued smoking which reduces to that of non-smokers with smoking cessation (Willigendael et al., 2005). These significant findings make smoking cessation a pre-requisite for any semi-elective or elective bypass surgery.

7.2 Exercise programs

In patients with intermittent claudication, supervised exercise programs have demonstrated clinical benefit in improving exercise performance (Stewart et al., 2002). It is likely that asymptomatic patients with PAD also benefit form exercise. In one prospective study, supervised exercise conducted for 3 months or longer, led to a clear increase in threadmill exercise performance and reduced the severity of claudication pain during exercise (Hiatt et al., 1994). There are multiple biological mechanisms underlying this clinical improvement, including the formation of collateral vessels and increased blood flow, changes in the microcirculation and endothelial function, changes in muscle metabolism and oxygen extraction, walking economy and systemic benefits of exercise including weight loss and improved cardiac function (Stewart et al., 2002).

Exercise sessions should be held three times per week, beginning with 30 minute sessions and then increasing to one-hour sessions. During each session, threadmill exercise is performed at a speed and grade that induces claudication within 3-5 minutes. The patient should continue to walk through the onset of claudication pain until it reaches moderate intensity and then stop until claudication resolves, after which exercise is resumed and the cycle repeated. The sessions are gradually increased to one hour duration as the patient becomes more comfortable with the exercise sessions, while avoiding excessive fatigue or leg discomfort. The speed or grade of the threadmill is increased as longer durations are required to induce claudication symptoms. An additional goal of the exercise program is to increase patient walking speed up to the normal 4.8 km/h from the average PAD patient walking speed of 2.4-3.2 km/h. This exercise prescription has been adapted from the TASC II guidelines (Norgren et al., 2007) and is summarised in table 6 below.

Exercise therapy in intermittent claudication

1. Supervised exercise should be made available as part of the initial treatment for all patients with PAD.

2. The most effective programs employ treadmill or track walking that is of sufficient intensity to bring on claudication, followed by rest, over the course of a 30-60 minute session.

3. Exercise sessions should typically be conducted three times a week for a minimum of three months.

Table 6. Exercise therapy for intermittent claudication (TASC II, 2007).

The benefits of an exercise program not only improve the patient's functional walking capacity, but also offer other benefits including improved overall cardiorespiratory function, a reduction in body weight, better lipid and glycemic profiles and lower blood pressure.

Unfortunately, there are some contraindications to participation in an effective exercise program. Some patients are unable to participate due to musculoskeletal disease, poor cardiac function or neurological impairment. Caution should be taken to ensure appropriate footwear for diabetic patients who are at increased risk of foot lesions due to peripheral neuropathy. The major limitation of exercise rehabilitation is the lack of availability of supervised settings to refer patients. Despite the proven benefits of exercise therapy, some patients lack the self motivation to persist with the program to maintain this benefit.

7.3 Optimising medical management of PAD patients

The medical optimisation of patients with peripheral arterial disease focuses primarily on reduction of cardiovascular risk. The goal of optimising medical therapy is to tackle each of the known cardiovascular risk factors and achieve specific targets with appropriate medical therapy. All patients with PAD commenced on secondary prevention of cardiovascular risk should be prescribed an antiplatelet, have a target LDL<2.59mmol/L and a blood pressure <140/90 mmHg. Diabetic patients have stricter targets, LDL< 1.81mmol/L and blood pressure <130/80 mmHg and have a taret HbA1c < 7.0% (Norgren et al., 2007). The medical therapy to achieve these targets are discussed below.

7.3.1 Antiplatelet therapy

The use of antiplatelets in arteriopathic patients is well established. The benefits of antiplatelets are best described in a meta-analysis of 129 RCCT published by the antiplatelet trialist's collaboration in the BMJ (1994a). The meta-analysis included >100,000 patients and demonstrated a 25% decrease in MI, stroke and death in arteriopathic patients on low dose prolonged antiplatelet treatment. Since this publication, the prescription of antiplatelet therapy has increased significantly, as is demonstrated in a recent study showing more than 96% of patients on some form of antiplatelet or anticoagulant therapy (Coveney et al., 2011). Antiplatelets are further indicated in PAD as they greatly reduce the risk of arterial or vascular graft occlusion (1994b). The use of the anticoagulant warfarin, is not indicated in PAD patients unless there is an increased risk of embolic events secondary to the presence of atrial fibrillation. However, the use of wafarin did deter the co-prescribing of an antiplatelet due to the increased risk of bleeding complications with only 3 of 17 patients on warfarin recieving aspirin also. (Coveney et al., 2011)

7.3.2 Lipid lowering therapy

Dietary modification should be the initial intervention to control abnormal lipid levels. All arteriopathic patients should be prescribed HMG CoA reductase inhibitors (statins). Arteriopathic patients should be aggressively treated with a lipid lowering therapy even if their baseline cholesterol levels are normal (2002b). LDL cholesterol should be the primary target of cholesterol lowering therapy as a 1% reduction in LDL levels reduces the relative risk of a major cardiovascular event by 1% over a five year period, independent of age, gender and baseline levels (Grundy et al., 2004). Statin therapy typically dropped LDL levels by 30-40% in all of the treatment arms of the major clinical trials (Shepherd et al., 2002, Sever et al., 2003, 1994c, 2002a, 2002b). The doses used are comparable to current clinical doses, representing a significant risk reduction benefit when used in arteriopathic patients. The

Prospective Study of Pravastatin in the Elderly at Risk (PROSPER) was a multicentre RCCT of Pravastatin use in 5,800 patients with vascular disease (Shepherd et al., 2002). Mortality from coronary artery disease fell by 24% in the pravastatin group. While the risk for stroke was unaffected, the hazard ratio for transient ischemic attacks was 0.75 in the treatment group compared to placebo. As well as improving overall survival, statins improve symptoms of PAD through pleiotropic effects, thought to be mediated through a reduction in endothelial dysfunction, plaque stabilisation and anti-inflammatory effects (Kinlay, 2005, Faggiotto and Paoletti, 1999). The Scandinavian Simvastatin Survival Study found a 38% decrease in "new or worsening claudication" over a 5.4 yr period in 4,444 patients treated with simvastatin (1994c). This further supports the use of statins in vascular patients.

7.3.3 Antihypertensive therapy

Hypertension is associated with a two- to three-fold increased risk for PAD. As mentioned above, hypertension guidelines support the aggressive treatment of blood pressure in patients with atherosclerotic PAD. In this high risk group, the TASC II recommendations set a target blood pressure of <140/90 mmHg, and <130/80 mmHg if the patient has diabetes or renal insufficiency. Achieving these blood pressure targets are more important than the choice of antihypertensive medication. Fortunately there are several effective antihypertensive medications available, including thiazide diuretics, ACE-inhibitors, angiotension receptor blockers, calcium channel blockers and Beta-adrenergic blocking drugs. Often more than one antihypertensive agent is required to achieve target blood pressure. Several of these antihypertensive agents provide additional benefits to the antihypertensive effects and should therefore be considered.

The use of beta-blockers is well established in coronary artery disease. A meta-analysis of 82 RCCTs incorporating >54,000 patients demonstrated the effect of beta-blockade in long-term secondary prevention after myocardial infarction with a proven reduction in mortality (Freemantle et al., 1999). Carotid artery disease, peripheral vascular disease and abdominal aortic aneurysms are termed coronary risk equivalents as they represent a comparable increased risk of developing new coronary events equivalent to patients with established coronary artery disease (>20% over 10 years). Patients with coronary risk equivalents should have the same target blood pressure as patients with coronary artery disease (2002c). The achievement of optimal blood pressure control appears more important than the antihypertensive agent used in overall risk reduction in patients without established coronary artery disease. One prospective observational study (Feringa et al., 2006), demonstrated a hazard ratio of 0.68 for patients with PAD receiving beta-blockers. In this study of 2,420 patients, beta-blockers were the second most benefical drug after statins in reducing long-term mortality.

Unfounded fears have existed with regard to the use of beta-blockers in patients with intermittent claudication. A recent Cochrane review of 6 RCCTs of beta-blocker vs. placebo in PAD showed no statistically significant worsening effect of beta-blockers on maximum walking distance, claudication distance, calf blood flow or skin temperature (Paravastu et al., 2008). An earlier meta-analysis of 11 RCCTs again showed no evidence of adverse effects on walking capacity or symptoms of intermittent claudication in patients with mild to moderate PAD (Feringa et al., 2006). Both of these publications support the use of beta-blockers in patients with coronary artery disease and PAD.

Angiotensin Converting Enzyme (ACE) inhibitors act on the renin-angiotensin-aldosterone system by inhibiting the ACE-mediated conversion of angiotensin I to angiotensin II. Angiotensin II is a potent vasoconstrictor. Within the kidneys, angiotensin II preferentially constricts the efferent arterioles leading to increased perfusion pressure in the glomeruli. It is a drop in this glomerular filtration pressure that initially stimulates renin release. Angiotensin II also stimulates the adrenal cortex to release aldosterone which causes retention of sodium and excretion of potassium in the kidneys which leads to increased water retention, blood volume and consequentially blood pressure. It also stimulates the release of anti-diuretic hormone from the posterior pituitary which again increases water retention and increases blood pressure. By blocking the conversion of angiotensin I to angiotensin II with ACE-inhibitors, antihypertensive effects are achieved.

However ACE–inhibitors have been shown to reduce the cardiovascular morbidity and mortality rates in patients with peripheral vascular disease by 25% regardless of the presence or absence of hypertension. This was demonstrated eloquently in the HOPE trial, a multicentre international RCCT with > 9,000 high risk vascular patients assigned to either a placebo group or a ramipril (10mg) group (Yusuf et al., 2000). In fact, the beneficial effects of ramipril were so evident that the trial was concluded after only 2yrs instead of the initially planned 4.5 years. The 2006 AHA/ACC guidelines state that it is reasonable to treat patients with peripheral vascular disease with ACE-inhibitors to reduce the risk of adverse cardiovascular events. As well as reducing mortality, a small double blind placebo controlled trial published by Ahimastos in 2006 demonstrated that ACE-inhibitors improve the symptoms of peripheral vascular disease, increasing walking time by >200%, although the patient numbers were small and patients with hypertension and diabetes were excluded (Ahimastos et al., 2006). Data from the same cohort of patients suggested that this improvement was due to reduced arterial wall stiffness caused by ACE-inhibitors in the treatment group (Ahimastos et al., 2008). Like Statins, ACE-inhibitors have pleiotropic vascular protective effects including plaque stabilisation, improved vasomotor dysfunction and many biochemical mechanisms including inhibition of platelet adhesion and aggregation, inhibition of platelet derived growth factor, endothelin, and stimulation of endothelial relaxation via stimulation of nitric oxide and prostacyclin (Faggiotto and Paoletti, 1999).

7.3.4 Glyceamic control

Diabetes increases the risk of PAD approximately three- to four-fold, the risk of claudication two-fold, and the risk of amputation five- to ten-fold. Studies of both type 1 and type 2 diabetic patients have demonstrated that aggressive blood-glucose lowering reduces the risk of microvascular complications, particularly retinopathy and nephropathy. However these findings have not be replicated in PAD, primarily because the studies have not been powered to examine the PAD endpoints (Norgren et al., 2007). The current American Diabetes Association guidelines recommend a HbA1c <7.0%. However its unclear whether achieving this goal will effectively protect the peripheral circulation or prevent amputation.

7.3.5 Adjuvant therapy

Cilostazol has been shown to significantly increase (35- 109%) walking distance in people with claudication in several large double blind placebo controlled randomized trials (Money et al., 1998, Elam et al., 1998). The precise role of cilostazol remains to be defined, but a trial of the drug is probably indicated in patients who have unacceptable symptoms despite three to six months of adherence to best medical treatment. No convincing evidence supports treatment with other drugs or vitamins.

8. When to refer to a vascular surgeon?

One of the principle roles of a general practitioner is to act as a gatekeeper to more resource intensive expert care available in teritary referral centres. General practitioners become skilled at recognising the signs and symptoms of serious pathology and referring patients with appropriate urgency. An indept knowledge of a patient's social, family and medical history helps to facilitate this important responsibility on general practitioners.

Due to the high prevalence of PAD, many PAD patients need to be diagnosed and treated by their general practitioner and never meet a vascular surgeon. Referral patterns vary considerably depending on local circumstances, such as the availability of teritary referral centres and the duration of vascular outpatient waiting lists.

If the primary care team is not confident of making the diagnosis, lacks the resources necessary to institute and monitor best medical treatment, or is concerned that the symptoms may have an unusual cause, then it is reasonable to make a referral to a vascular surgical service. Equally, if a patient has unacceptable symptoms despite a reasonable trial of, and adherence to, best medical treatment, then expert vascular surgical assessment and advice is appropriate. Patients who have a weak or absent femoral pulse should be sent to a vascular surgeon for further investigation of aortoiliac disease.

Patients with critical limb ischaemia should be referred urgently to a vascular surgical service. These will include patients with rest pain, gangrene and ulceration. Patients with a clinically suspected abdominal aortic aneurysm or a carotid territory transient ischemic attack should also be referred on an urgent basis to a vascular service.

9. Vascular surgical interventions for PAD

Despite best medical management approximately 25% of patients with intermittent claudication will suffer a deterioration in their PAD. Many of these patient will require a re-vascularisation procedure to improve their symptoms and prolong the functional use of their leg. Unfortunately, even with the current available re-vascularisation procedures, patients with severe PAD may ultimately require amputation for relief of symptoms and to prevent death from sepsis. In general the risk of surgery outweighs the benefit, except in cases of critical limb ischeamia, where the limb is at risk. Intermittent claudication is generally not an indication for re-vascularisation.

Re-vascularisation procedures can be classified into endovascular procedures and open surgical procedures. Often a combination of both are utilised and close co-operation between interventional radiologists and vascular surgeons is essential. Complete smoking cessation and best medical therapy are essential to maximise the durability of any re-vascularisation procedure.

Endovascular procedures use balloon angioplasty to dilate discrete arterial stenoses, typically seen in the superficial femoral artery. It necessitates arterial puncture at the femoral artery, which is not without its risks as discussed with diagnostic angiography. An example of a successful angioplasty is shown below in figure 2. Placement of endovascular stents is also feasible in larger calibre arteries, which in practice implies suprainguinal arteries.

Open surgical interventions include endarterectomy which involves opening up the diseased artery and removing the atherosclerotic plaque to restore blood flow. With severe long segment disease a bypass procedure can be performed, such as a femoral-popliteal bypass for an occluded superfical femoral artery or an aorto-bifemoral bypass for occlusive iliac disease. Endogenous graft material is significantly more superior to exogenous synthetic grafts with significantly better 5 year patency rates. The long saphenous vein or cephalic vein are the most commonly used vessels for endogenous grafts.

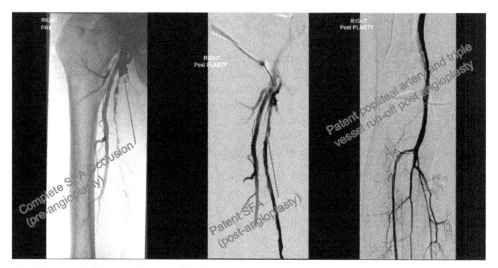

Fig. 2. Successful 5mm subintimal balloon angioplasty of an occluded superficial femoral artery of a 65 yr old male.

10. Summary

The prevalence of PAD is increasing with an aging global population. PAD is a marker of systemic atherosclerotic disease. Patients diagnosed early with PAD can be initiated on appropriate secondary preventative meaures to reduce the significantly increased cardiovascular risk associated with PAD, as well as preventing progression of their PAD. More than two thirds of patients with PAD are asymptomatic, which highlights the major role primary care physicians can play in identifying, screening and diagnosing patients with PAD. Optimal secondary preventative treatment for PAD, requires complete smoking cessation, a supervised exercise program, cholesterol reduction, antihypertensive therapy, tight glyceamic control (in diabetics) and antiplatelet therapy.

11. References

1994a. Collaborative overview of randomised trials of antiplatelet therapy--I: Prevention of death, myocardial infarction, and stroke by prolonged antiplatelet therapy in various categories of patients. Antiplatelet Trialists' Collaboration. *BMJ,* 308, 81-106.

1994b. Collaborative overview of randomised trials of antiplatelet therapy--II: Maintenance of vascular graft or arterial patency by antiplatelet therapy. Antiplatelet Trialists' Collaboration. *BMJ,* 308, 159-68.

1994c. Randomised trial of cholesterol lowering in 4444 patients with coronary heart disease: the Scandinavian Simvastatin Survival Study (4S). *Lancet,* 344, 1383-9.

2002a. Major outcomes in moderately hypercholesterolemic, hypertensive patients randomized to pravastatin vs usual care: The Antihypertensive and Lipid-Lowering Treatment to Prevent Heart Attack Trial (ALLHAT-LLT). *JAMA,* 288, 2998-3007.

2002b. MRC/BHF Heart Protection Study of cholesterol lowering with simvastatin in 20,536 high-risk individuals: a randomised placebo-controlled trial. *Lancet,* 360, 7-22.

2002c. Third Report of the National Cholesterol Education Program (NCEP) Expert Panel on Detection, Evaluation, and Treatment of High Blood Cholesterol in Adults (Adult Treatment Panel III) final report. *Circulation,* 106, 3143-421.

2003. Peripheral arterial disease in people with diabetes. *Diabetes Care,* 26, 3333-41.

AHIMASTOS, A. A., DART, A. M., LAWLER, A., BLOMBERY, P. A. & KINGWELL, B. A. 2008. Reduced arterial stiffness may contribute to angiotensin-converting enzyme inhibitor induced improvements in walking time in peripheral arterial disease patients. *J Hypertens,* 26, 1037-42.

AHIMASTOS, A. A., LAWLER, A., REID, C. M., BLOMBERY, P. A. & KINGWELL, B. A. 2006. Brief communication: ramipril markedly improves walking ability in patients with peripheral arterial disease: a randomized trial. *Ann Intern Med,* 144, 660-4.

ANTHONISEN, N. R., SKEANS, M. A., WISE, R. A., MANFREDA, J., KANNER, R. E. & CONNETT, J. E. 2005. The effects of a smoking cessation intervention on 14.5-year mortality: a randomized clinical trial. *Ann Intern Med,* 142, 233-9.

BANERJEE, A., FOWKES, F. G. & ROTHWELL, P. M. 2010. Associations between peripheral artery disease and ischemic stroke: implications for primary and secondary prevention. *Stroke,* 41, 2102-7.

BEKS, P. J., MACKAAY, A. J., DE NEELING, J. N., DE VRIES, H., BOUTER, L. M. & HEINE, R. J. 1995. Peripheral arterial disease in relation to glycaemic level in an elderly Caucasian population: the Hoorn study. *Diabetologia,* 38, 86-96.

BIANCARI, F., D'ANDREA, V., DI MARCO, C., SAVINO, G., TIOZZO, V. & CATANIA, A. 2010. Meta-analysis of randomized trials on the efficacy of vascular closure devices after diagnostic angiography and angioplasty. *Am Heart J,* 159, 518-31.

BOUSHEY, C. J., BERESFORD, S. A., OMENN, G. S. & MOTULSKY, A. G. 1995. A quantitative assessment of plasma homocysteine as a risk factor for vascular disease. Probable benefits of increasing folic acid intakes. *JAMA,* 274, 1049-57.

BOWERS, B. L., VALENTINE, R. J., MYERS, S. I., CHERVU, A. & CLAGETT, G. P. 1993. The natural history of patients with claudication with toe pressures of 40 mm Hg or less. *J Vasc Surg,* 18, 506-11.

CACOUB, P., CAMBOU, J. P., KOWNATOR, S., BELLIARD, J. P., BEREGI, J. P., BRANCHEREAU, A., CARPENTIER, P., LEGER, P., LUIZY, F., MAIZA, D., MIHCI, E., HERRMANN, M. A. & PRIOLLET, P. 2009. Prevalence of peripheral arterial disease in high-risk patients using ankle-brachial index in general practice: a cross-sectional study. *Int J Clin Pract,* 63, 63-70.

COLE, C. W., HILL, G. B., FARZAD, E., BOUCHARD, A., MOHER, D., RODY, K. & SHEA, B. 1993. Cigarette smoking and peripheral arterial occlusive disease. *Surgery,* 114, 753-6; discussion 756-7.

COVENEY, A. P., O'BRIEN, G. C. & FULTON, G. J. 2011. ACE up the sleeve - are vascular patients medically optimized? *Vasc Health Risk Manag,* 7, 15-21.

CRIQUI, M. H., DENENBERG, J. O., LANGER, R. D. & FRONEK, A. 1997. The epidemiology of peripheral arterial disease: importance of identifying the population at risk. *Vasc Med,* 2, 221-6.

CRIQUI, M. H., FRONEK, A., KLAUBER, M. R., BARRETT-CONNOR, E. & GABRIEL, S. 1985. The sensitivity, specificity, and predictive value of traditional clinical evaluation of peripheral arterial disease: results from noninvasive testing in a defined population. *Circulation,* 71, 516-22.

DORMANDY, J. A. & MURRAY, G. D. 1991. The fate of the claudicant--a prospective study of 1969 claudicants. *Eur J Vasc Surg,* 5, 131-3.

ELAM, M. B., HECKMAN, J., CROUSE, J. R., HUNNINGHAKE, D. B., HERD, J. A., DAVIDSON, M., GORDON, I. L., BORTEY, E. B. & FORBES, W. P. 1998. Effect of the novel antiplatelet agent cilostazol on plasma lipoproteins in patients with intermittent claudication. *Arterioscler Thromb Vasc Biol,* 18, 1942-7.

FAGGIOTTO, A. & PAOLETTI, R. 1999. State-of-the-Art lecture. Statins and blockers of the renin-angiotensin system: vascular protection beyond their primary mode of action. *Hypertension,* 34, 987-96.

FEIGELSON, H. S., CRIQUI, M. H., FRONEK, A., LANGER, R. D. & MOLGAARD, C. A. 1994. Screening for peripheral arterial disease: the sensitivity, specificity, and predictive value of noninvasive tests in a defined population. *Am J Epidemiol,* 140, 526-34.

FERINGA, H. H., VAN WANING, V. H., BAX, J. J., ELHENDY, A., BOERSMA, E., SCHOUTEN, O., GALAL, W., VIDAKOVIC, R. V., TANGELDER, M. J. & POLDERMANS, D. 2006. Cardioprotective medication is associated with improved survival in patients with peripheral arterial disease. *J Am Coll Cardiol,* 47, 1182-7.

FOWKES, F. G. 1988. The measurement of atherosclerotic peripheral arterial disease in epidemiological surveys. *Int J Epidemiol,* 17, 248-54.

FOWKES, F. G., HOUSLEY, E., CAWOOD, E. H., MACINTYRE, C. C., RUCKLEY, C. V. & PRESCOTT, R. J. 1991. Edinburgh Artery Study: prevalence of asymptomatic and symptomatic peripheral arterial disease in the general population. *Int J Epidemiol,* 20, 384-92.

FOWKES, F. G., HOUSLEY, E., RIEMERSMA, R. A., MACINTYRE, C. C., CAWOOD, E. H., PRESCOTT, R. J. & RUCKLEY, C. V. 1992. Smoking, lipids, glucose intolerance, and blood pressure as risk factors for peripheral atherosclerosis compared with ischemic heart disease in the Edinburgh Artery Study. *Am J Epidemiol,* 135, 331-40.

FOWKES, F. G., MURRAY, G. D., BUTCHER, I., HEALD, C. L., LEE, R. J., CHAMBLESS, L. E., FOLSOM, A. R., HIRSCH, A. T., DRAMAIX, M., DEBACKER, G., WAUTRECHT, J. C., KORNITZER, M., NEWMAN, A. B., CUSHMAN, M., SUTTON-TYRRELL, K., LEE, A. J., PRICE, J. F., D'AGOSTINO, R. B., MURABITO, J. M., NORMAN, P. E., JAMROZIK, K., CURB, J. D., MASAKI, K. H., RODRIGUEZ, B. L., DEKKER, J. M., BOUTER, L. M., HEINE, R. J., NIJPELS, G., STEHOUWER, C. D., FERRUCCI, L., MCDERMOTT, M. M., STOFFERS, H. E., HOOI, J. D., KNOTTNERUS, J. A., OGREN, M., HEDBLAD, B., WITTEMAN, J. C., BRETELER, M. M., HUNINK, M. G., HOFMAN, A., CRIQUI, M. H., LANGER, R. D., FRONEK,

A., HIATT, W. R., HAMMAN, R., RESNICK, H. E. & GURALNIK, J. 2008. Ankle brachial index combined with Framingham Risk Score to predict cardiovascular events and mortality: a meta-analysis. *JAMA*, 300, 197-208.

FREEMANTLE, N., CLELAND, J., YOUNG, P., MASON, J. & HARRISON, J. 1999. beta Blockade after myocardial infarction: systematic review and meta regression analysis. *BMJ*, 318, 1730-7.

GRAHAM, I. M., DALY, L. E., REFSUM, H. M., ROBINSON, K., BRATTSTROM, L. E., UELAND, P. M., PALMA-REIS, R. J., BOERS, G. H., SHEAHAN, R. G., ISRAELSSON, B., UITERWAAL, C. S., MELEADY, R., MCMASTER, D., VERHOEF, P., WITTEMAN, J., RUBBA, P., BELLET, H., WAUTRECHT, J. C., DE VALK, H. W., SALES LUIS, A. C., PARROT-ROULAND, F. M., TAN, K. S., HIGGINS, I., GARCON, D., ANDRIA, G. & ET AL. 1997. Plasma homocysteine as a risk factor for vascular disease. The European Concerted Action Project. *JAMA*, 277, 1775-81.

GRUNDY, S. M., CLEEMAN, J. I., MERZ, C. N., BREWER, H. B., JR., CLARK, L. T., HUNNINGHAKE, D. B., PASTERNAK, R. C., SMITH, S. C., JR. & STONE, N. J. 2004. Implications of recent clinical trials for the National Cholesterol Education Program Adult Treatment Panel III guidelines. *Circulation*, 110, 227-39.

HIATT, W. R., HOAG, S. & HAMMAN, R. F. 1995. Effect of diagnostic criteria on the prevalence of peripheral arterial disease. The San Luis Valley Diabetes Study. *Circulation*, 91, 1472-9.

HIATT, W. R., WOLFEL, E. E., MEIER, R. H. & REGENSTEINER, J. G. 1994. Superiority of treadmill walking exercise versus strength training for patients with peripheral arterial disease. Implications for the mechanism of the training response. *Circulation*, 90, 1866-74.

HIRSCH, A. T., CRIQUI, M. H., TREAT-JACOBSON, D., REGENSTEINER, J. G., CREAGER, M. A., OLIN, J. W., KROOK, S. H., HUNNINGHAKE, D. B., COMEROTA, A. J., WALSH, M. E., MCDERMOTT, M. M. & HIATT, W. R. 2001. Peripheral arterial disease detection, awareness, and treatment in primary care. *JAMA*, 286, 1317-24.

HIRSCH, A. T., HASKAL, Z. J., HERTZER, N. R., BAKAL, C. W., CREAGER, M. A., HALPERIN, J. L., HIRATZKA, L. F., MURPHY, W. R., OLIN, J. W., PUSCHETT, J. B., ROSENFIELD, K. A., SACKS, D., STANLEY, J. C., TAYLOR, L. M., JR., WHITE, C. J., WHITE, J., WHITE, R. A., ANTMAN, E. M., SMITH, S. C., JR., ADAMS, C. D., ANDERSON, J. L., FAXON, D. P., FUSTER, V., GIBBONS, R. J., HUNT, S. A., JACOBS, A. K., NISHIMURA, R., ORNATO, J. P., PAGE, R. L. & RIEGEL, B. 2006. ACC/AHA 2005 Practice Guidelines for the management of patients with peripheral arterial disease (lower extremity, renal, mesenteric, and abdominal aortic): a collaborative report from the American Association for Vascular Surgery/Society for Vascular Surgery, Society for Cardiovascular Angiography and Interventions, Society for Vascular Medicine and Biology, Society of Interventional Radiology, and the ACC/AHA Task Force on Practice Guidelines (Writing Committee to Develop Guidelines for the Management of Patients With Peripheral Arterial Disease): endorsed by the American Association of Cardiovascular and Pulmonary Rehabilitation; National Heart, Lung, and Blood Institute; Society for Vascular Nursing; TransAtlantic Inter-Society Consensus; and Vascular Disease Foundation. *Circulation*, 113, e463-654.

HOFFMAN, M. 2011. Hypothesis: Hyperhomocysteinemia is an indicator of oxidant stress. *Med Hypotheses*, 77, 1088-93.

HOOI, J. D., KESTER, A. D., STOFFERS, H. E., RINKENS, P. E., KNOTTNERUS, J. A. & VAN REE, J. W. 2004. Asymptomatic peripheral arterial occlusive disease predicted cardiovascular morbidity and mortality in a 7-year follow-up study. *J Clin Epidemiol,* 57, 294-300.

HOOI, J. D., STOFFERS, H. E., KESTER, A. D., RINKENS, P. E., KAISER, V., VAN REE, J. W. & KNOTTNERUS, J. A. 1998. Risk factors and cardiovascular diseases associated with asymptomatic peripheral arterial occlusive disease. The Limburg PAOD Study. Peripheral Arterial Occlusive Disease. *Scand J Prim Health Care,* 16, 177-82.

INGOLFSSON, I. O., SIGURDSSON, G., SIGVALDASON, H., THORGEIRSSON, G. & SIGFUSSON, N. 1994. A marked decline in the prevalence and incidence of intermittent claudication in Icelandic men 1968-1986: a strong relationship to smoking and serum cholesterol--the Reykjavik Study. *J Clin Epidemiol,* 47, 1237-43.

KANNEL, W. B. & MCGEE, D. L. 1985. Update on some epidemiologic features of intermittent claudication: the Framingham Study. *J Am Geriatr Soc,* 33, 13-8.

KANNEL, W. B. & SHURTLEFF, D. 1973. The Framingham Study. Cigarettes and the development of intermittent claudication. *Geriatrics,* 28, 61-8.

KATSILAMBROS, N. L., TSAPOGAS, P. C., ARVANITIS, M. P., TRITOS, N. A., ALEXIOU, Z. P. & RIGAS, K. L. 1996. Risk factors for lower extremity arterial disease in non-insulin-dependent diabetic persons. *Diabet Med,* 13, 243-6.

KINLAY, S. 2005. Potential vascular benefits of statins. *Am J Med,* 118 Suppl 12A, 62-7.

LENG, G. C., LEE, A. J., FOWKES, F. G., WHITEMAN, M., DUNBAR, J., HOUSLEY, E. & RUCKLEY, C. V. 1996. Incidence, natural history and cardiovascular events in symptomatic and asymptomatic peripheral arterial disease in the general population. *Int J Epidemiol,* 25, 1172-81.

LONN, E. 2008. Homocysteine-lowering B vitamin therapy in cardiovascular prevention--wrong again? *JAMA,* 299, 2086-7.

MCDANIEL, M. D. & CRONENWETT, J. L. 1989. Basic data related to the natural history of intermittent claudication. *Ann Vasc Surg,* 3, 273-7.

MCDERMOTT, M. M., GREENLAND, P., LIU, K., GURALNIK, J. M., CELIC, L., CRIQUI, M. H., CHAN, C., MARTIN, G. J., SCHNEIDER, J., PEARCE, W. H., TAYLOR, L. M. & CLARK, E. 2002. The ankle brachial index is associated with leg function and physical activity: the Walking and Leg Circulation Study. *Ann Intern Med,* 136, 873-83.

MCDERMOTT, M. M., GREENLAND, P., LIU, K., GURALNIK, J. M., CRIQUI, M. H., DOLAN, N. C., CHAN, C., CELIC, L., PEARCE, W. H., SCHNEIDER, J. R., SHARMA, L., CLARK, E., GIBSON, D. & MARTIN, G. J. 2001. Leg symptoms in peripheral arterial disease: associated clinical characteristics and functional impairment. *JAMA,* 286, 1599-606.

MEIJER, W. T., HOES, A. W., RUTGERS, D., BOTS, M. L., HOFMAN, A. & GROBBEE, D. E. 1998. Peripheral arterial disease in the elderly: The Rotterdam Study. *Arterioscler Thromb Vasc Biol,* 18, 185-92.

MOLGAARD, J., MALINOW, M. R., LASSVIK, C., HOLM, A. C., UPSON, B. & OLSSON, A. G. 1992. Hyperhomocyst(e)inaemia: an independent risk factor for intermittent claudication. *J Intern Med,* 231, 273-9.

MONEY, S. R., HERD, J. A., ISAACSOHN, J. L., DAVIDSON, M., CUTLER, B., HECKMAN, J. & FORBES, W. P. 1998. Effect of cilostazol on walking distances in patients with intermittent claudication caused by peripheral vascular disease. *J Vasc Surg,* 27, 267-74; discussion 274-5.

MOST, R. S. & SINNOCK, P. 1983. The epidemiology of lower extremity amputations in diabetic individuals. *Diabetes Care,* 6, 87-91.

MOYSIDIS, T., NOWACK, T., EICKMEYER, F., WALDHAUSEN, P., BRUNKEN, A., HOCHLENERT, D., ENGELS, G., SANTOSA, F., LUTHER, B. & KROGER, K. 2011.

Trends in amputations in people with hospital admissions for peripheral arterial disease in Germany. *Vasa*, 40, 289-95.

MURABITO, J. M., D'AGOSTINO, R. B., SILBERSHATZ, H. & WILSON, W. F. 1997. Intermittent claudication. A risk profile from The Framingham Heart Study. *Circulation*, 96, 44-9.

MURABITO, J. M., EVANS, J. C., NIETO, K., LARSON, M. G., LEVY, D. & WILSON, P. W. 2002. Prevalence and clinical correlates of peripheral arterial disease in the Framingham Offspring Study. *Am Heart J*, 143, 961-5.

MURRAY, C. J. & LOPEZ, A. D. 1997. Mortality by cause for eight regions of the world: Global Burden of Disease Study. *Lancet*, 349, 1269-76.

NEWMAN, A. B., SISCOVICK, D. S., MANOLIO, T. A., POLAK, J., FRIED, L. P., BORHANI, N. O. & WOLFSON, S. K. 1993. Ankle-arm index as a marker of atherosclerosis in the Cardiovascular Health Study. Cardiovascular Heart Study (CHS) Collaborative Research Group. *Circulation*, 88, 837-45.

NORGREN, L., HIATT, W. R., DORMANDY, J. A., NEHLER, M. R., HARRIS, K. A., FOWKES, F. G., BELL, K., CAPORUSSO, J., DURAND-ZALESKI, I., KOMORI, K., LAMMER, J., LIAPIS, C., NOVO, S., RAZAVI, M., ROBBS, J., SCHAPER, N., SHIGEMATSU, H., SAPOVAL, M., WHITE, C., WHITE, J., CLEMENT, D., CREAGER, M., JAFF, M., MOHLER, E., 3RD, RUTHERFORD, R. B., SHEEHAN, P., SILLESEN, H. & ROSENFIELD, K. 2007. Inter-Society Consensus for the Management of Peripheral Arterial Disease (TASC II). *Eur J Vasc Endovasc Surg*, 33 Suppl 1, S1-75.

NOVO, S., AVELLONE, G., DI GARBO, V., ABRIGNANI, M. G., LIQUORI, M., PANNO, A. V. & STRANO, A. 1992. Prevalence of risk factors in patients with peripheral arterial disease. A clinical and epidemiological evaluation. *Int Angiol*, 11, 218-29.

PARAVASTU, S. C., MENDONCA, D. & DA SILVA, A. 2008. Beta blockers for peripheral arterial disease. *Cochrane Database Syst Rev*, CD005508.

POWELL, J. T., EDWARDS, R. J., WORRELL, P. C., FRANKS, P. J., GREENHALGH, R. M. & POULTER, N. R. 1997. Risk factors associated with the development of peripheral arterial disease in smokers: a case-control study. *Atherosclerosis*, 129, 41-8.

PRICE, J. F., MOWBRAY, P. I., LEE, A. J., RUMLEY, A., LOWE, G. D. & FOWKES, F. G. 1999. Relationship between smoking and cardiovascular risk factors in the development of peripheral arterial disease and coronary artery disease: Edinburgh Artery Study. *Eur Heart J*, 20, 344-53.

REUNANEN, A., TAKKUNEN, H. & AROMAA, A. 1982. Prevalence of intermittent claudication and its effect on mortality. *Acta Med Scand*, 211, 249-56.

ROTHWELL, P. M. 2000. Carotid artery disease and the risk of ischaemic stroke and coronary vascular events. *Cerebrovasc Dis*, 10 Suppl 5, 21-33.

SANNA, G., ALESSO, D., MEDIATI, M., CIMMINIELLO, C., BORGHI, C., FAZZARI, A. L. & MANGRELLA, M. 2011. Prevalence of peripheral arterial disease in subjects with moderate cardiovascular risk: Italian results from the PANDORA study Data from PANDORA (Prevalence of peripheral Arterial disease in subjects with moderate CVD risk, with No overt vascular Diseases nor Diabetes mellitus). *BMC Cardiovasc Disord*, 11, 59.

SELVIN, E. & ERLINGER, T. P. 2004. Prevalence of and risk factors for peripheral arterial disease in the United States: results from the National Health and Nutrition Examination Survey, 1999-2000. *Circulation*, 110, 738-43.

SEVER, P. S., DAHLOF, B., POULTER, N. R., WEDEL, H., BEEVERS, G., CAULFIELD, M., COLLINS, R., KJELDSEN, S. E., KRISTINSSON, A., MCINNES, G. T., MEHLSEN, J., NIEMINEN, M., O'BRIEN, E. & OSTERGREN, J. 2003. Prevention of coronary and stroke events with atorvastatin in hypertensive patients who have average or lower-than-average cholesterol concentrations, in the Anglo-Scandinavian Cardiac Outcomes Trial--Lipid Lowering Arm (ASCOT-LLA): a multicentre randomised controlled trial. *Lancet*, 361, 1149-58.

SHEPHERD, J., BLAUW, G. J., MURPHY, M. B., BOLLEN, E. L., BUCKLEY, B. M., COBBE, S. M., FORD, I., GAW, A., HYLAND, M., JUKEMA, J. W., KAMPER, A. M., MACFARLANE, P. W., MEINDERS, A. E., NORRIE, J., PACKARD, C. J., PERRY, I. J., STOTT, D. J., SWEENEY, B. J., TWOMEY, C. & WESTENDORP, R. G. 2002. Pravastatin in elderly individuals at risk of vascular disease (PROSPER): a randomised controlled trial. *Lancet*, 360, 1623-30.

SMITH, G. D., SHIPLEY, M. J. & ROSE, G. 1990. Intermittent claudication, heart disease risk factors, and mortality. The Whitehall Study. *Circulation*, 82, 1925-31.

SONG, Y., COOK, N. R., ALBERT, C. M., VAN DENBURGH, M. & MANSON, J. E. 2009. Effect of homocysteine-lowering treatment with folic Acid and B vitamins on risk of type 2 diabetes in women: a randomized, controlled trial. *Diabetes*, 58, 1921-8.

STEAD, L. F. & LANCASTER, T. 2000. Group behaviour therapy programmes for smoking cessation. *Cochrane Database Syst Rev*, CD001007.

STEWART, K. J., HIATT, W. R., REGENSTEINER, J. G. & HIRSCH, A. T. 2002. Exercise training for claudication. *N Engl J Med*, 347, 1941-51.

TAYLOR, L. M., JR., DEFRANG, R. D., HARRIS, E. J., JR. & PORTER, J. M. 1991. The association of elevated plasma homocyst(e)ine with progression of symptomatic peripheral arterial disease. *J Vasc Surg*, 13, 128-36.

TONSTAD, S., FARSANG, C., KLAENE, G., LEWIS, K., MANOLIS, A., PERRUCHOUD, A. P., SILAGY, C., VAN SPIEGEL, P. I., ASTBURY, C., HIDER, A. & SWEET, R. 2003. Bupropion SR for smoking cessation in smokers with cardiovascular disease: a multicentre, randomised study. *Eur Heart J*, 24, 946-55.

TOOLE, J. F., MALINOW, M. R., CHAMBLESS, L. E., SPENCE, J. D., PETTIGREW, L. C., HOWARD, V. J., SIDES, E. G., WANG, C. H. & STAMPFER, M. 2004. Lowering homocysteine in patients with ischemic stroke to prevent recurrent stroke, myocardial infarction, and death: the Vitamin Intervention for Stroke Prevention (VISP) randomized controlled trial. *JAMA*, 291, 565-75.

TOUZE, E., VARENNE, O., CHATELLIER, G., PEYRARD, S., ROTHWELL, P. M. & MAS, J. L. 2005. Risk of myocardial infarction and vascular death after transient ischemic attack and ischemic stroke: a systematic review and meta-analysis. *Stroke*, 36, 2748-55.

WHYMAN, M. R., FOWKES, F. G., KERRACHER, E. M., GILLESPIE, I. N., LEE, A. J., HOUSLEY, E. & RUCKLEY, C. V. 1997. Is intermittent claudication improved by percutaneous transluminal angioplasty? A randomized controlled trial. *J Vasc Surg*, 26, 551-7.

WILLIGENDAEL, E. M., TEIJINK, J. A., BARTELINK, M. L., PETERS, R. J., BULLER, H. R. & PRINS, M. H. 2005. Smoking and the patency of lower extremity bypass grafts: a meta-analysis. *J Vasc Surg*, 42, 67-74.

WILSON, J. M. G. & JUNGNER, G. 1968. Principles and practice of screening for disease. *Public Health papers*. Geneva: World Health Organisation.

YUSUF, S., SLEIGHT, P., POGUE, J., BOSCH, J., DAVIES, R. & DAGENAIS, G. 2000. Effects of an angiotensin-converting-enzyme inhibitor, ramipril, on cardiovascular events in high-risk patients. The Heart Outcomes Prevention Evaluation Study Investigators. *N Engl J Med*, 342, 145-53.

6

The Role of Fracture Liaison Services in Re-Fracture Prevention

Kirtan Ganda and Markus J. Seibel
Bone Research Program, ANZAC Research Institute
The University of Sydney at Concord Campus, Sydney,
Australia

1. Introduction

1.1 The burden of osteoporotic fractures

Osteoporosis is a disorder of low bone mass and micro-architectural deterioration in bone, resulting in increased bone fragility and susceptibility to fractures even after minimal or inadequate trauma [Anonymous, Consensus conference, 1993]. On statistical grounds, more than 50% of postmenopausal women, and approximately 30% of men over the age of 60 years will suffer at least one minimal trauma fracture during their remaining lifetime [Kanis et al. 2000]. However, any osteoporotic fracture predisposes to further fractures, significant morbidity, and premature death. There is a 2-3 fold increase in the risk of repeat fractures after a first minimal trauma fracture. This is true for both men and women in all age categories [Langsetmo et al. 2009]. In the year 2000, there were about 8.9 million fractures worldwide [Johnell et al. 2006], of which 1.6 million were hip fractures. The number of hip fractures is expected to increase worldwide to 6.26 million by 2050 in the context of an ageing population, and longer life expectancy in the developing world [Sambrook P, Cooper C. 2006]. In Australia, the annual number of fractures is projected to increase by 250%, from 83,238 in 1996 to 207,657 fractures in 2051 as a result of the ageing population. Hip fractures are expected to quadruple over the same period of time [Sanders et al. 1999]. There is significant economic burden associated with minimal trauma fractures. In the USA the cost of minimal trauma fractures was estimated at US $17 billion in 2005, with the annual cost predicted to increase by 50% in 2025 [Burge et al. 2007]. In Australia the cost of fragility fractures was AU$ 7.4 billion in 2001 [Sambrook et al. 2002].

1.2 The treatment gap in osteoporosis

Despite the availability of advanced medical care and medications that reduce the risk of re-fracture by 30–90% [Giangregorio et al., 2006], the majority of patients with incident osteoporotic fractures are neither investigated nor treated for their underlying condition. This is referred to as the 'treatment gap in osteoporosis', which has been extensively documented in the international literature [Bliuc et al., 2005; Panneman et al., 2004; Shibli-Rahhal et al., 2011]. A systematic review [Giangregorio et al. 2006] revealed that following a minimal trauma fracture the median rate of bone mineral density (BMD) testing was as low as 10%, as was the initiation of treatment (Figs. 1, 2).

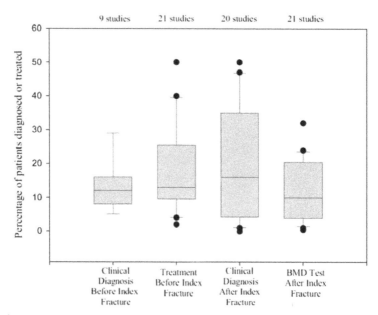

Fig. 1. The diagnostic gap: Low rate of investigations after a minimal trauma fracture. (Reproduced from Giangregorio et al., 2006, with permission.)

A thorough understanding of the factors contributing to the care gap in osteoporosis is pivotal to finding effective solutions. Generally speaking, significant deficits exist on three different levels: patient, doctor, and system level. On a patient and doctor level, a lack of awareness and understanding that a minimal trauma fracture should prompt a thorough evaluation for osteoporosis has been well documented [The Burden of Brittle Bones, 2007]. Patients may be reluctant to be evaluated due to perceived medication side effects, time constraints, costs, and language barriers. A desire to avoid polypharmacy may also contribute to the reluctance of elderly patients and their carers to initiate treatment. Doctors may have the misconception that the current treatments available for osteoporosis are ineffective or fraught with side effects, or they may not have the resources (e.g. for bone mineral density testing) or time to evaluate patients for osteoporosis, especially in an acute hospital setting. On a systems level, fragmentation of care further contributes to the "care gap", in that no single care provider (primary care physician, orthopaedic surgeon, specialist physician, or primary care physician) takes responsibility for osteoporosis management. Furthermore, a lack of funding for osteoporosis may be a consequence of low priority of osteoporosis in the public mind. For instance, osteoporosis has to compete for funding with diseases such as breast cancer and leukaemia which have more 'prestige' and therefore lobbying power, probably because they are associated with death at a younger age. According to the National Institutes of Health in the US [http://report.nih.gov/rcdc/categories/], estimated funding for breast cancer research for the 2011 financial year was quadruple that for osteoporosis, despite a higher incidence of osteoporosis. That is, 12.5% of women in the US will develop breast cancer during their lifetime, whereas 50% of women will suffer from a minimal trauma fracture after the age of 60 years.

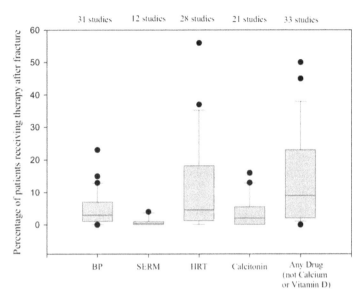

Fig. 2. The therapeutic gap: Low rate of osteoporosis treatment after a minimal trauma fracture. Key: BP = bisphosphonate, SERM = Selective Estrogen Receptor Modulator, HRT = Hormone Replacement Therapy. (Reproduced from Giangregorio et al., 2006, with permission.)

2. Fracture liaison services

2.1 Bridging the gap in osteoporosis care through fracture liaison services

The acute presentation of a patient with a minimal trauma fracture to a health care facility (usually an emergency department) is an easily identifiable clinical event. Care of these patients is then transferred to an orthopaedic service, either in an inpatient or an outpatient setting. This process represents a unique window of opportunity to identify, investigate and appropriately treat patients with osteoporosis [Gallacher, 2005]. Thus, over the last 10 years several groups across the world, including Australia, Canada, Europe and the USA have attempted to address the osteoporosis care gap via the development and clinical implementation of what is now generally known as "Fracture Liaison Services" (FLS). However, the published literature on FLS, while substantial and often of good quality, is characterized by enormous heterogeneity in the methods of patient identification, patient capture, and intensity of intervention. Thus, there is significant variation in the type of studies, patient characteristics, methodology and criteria of patient identification. The extent of engagement of the service in the investigation and treatment of the patient also varies significantly, together with outcomes in relation to bone mineral density (BMD) testing, treatment initiation, adherence, and re-fracture rates. This chapter will review the existing literature on FLS to provide a coherent overview of their methodology and outcomes.

2.2 Models of Care based upon intervention intensity

The spectrum of possible interventions prompted by a patient presenting to hospital with a minimal trauma fracture can be summarized as follows:

i.   Provision of specific "osteoporosis protocols" to staff at inpatient wards, orthopaedic fracture clinics and emergency departments;
ii. Education of patients through letter (information sheet), or direct communication either 'face-to-face' or via telephone;
iii. Alerting the Primary Care Physician (PCP) of the need to evaluate and treat their patient for osteoporosis via direct communication, letter, or email;
iv. Assessment of clinical risk factors for osteoporosis;
v.   Offering BMD testing (osteodensitometry);
vi. Investigation for secondary causes of osteoporosis;
vii. Initiating treatment (both non-pharmacological and pharmacological);
viii. Monitoring with regular follow-up, using a dedicated database to evaluate effectiveness of intervention.

Depending on the model of care implemented at any given site, the actual intervention can range from a simple, education-based model with high patient capture and turnover to more complex models involving most or all components listed above. More complex, intensive models typically incorporate patient education and risk assessment, with on-site bone densitometry testing, as well as treatment initiation. In these complex models of care it is often the fracture liaison co-coordinator who plays a pivotal role in orchestrating and co-ordinating care, after the minimal trauma fracture.

Given the heterogeneity in models of care and their reporting of outcomes, the following classification of FLS from 'type A' to 'type D' models of care, based upon the type and intensity of the intervention has been suggested (Table 1). 'Type E' model of care is a category unrelated to intervention intensity, representing inpatient intervention only:

Model of Care	Description
A	Identification, Assessment (risk factors, pathology testing, BMD), Treatment initiation
B	Identification, Assessment, Treatment recommendation only
C	Education of patient and Primary Care Physician
D	Education of patient only
E	Inpatient specialist consultation

Table 1. Categorical types of FLS according to Model of Care

This categorization of intervention types is graded from A through to D, with A representing the most intensive, all-encompassing intervention. Although each model of care is unique, there are significant variations in details of the intervention, and reporting of outcomes between each study. It is also important to note that health care environments and resources differ with countries, leading to the development of unique models of care.

2.3 'Type A' models of care

Since 2000, there have been thirteen studies published describing a 'type A' model of care, heralding from Australia (four studies – Kuo et al., 2007; Vaile et al., 2007; Giles et al., 2010;

Lih et al., 2011), US (three studies – Edwards et al., 2005; Dell et al., 2008; Navarro et al., 2011), Canada (three studies – Bogoch et al., 2006; Majumdar et al., 2007 & 2011; Morrish et al., 2009) and Europe (two studies – Clunie et al., 2008; Boudou et al., 2011). A further two studies focused on the cost analysis of individual FLS (Sander et al., 2008; Cooper et al., 2011).

These clinical studies are unique in describing a co-ordinated model of care through which patients are identified, assessed and treated following a minimal trauma fracture as part of an all-encompassing service. Assessment includes evaluation of clinical risk factors for osteoporosis, a bone mineral density scan, radiographic or other imaging as required, and various pathology tests to exclude secondary causes of osteoporosis. This assessment is then followed by the initiation of appropriate non-pharmacological and pharmacological interventions. An example of a classical 'type A' model of care is the Concord Hospital FLS (Figure 3). Table 2 illustrates the summary of outcomes for 'Type A' model of care. For a more analytical evaluation of the cited studies see Appendix A.

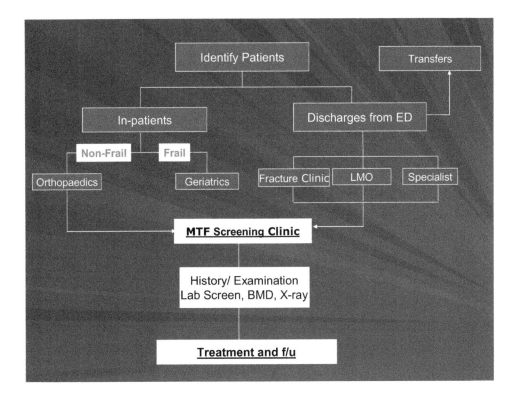

Fig. 3. An example of the structure of a 'Type A' FLS. Key: MTF = Minimal Trauma Fracture; f/u = follow-up; LMO=Local Medical Officer or primary care physician

Country	Study	Study Type	BMD/Rx	BMD	Rx	Rx Adherence	Refractures	Cost Effectiveness
Australia	Vaile et al., 2007	Before & After	NA	All	51% v 11%	95%@12/12	NA	Y
	Lih et al. 2011	Prospective Controlled	NA	All	79% v 31%	NA	4.1 v 19.7% @4yr	Y
	Giles et al. 2010	Cross Sectional	NA	NA	NA	NA	NA	NA
	Kuo et al. 2007	Before & After	NA	83% v 10%	NA	10 months 80%	NA	NA
United States	Navarro et al. 2011	Cross Sectional	F 92%,M 75%, nil racial disparity	NA	NA	NA	NA	NA
	Dell et al. 2008	Prospective Observational	NA	58% in 2006, 16% in 2002 to	60% v 24%	NA	37.2% RRR in hip fractures	NA
	Edwards et al. 2005	Before & After	NA	100%	hip 28% v 70% @ 6 months v 25% @12 months	NA	NA	NA
	Majumdar et al. 2011	RCT	Appro Rx 57%('A') v 28%('C')	81% v 52%	43% v 12%	NA	NA	NA
Canada	Majumdar et al. 2007; Morrish et al 2009	RCT	67%('A') vs 45%('B') vs 26%('D')	80% vs 68% vs 29% (@6 months)	51% v 38% v 22% at 6 months	NA	No difference @12months	Y
	Sander et al. 2008	Cost analysis of Bogoch						Y
	Bogoch et al. 2006	Cross Sectional	97%(inlcuding referral)	NA	NA	NA	NA	NA
	Clunie et al. 2008	Cross Sectional	NA	91.2% (50-69yo)	NA	NA	NA	NA
EU	Boudou et al. 2011	Cross Sectional	NA	NA	90.3% initiated	80% on Rx after one yr, after 27.4 months, 68% persistent w Rx	11.40%	NA

Table 2. 'Type A' Model of Care Fracture Liaison Services – Summary of Outcomes; Key: The first % figure in each cell represents the intervention group result and the second % figure represents the control group. 'v' =versus. F=female, M=male, BMD/Rx=BMD testing and/or treatment rates; RRR= relative risk reduction, BMD=BMD testing rates; Rx=treatment rates; See Appendix A for further details.

'Type A' model of care fracture liaison services – Summary of outcomes

The twelve studies evaluating a 'type A' model of care reviewed here varied greatly in regards to study design, ranging from randomised controlled trials to simple cross-sectional analyses. All except one study [Boudou et al., 2011] evaluated male and female patients, with information on racial background being reported in 3 out of 11 studies [Majumdar et al., 2007 & 2011; Navarro et al., 2011]. The number of patients ranged from 46 to 620,000, but most studies included between 200 to 400 subjects. Most studies included all fracture types. So far, only two FLS were analysed in regards to their cost-effectiveness but in both cases cost-effectiveness of the service was clearly established.

In terms of outcomes, all 'type A' FLS resulted in increased assessment, testing and treatment rates. In the four studies that included valid control groups, the average rate of BMD testing increased from 40.5% in the controls to 80.5% in the intervention groups [Majumdar et al., 2007 & 2011; Morrish et al., 2009 & Lih et al., 2011]. In the same studies, the average rate of anti-osteoporosis treatment initiation rose from 22% in the control groups to 58% in the intervention groups. Re-fracture rates were reported in only four studies. Lih and colleagues (2011) reported a significant improvement in re-fracture rate from 19.7% in the control group to 4.1% in the intervention group. Dell and colleagues (2008) reported a relative risk reduction of 37.2% for hip fractures, using historical data for comparison. Boudou and colleagues (2011) reported an 11.4% re-fracture rate after a mean follow-up period of 27.4 months, while the study by Morrish et al. (2009) was underpowered to demonstrate any significant changes in re-fracture rates after one year of follow-up.

A 'type A' intervention represents the most intensive and costly model of care, where patients are identified, assessed and treated for their osteoporosis after minimal trauma fracture. Central to the success of this model is the Fracture Liaison Co-ordinator (FLC), who orchestrates the identification, assessment and treatment of eligible patients. Thus, the barriers of patient education, primary care physician inertia and lack of a single care provider are addressed in one all-encompassing service. As expected, most 'type A' fracture liaison services differ by region due to the fact that they are embedded within different health care systems. This difference is primarily apparent if one compares the United States with Australia. While successful FLS have been developed in Australia, all of the services are based upon individual initiatives with no systemic support by the Area Health Service. As a result, patient numbers are relatively small. In contrast, the US system exemplified by the Kaiser Permanente group has the advantage of integrated, electronic health care delivery network, enabling the FLS to serve larger numbers of patients. In addition, there is a process of continual feedback to stimulate improvements in care over time. Non-electronic based intervention models have the disadvantage of being more labour-intensive. Overall, the critical component of these services is streamlining the transition from acute fracture care to osteoporosis care, targeted at reducing the risk of future fractures.

As a general observation, most 'type A' fracture liaison services identified patients from a number of sources, including emergency departments, outpatients clinics and inpatient wards. The setting in which assessment, treatment and follow-up occurs is generally on an outpatient basis, which requires patients to be ambulatory and not institutionalised. This is reflected by a comparatively "young" mean age of 68 years in 'type A' studies, as well as a predilection for the recruitment of patients with non-hip fractures. Thus the care of patients with minimal trauma fractures can be conceptualised as having two arms – one arm for the frail elderly who constitute most patients with hip fractures, and the other arm for the younger, more ambulatory patients who tend to have non-hip fractures. Although it is important to treat the frail elderly patient for osteoporosis after a minimal trauma fracture, these patients are streamlined to the realm of the geriatricians who need to prioritise osteoporosis treatment in the context of multiple competing co-morbidities. On the other hand, the 'type A' fracture liaison service is ideally suited to younger patients with minimal trauma fractures because it is easier for them to attend outpatient clinics. In addition, identifying osteoporosis and treating osteoporosis early will reduce the risk of future fractures for those with a likely life expectancy beyond twenty years. Thus, the short term expenditure of a health care system on a 'type A' FLS, will have substantial health and economic benefits for the population as a whole, in any country or region of the world.

2.4 'Type B' models of care

'Type B' models of intervention are slightly less intensive compared to 'type A' models of care in that treatment initiation is the responsibility of the primary care physician. That is, 'type B' interventions identify and assess patients with a minimal trauma fracture, then make treatment recommendations to the primary care physician. There have been eleven studies describing a 'type B' intervention, including New Zealand (one study – Sidwell et al., 2004) and Canada (one study – Morrish et al., 2009), the United States (two studies – Cuddihy et al., 2004 & Johnson et al., 2005), the United Kingdom (four studies – Charalambous et al., 2002; McLellan et al., 2003; Langridge et al., 2007 & McLellan et al., 2011) and the Netherlands (three studies – Chevalley et al., 2002; Astrand et al., 2006 & Huntjens et al., 2010). Table 3 illustrates the summary of outcomes for 'Type B' model of care. For a more analytical evaluation of the cited studies see Appendix B.

'Type B' model of care fracture liaison services – Summary of outcomes

We have identified eleven publications describing a 'Type B' intervention. One of these was a review of five different fracture liaison services in the Netherlands. Thus there are a total of 15 'Type B' models of care described from New Zealand (n= 1), the United States (n =2), Canada (n = 1), and Europe (n= 11). Study types varied between randomised controlled / case control studies (n= 1 each), 'before and after' studies (n= 4) and cross-sectional analyses (n= 9). The average proportion of females was 72%, with one study recruiting only female patients, and another including 96% males. Racial background was reported in only one study, at 86% white Caucasian. The number of subjects varied from 96 to 11,096 with a median number of subjects per study of 934. The mean age across all studies was 68 years and the wrist was the most frequent site of fracture. This is in keeping with the fact that most patients were identified in an outpatient setting, and patients with dementia, or frail patients were excluded. All services apart from two [Sidwell et al., 2004 & Charalambous et al., 2002] utilized a fracture liaison co-ordinator.

In terms of outcomes, the overall rate of BMD testing and/or treatment reported in two studies was about 76% [Charalambous et al., 2002 & McLellan et al., 2003]. In four studies with control group outcomes, the average rate of bone mineral density testing in controls was 12.5%, and 57.5% in the intervention groups [McLellan et al., 2003; Cuddihy et al., 2004; Sidwell et al., 2004 & Johnson et al., 2005]. In three cross-sectional studies, the average rate of

Country	Study	Study Type	BMD/Rx	BMD	Rx	Rx Adherence	Refractures	Cost Effectiveness
New Zealand	Sidwell et al 2004	Before & After	NA	78% vs 11%	34% vs 10% (@9 months)	NA	NA	NA
United States	Cuddihy et al 2004	Before & After	NA	45% vs 16%	NA	36% v 9% (@6 months)	NA	NA
	Johnson et al 2005	Before & After	NA	63% vs 13%	Recommended (if OP on BMD): 19 v 7%	6-7mnth: 13% v 6% (@ 6months)	NA	NA
Canada	Morrish et al 2009	RCT			(see Majumdar et al 2007, Table 2)			
	Langridge et al 2007	Case control	NA	NA	37% (of 129)	NA	see McLellan et al 2011	see McLellan et al 2011
	Charalambous et al 2002	Before & After	79% v 11%	NA	NA	NA	NA	NA
EU (UK)	McLellan et al 2003	Cross Sectional	73.50%	44% (vs 10% historical control)	27% Rx wout BMD; 20% no Rx needed; no other outcomes	NA	NA	NA
	McLellan et al 2011	Cross sectional	NA	49%	54% (11% on Rx previously)	12mnth 86%	12% (4yr f/u)	see text of chapter
	Chevalley et al 2002	Cross Sectional	NA	63%	63%	6months: 67% of initiated	NA	NA
	Astrand et al 2006	Cross Sectional	NA	93%	NA	NA	NA	NA
EU	Huntjens et al 2010	Cross Sectional	NA	Y	NA	NA	NA	NA
	Huntjens et al 2010	Cross Sectional	NA	Y	NA	NA	NA	NA
	Huntjens et al 2010	Cross Sectional	NA	Y	NA	NA	NA	NA
	Huntjens et al 2010	Cross Sectional	NA	Y	NA	NA	NA	NA
	Huntjens et al 2010	Cross Sectional	NA	Y	NA	NA	NA	NA

Table 3. 'Type B' Model of Care Fracture Liaison Services – Summary of Outcomes.
Key: The first % figure in each cell represents the intervention group result and the second % figure represents the control group. 'v' =versus. BMD/Rx=BMD testing and/or treatment rates; BMD=BMD testing rates; Rx=treatment rates; See Appendix B for further details.

BMD testing was 68% [Chevalley et al., 2002; Astrand et al., 2006 & McLellan et al., 2011]. In three studies with control group outcomes for treatment rates, the average rate of initiation of anti-osteoporosis medications in controls was 9%, compared to 35% in the intervention groups [Sidwell et al., 2004; Johnson et al., 2005 & McLellan et al., 2011]. Cuddihy et al., 2004 and Johnson et al., 2005 reported adherence rates at six months, of 7.5% in the control group versus 24.5% in the intervention group. The Glasgow Fracture Liaison Service, reported re-fractures rates of 5.1% at 3.5 years follow-up, and 12% at 8 years follow-up [McLellan et al., 2011]. In the same study, the Glasgow service was been shown to be cost-effective.

Taken together, 'Type B' interventions appear to be nearly as effective as a 'Type A' interventions if implemented in the right setting. On the other hand, as shown by Majumdar and Morrish in a randomised controlled trial, there is an incremental benefit in BMD testing and treatment rates with 'Type A' versus 'Type B' models of care. Another interesting point is the high number of patients identified with this form of intervention – that is, a high turnover rate, which does not necessarily translate to anti-fracture benefits in the long term. This is illustrated by comparing the re-fracture rate of 4.1% (over 4 years) in the 'Type A' Concord Hospital service, with the re-fracture rate of 12% over 4 years in the 'Type B' Glasgow service. While both services differ in some aspects they are similar enough to allow a comparison of fracture outcomes. Therefore, the lower re-fracture rate in 'Type A' services may be related to greater attention given to patient follow-up and compliance within the service itself, rather than relying on external follow-up by the PCP. 'Type B' services seem to be most effective if there is a good rapport and communication between the primary care physician and the fracture liaison service.

2.5 'Type C' models of care

'Type C' models of care are characterised by a less intensive intervention, compared to 'A' and 'B' designs. Once patients are identified after their minimal trauma fracture they receive education regarding osteoporosis in general, risk factors for osteoporosis, lifestyle advice (including falls prevention) and the need for further assessment and treatment. The second component of this model of care involves engaging and alerting the primary care physician regarding the minimal trauma fracture, and the need for further assessment and treatment to reduce the risk of further fractures. Communication with patient or primary care physician is performed either 'face-to-face', via personalised letter, or a telephone call. No further assessment is performed with respect to bone mineral density testing or specific treatment for osteoporosis by the FLS.

Table 4 summarises the outcomes from a total of twelve studies describing a 'type C' model of care: one from Australia, six from the United States, and five from Canada. For a more analytical evaluation of the cited studies see Appendix C.

'Type C' Model of care fracture liaison services – Summary of outcomes

There are twelve published studies describing 'type C' interventions, including four randomised controlled trials [Gardner et al., 2005; Feldstein et al., 2006; Solomon et al., 2007; Majumdar et al., 2008], four 'before and after' analyses [Inderjeeth et al., 2010; Harrington et al., 2005 (two studies); Hawker et al., 2003], two prospective controlled trials [Ashe et al., 2004; Majumdar et al., 2004], one cross sectional study [Skedros, 2004], and one cluster randomised trial [Cranney et al., 2008]. Patients were identified from wards, outpatient

departments and the emergency departments by a fracture liaison nurse in all but four studies, in which existing staff were utilized, such as orthopaedic surgeons [Cranney et al., 2008; Hawker et al., 2003; Skedros, 2004; Inderjeeth et al., 2010]. To determine outcomes, most patients were followed-up at six months after the intervention, apart from two studies which involved 10 and 18 month follow-up periods [Solomon et al., 2007 & Harrington et al., 2005 respectively]. The average rate of BMD testing and/or treatment for osteoporosis was reported in seven studies [Gardner et al., 2005; Feldstein et al., 2006; Harrington et al., 2005; Solomon et al., 2007; Majumdar et al., 2004 & 2008], with a rate in the control group of 11.7 %(range 5%-21%), compared to 39.2% (range 14%-71%) in the intervention group. This translated to a 27.5% improvement with the intervention. Derived from six studies [Inderjeeth et al., 2010; Majumdar et al., 2004 & 2008; Ashe et al., 2004; Hawker et al., 2003; Cranney et al., 2008], the average rate of BMD testing was 18% (range 3%-28%) in the control group and 59% (range 43%-92%) in the intervention group. This represents a risk difference of 41% with the intervention. Amongst the five studies reporting on anti-osteoporosis treatment [Inderjeeth et al., 2010; Feldstein et al., 2006; Majumdar et al., 2004 & 2008; Hawker et al., 2003], the average rate was 7.6% (range 5%-10%) in the control group, and 24.4% (range 11%-40%) in the intervention group. This translates to a 16.8% absolute improvement with intervention 'type C'.

The provision of information to patients and physicians was the key component of all 'type C' services. Despite this, there was still significant variability in the results with different studies. For instance the study by Solomon et al. (2007) only improved BMD testing and/or treatment by 4% (baseline of 10%). There may be a number of factors contributing to this poor result, such as the non-patient specific nature of the educational intervention for the primary care physicians in this study, whereby a list of patients was provided during a visit to the primary care physician by a pharmacist, who then provided general information about osteoporosis to the physician. Secondly, patient education took the form of an automated phone call to the patient, which is probably not as effective as personal "one-on-one" contact over the phone or face-to-face. Thirdly, there may have been resistance from physicians to the intervention, as pharmacists may not have as much impact on practice as a "respected opinion leader". This is in contrast to other studies which provided information to primary care physicians with the endorsement of a "respected opinion leader".

2.6 'Type D' models of care

'Type D' interventions represent a model of care in which patients receive specific osteo-porosis education following a minimal trauma fracture. Patient education can take the form of a patient-specific letter, educational pamphlet, video, or personal communication to the patient via a telephone or 'face-to-face' interaction. Table 5 summarises the major outcomes reported in the three publications describing a 'Type D' model of care. For a more analytical evaluation of the cited studies see Appendix D.

'Type D' model of care fracture liaison services – Summary of outcomes

As illustrated in Table 5, patient education alone has little or no impact on rates of treatment initiation, despite an increase in the rate of BMD testing. Thus, it is unlikely that this form of intervention has any impact, unless combined with other components such assessment and treatment for osteoporosis.

Country	Study	Study Type	BMD/Rx	BMD	Rx	Rx Adherence	Refractures	Cost Effectiveness
Australia	Inderjeeth et al. 2010	Before & After	NA	51% vs 3%	29% vs 6% (@10 to 13 mnth f/u)	NA	NA	NA
	Gardner et al. 2005	RCT	42% vs 19% (@6 months)	NA	NA	NA	NA	NA
	Feldstein et al. 2006	RCT	51.5% vs 43.1% v 5.9% (@6 months)	NA	6mnth: 27.7% vs 20.2% v 5.0% (@6 months)	NA	NA	NA
United States	Harrington et al. 2005	Before & After	20% vs 5% (@6 months)	NA	NA	NA	NA	NA
	Harrington et al. 2005	Before & After	46% vs <10% (up to 18months)	58% @18months	NA	NA	NA	NA
	Skedros, 2004	Cross sectional	NA	NA	30% (@3months)	NA	NA	NA
	Solomon et al. 2007	RCT	14% vs 10% (@10 months)	NA	NA	NA	No difference	NA
	Majumdar et al. 2004	Prospective Controlled	71% v 21% (@6 months)	62% v 17% 6months	40% vs 10% (@6months)	NA	NA	NA
	Ashe et al. 2004	Prospective Controlled	NA	92% v 23%	NA	NA	NA	NA
Canada	Hawker et al. 2003	Before & After		Ordered 43% v 18%	11% vs 10%	NA	NA	NA
	Majumdar et al. 2008	RCT	38% vs 11%	52% vs 18%	22% vs 7%	NA	NA	NA
	Cranney et al. 2008	Cluster Randomized	NA	53% vs 28%	NA	NA	NA	NA

Table 4. 'Type C' Model of Care Fracture Liaison Services – Summary of Outcomes.
Key: The first % figure in each cell represents the intervention group result and the second % figure represents the control group. 'v' =versus. BMD/Rx=BMD testing and/or treatment rates; BMD=BMD testing rates; Rx=treatment rates; Y = Yes. See Appendix C for further details.

Country	Study	Study Type	BMD/Rx	BMD	Rx	Rx Adherence	Refractures	Cost Effectiveness
Australia	Bliuc et al. 2006	RCT	38% vs 11%	38% vs 6%	6% vs 5%	NA	NA	NA
	Diamond T, Lindenberg M. 2002	Cross Sectional	NA	51%	29%	NA	NA	NA
Canada	Bessette et al., 2011	RCT	NA	15%(D) vs 12%(control)	14% vs 8%	NA	NA	NA

Table 5. 'Type D' Model of Care Fracture Liaison Services – Summary of Outcomes; *Key: The first % figure in each cell represents the intervention group result and the second % figure represents the control group. 'v' =versus. BMD/Rx=BMD testing and/or treatment rates; BMD=BMD testing rates; Rx=treatment rates; see Appendix D for further details.*

2.7 'Type E' models of care

'Type E' interventions are limited to inpatient specialist consultations. This intervention does not include any outpatient component and is the most heterogenous model as inpatient consultations vary significantly in the degree of intervention at each site. Table 6 illustrates the summary of outcomes for 'Type E' model of care. For a more analytical evaluation of the cited studies see Appendix E.

Country	Study	Study Type	BMD/Rx	BMD	Rx	Rx Adherence	Refractures	Cost Effectiveness
Australia	Chong et al. 2008	Cross Sectional	NA	NA	NA	NA	NA	NA
	Jones et al. 2005	Before & After	NA	NA	24% vs 5%	NA	NA	NA
	Streeten et al. 2006	Cross Sectional	NA	66%	68% vs 3%	NA	NA	NA
United States	Jachna et al. 2003	Cross Sectional	NA	NA	No significant impact	NA	NA	NA
	Kamel et al. 2000	Cross Sectional	NA	3%	<10% (93% medical consultant)	NA	NA	NA
EU - UK	Wallace et al. 2011	Cross Sectional	NA	NA	90.5% vs 60.5%	NA	NA	NA

Table 6. 'Type E' Model of Care Fracture Liaison Services – Summary of Outcomes.
Key: The first % figure in each cell represents the intervention group result and the second % figure represents the control group. 'v' =versus.BMD/Rx=BMD testing and/or treatment rates; BMD=BMD testing rates; Rx=treatment rates. See Appendix E for further details.

'Type E' model of care fracture liaison services - Summary of outcomes

Taken together, inpatient protocols together with ortho-geriatric and fracture liaison services improved treatment outcomes. However, inpatient physician consultation alone appeared to be ineffective. This is likely due to the fact that a specific osteoporosis consultation was not asked for in these studies. Summary statistics were not performed due to marked variability in the reporting of outcomes, making interpretation relative to other models of care less reliable. It is important to bear in mind that most of the studies published on fracture liaison services excluded frail, demented patients, often living in assisted accommodation. A separate assessment pathway is required, as their needs are very different from those who are still living at home. Perhaps a greater focus needs to be placed on falls prevention strategies in this sub-group.

3. Conclusions

In this chapter, an attempt has been made to collate, compare and discuss the methodology and outcomes of different types of fracture liaison services around the world. Comparisons between models, and even within the same intervention model are generally difficult due to a lack of standardised outcome measures. Nevertheless, Table 7 represents a summary of relevant outcome data (rates of BMD testing, rates of treatment initiation), categorised according to the model of care. Figure 4 illustrates the same outcome measures without correction against controls, which are often not valid (e.g. historical controls), or not reported. It is clear from this summary that the effectiveness of a fracture liaison service is related to the intensity of the intervention. Thus, 'type A' models of care are more effective than 'type B' models of care, and 'type B' models of care produce better outcomes than 'type C', or 'D' models of care. This relationship is also evident from a number of randomised controlled trials [Gardner et al., 2005; Bliuc et al., 2006; Feldstein et al., 2006; Majumdar et al., 2007 & 2008; Solomon et al., 2007; Morrish et al., 2009]. Clearly, the specific health care system in which a FLS is embedded is of pivotal importance. For example, a 'type B' model of care has been shown to be extremely effective in the UK due to the strong structural integration between primary care physicians and public hospitals. As would be expected, educational interventions alone (type C and D interventions) were less effective than types A and B interventions. An educational intervention system still had some limited benefits, and may be an option in resource poor areas.

Intervention Type	BMD (%)	Rx (%)
A	85 (58-100)	57 (45-90)
B	62 (44-93)	42 (27-63)
C	59 (43-92)	27 (11-40)
D	35 (15-51)	16 (6-29)

Table 7. Outcome measures according to intervention model of care, including the ranges of outcome rates (%) across studies.

A further factor which is likely to have a significant impact on the effectiveness of any intervention is the length of time between the fracture and the intervention. For example, treatment rates at six months with the same 'type C' intervention was 22% if the intervention occurred immediately after the fracture [Majumdar et al., 2008], compared to 11% if the same intervention occurred one year after the fracture [Majumdar et al, 2011]. Perhaps the short period of pain associated with the fracture provides a 'window of opportunity' to instigate behavioural change in the patient.

A major deficit in the published literature on models of post-fracture care is the inconsistent reporting of results. This covers a spectrum of outcomes such as the identification rate of potentially eligible patients, the length of time between fracture and FLS evaluation, the extent of risk factor evaluation, the assessment for secondary causes for osteoporosis, the rate of BMD testing, the rate of treatment, adherence to anti-osteoporosis therapy, the definition of the term "appropriate care", re-fracture rates, and formal cost-effectiveness evaluations. All of these measures would be important for quality assurance and to benchmark performance. Thus, guidelines on reporting outcomes may be of benefit in the future.

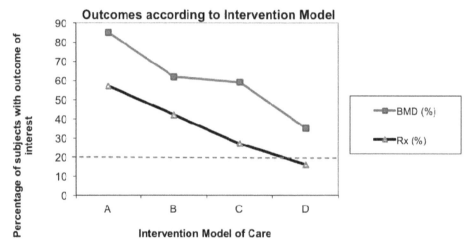

Fig. 4. Relationship between intervention intensity and outcomes. The dotted line represents the proportion of patients on treatment without any intervention.
Key: Rx = anti-osteoporosis treatment; BMD = bone mineral density testing.

Not only is their heterogeneity in outcomes, but also the very definition of a minimal trauma. Although the vast majority of studies define it as a fall from standing height or less, one study defined minimal trauma as the impact from a fall less than one metre in height [Bessette et al. 2011[. It is questionable if a fall from two or three steps, or inversion of the ankle should be defined as minimal trauma.

The vast majority of studies (91%) included both males and females, with the mean proportion of females in each study of 72%. Four studies (9%) included females only. Many studies confirm the well-known gender disparity in the evaluation and treatment of osteoporosis [Bogoch et al., 2006; Cuddihy et al., 2004; Dell et al 2008; Diamond and Lindenberg 2002; Kuo et al., 2007; Navarro et al., 2011].

The under-recognition of osteoporosis in men is illustrated by Cuddihy and colleagues, who noted amongst those who had a prior fracture, none of the men had a diagnosis of osteoporosis, whereas 79% of women did. Similarly, Bogoch and co-workers noticed that baseline osteoporosis treatment rates were lower in men (15.5%) than in women (39%). Kuo and colleagues also found the baseline osteoporosis management rates were lower in men (9%) compared with women (34%).

Furthermore, after institution of the Healthy Bones Program, the Kaiser Permanente group reported a significant gender disparity, with a higher treatment rate amongst women (92.1%) compared to men (75.2%) [Navarro et al. 2011]. In the same study, amongst those who sustained a further hip fracture, 73.5% of women and 30.7% of men were on osteoporosis treatment at the time of the fracture. With the institution of the Healthy Bones Program, Dell et al. (2008) reported an increase in the proportion of all BMD scans performed for men from 7.2% in 2002, to 14.5% in 2006. The proportion of all osteoporosis therapy dispensed for men went from 8% (2002) to 10% (2006), which is much lower than expected from the gender distribution in the studies (i.e., 25% were men).

The factors contributing to the gender disparity include men being less proactive with their health than women, due to lack of interest or awareness. Physicians may be more complacent with men due to a misperception that osteoporosis only affects women. Bliuc and colleagues (2006) found that men were less likely than women to respond to an information based intervention by going to their PCP for osteoporosis assessment. Amongst those who did see their PCP, men were less likely to have anti-resorptives recommended, indicating a physician-related barrier to treatment. Diamond and Lindenberg also reported lower treatment uptake rates amongst men who sustained a minimal trauma fracture and were found to have an osteoporotic range BMD T-score.

These studies indicate that the gender disparity needs to be addressed on different levels: patient, health care professional, and system level. Awareness of the gender disparity in recognition and treatment of osteoporosis may help clinicians target this group more effectively.

Ethnicity was only reported in five of forty two studies. Despite documented racial disparities in osteoporosis management in the United States [Wei et al., 2003; Epstein et al., 2010], it is reassuring to see an absence of racial disparity in the Kaiser Permanente system of care [Navarro et al. 2011].

Treatment rates may vary between health networks and countries due to different diagnostic and treatment thresholds. For example, in the South Glasgow service, patients with hip fractures were treated without a prior BMD scan, whereas in the West Glasgow service a BMD study was routinely preformed in all patients and pharmacotherapy was initiated if the T-score was less than -2.0 SD. This threshold, however, differs from that of other centres (e.g. Majumdar et al., 2007: T-score of less than -1.5 SD). In the UK studies, only oral bisphosphonates were initiated, mostly due to cost considerations. Those patients who could not tolerate or receive oral bisphosphonates were treated with calcium and vitamin D only, a strategy which would certainly differ between countries.

Treatment rates are still suboptimal, even in 'type A' services. In order to improve capture rates, fracture liaison services will need to utilize integrated electronic health system databases. There is no doubt that there is a paucity of data on re-fracture rates, adherence, and cost-effectiveness of intensive models of care, although initial results are promising. Attempts should be made at collaboration between centres, especially in fragmented health care networks within countries. Unfortunately, there is a paucity of data on FLS in the majority of the world's population. That is, the populations of the US, Canada, Australia, New Zealand and Europe only constitute 17% of the world's population. We need to ensure that treatment disparities between regions, genders, as well as race, are addressed. Therefore, although fracture liaison services have contributed significantly towards closing the care gap in osteoporosis management in patients after a minimal trauma fracture, there is room for significant improvements in post-fracture management of patients with osteoporosis.

4. Acknowledgements

Lyn March and Michele Puech for beginning the process of reviewing fracture liaison services, and for the categorisation of intervention types A through to E.

Kaye Lee for help with the literature search.

Benchao Feng for assisting with the summary tables.

5. Appendices

5.1 Appendix A

5.1.1 'Type A' fracture liaison services in Australia

There have been four publications from Australia describing a 'Type A' intervention [Kuo et al., 2007; Vaile et al., 2007; Giles et al., 2010; Lih et al., 2011]. Individual hospital Fracture Liaison Services have grown over the last decade, out of individuals "championing" the cause of patients after a minimal trauma fracture. Each hospital has tailored their approach according to their resources and experience.

Australian residents fall under the umbrella of Medicare, a comprehensive health care system whereby free public hospital care is provided. Medicare Australia also funds the Pharmaceutical Benefits Scheme (PBS), whereby a comprehensive list of pharmaceuticals are subsidized. This system provides an ideal environment for fracture liaison services because medical practitioner consultation, osteodensitometry, and pathology testing are performed at no expense to the patient. A comprehensive list of specific anti-osteoporosis therapy is subsidized by the PBS, thus allowing patients to commence (and continue) treatment at minimal expense. Notably, calcium and vitamin D supplementation is not subsidized under this scheme.

Despite universal health care coverage in Australia, there is limited integration of health care information and collaboration between hospitals, probably due to historical precedent in funding structure of individual hospitals. Therefore various FLS have developed independently in individual hospitals, leading to smaller numbers of patients in each study (hundreds), in contrast to the Kaiser Permanente group in the US (thousands of patients) which is characterized by an integrated electronic medical record system spanning wide geographic areas.

The New South Wales (NSW) government is currently attempting to integrate and standardize post-fracture care in NSW, through the Agency for Clinical Innovation (ACI).

The ACI is focused on an agenda to develop FLS in all hospitals across NSW to address the care gap in osteoporosis. Ideally, this system would allow integration of all data in a central database to help benchmark performance.

Study types and patient characteristics

There have been two 'before and after' type studies [Kuo et al., 2007; Vaille et al., 2007], one cross-sectional study [Giles et al., 2010], and one prospective controlled study [Lih et al., 2011]. All studies were from Eastern New South Wales. Three studies had control groups: in in the study by Lih and colleagues (2011), the control group was concurrent. That is, the control group was derived from eligible patients who presented to hospital with a minimal trauma fracture but for various reasons were not seen by the FLS. The other two studies reported historical control groups, which therefore provide less robust outcome data [Kuo et al., 2007; Vaile et al., 2007].

All studies recruited male and female patients, with the proportion of females varying from 71% to 79%. Race or ethnicity was not described in any of the four studies but given the demographics of Eastern New South Wales, it is likely that the majority of patients were of Caucasian ethnicity. The numbers of patients identified by each FLS ranged from 155 to 2049. All four studies included patients who sustained symptomatic fractures at any site although three studies excluded skull fractures [Kuo et al., 2007; Giles e al., 2010; Lih et al., 2011], and Kuo et al. (2007) excluded fractures of fingers and toes, whilst Lih and colleagues excluded vertebral fractures. In the three studies reporting on fracture sites, the proportion of patients with wrist fractures varied from 22-45%. The lower age limit was 50 years in two studies [Vaile et al., 2007; Giles et al., 2010], 45 years [Lih et al, 2011], and 20 years [Kuo et al, 2007]. The mean age of patients varied from 60 years to 75 years. The reason for the older demographic in the study by Giles and colleagues (2010) was the inclusion of patients residing in nursing homes, who were excluded from the other studies.

Patient identification methods and capture rates

The fracture liaison co-coordinator played a pivotal role in identifying eligible patients in all studies. This was performed in close collaboration with the staff of orthopaedic and emergency departments, including secretaries, nurses, allied health, and doctors. In the study by Giles and co-workers (2010), the successful utilization of an electronically derived patient list of relevant emergency department presentations, together with electronic prompts for referral on discharge letters, lead to the identification of all potentially eligible patients. Kuo and colleagues, recruited orthopaedic outpatients only. The other three studies recruited patients from varying combinations of orthopaedic ward, orthopaedic clinic, and the emergency department.

The 'capture rate', refers to the proportion of eligible patients who underwent some form of intervention. Remarkably, Giles and co-workers (2010) reported 100% capture, because everyone with a minimal trauma fracture was identified and given some form of intervention, such as letter to the patient and PCP indicating the importance of osteoporosis assessment, which is a model C intervention (see below). In the same study, about 38% of patients underwent a 'type A' intervention by attending the osteoporosis clinic. Lih and colleagues (2011) reported a capture rate of 41%, while in the remaining two studies no information of capture rates was provided. Although not specifically addressed in the studies, streamlining the process of referral to the FLS from the orthopaedic surgeon or primary care physician is paramount if a service is to improve capture and assessment rates.

Interventions

There are minor variations in the reporting of the intervention applied. In all studies, the FLS was an outpatient clinic run by a fracture liaison co-ordinator. The intervention included the following components: (i) Patient education, (ii) Assessment and investigation; and (iii) treatment initiation. Education components included aspects of nutrition and diet, exercise, risk factor reduction and falls prevention. A full risk factor assessment occurred in two of the four studies [Kuo et al, 2007; Lih et al, 2011]. Patients were assessed by bone mineral density and pathology testing in all studies, while routine thoraco-lumbar spine X-rays were part of the evaluation in all but one study [Kuo et al., 2007]. Follow-up occurred annually in two studies [Vaile et al., 2007; Lih et al., 2011] but was not described in the remaining two reports.

Outcomes

a. Risk factor analysis and pathology testing for secondary causes

Osteoporosis risk factor analysis was specifically described in two studies [Kuo et al., 2007; Lih et al., 2011]. For instance, Lih and co-workers reported 6.5% of patients had a prior non-vertebral fracture, whilst Kuo and co-workers reported that half of patients had sustained prior fractures. Pathology testing for secondary causes of osteoporosis was reported in three studies [Kuo et al, 2007; Vaile et al., 2007; Lih et al, 2011]. Vaile and colleagues reported a positive coeliac screen in 0.2% of patients. Kuo and co-workers (2007) found new diagnoses of hyperthyroidism in 2.1% of patients, primary hyperparathyroidism in 1.4%, and hypovitaminosis D in 41% (i.e. 25-OH-vitamin D level < 50 nmol/L).

b. BMD testing

The rate of BMD testing in those attending the service ranged from 83% to 100%, although Giles and co-workers (2010) have not included this data in their report. The reported rates for BMD assessment contrast with a 10% uptake rate of BMD testing in an information-based intervention ('type D') as per Kuo et al. 2007.

c. Pharmacological treatment

Lih and colleagues (2011) reported treatment rates of 79% in the intervention group compared to 31% in the control group. Vaile and colleagues (2007) revealed treatment rates were 51% in the intervention group compared to 11% in a historical control group. In this study, self-reported adherence at twelve months was 95%. In the study by Kuo and co-workers (2007), 80% of patients were adherent to treatment at a mean follow-up of 10 months with female gender and a diagnosis of osteoporosis being predictors of adherence.

d. Re-fracture rates

The only study describing re-fracture rates was by Lih and colleagues (2011). At four years of follow-up, a highly significant difference in re-fracture rates was reported: 4.1% in the group attending the fracture liaison service compared to 19.7% in the control group (Fig. 5). This difference corresponds to an 80% reduction in re-fracture rates in patients managed by a FLS.

e. Cost-effectiveness

An informal evaluation of cost-effectiveness of a 'type A' intervention was described by Vaile et al. (2007), estimating that if one hip fracture is prevented, savings of AUD23,000 could pay for the salary of a fracture liaison co-coordinator for six months, or for the osteoporosis evaluation of 54 patients with minimal trauma fractures.

A formal and more comprehensive cost-effectiveness analysis of the Concord Hospital Fracture Liaison service by Cooper et al. (2011) revealed that the service was highly cost effective with a cost of around AUD 20,000 – 30,000 per QALY gained, depending on the model examined. As the Concord Hospital FLS is a typical 'type A' model, it can be safely assumed that most, if not all, comprehensive FLS are cost-effective interventions.

f. Other outcome measures

A further outcome measure reported Giles and colleagues (2010) was an improvement in referral of eligible patients by orthopaedic surgeons, physicians and general practitioners, to the osteoporosis clinic. Referral rates improved from 9% prior to the fracture liaison service, to 34% after commencement of the fracture liaison service. Furthermore, the period of time from fracture occurrence to attendance at the osteoporosis clinic decreased from 68 days to 44 days.

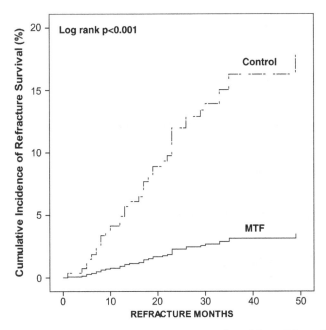

Fig. 5. Cumulative re-fracture incidence by groups (reproduced from Lih et al., 2011 with permission)

5.1.2 'Type A' fracture liaison services in the United States

In the United States, orthopaedic surgeons have been the "champions" at the forefront of co-ordinating osteoporosis care of patients after a minimal trauma fracture. In contrast to

Australia, some of the studies emanate from large, integrated health care networks, rather than individual hospitals. A good example is the Kaiser Permanente Group. This group is a health maintenance organization with 3.1 million members, spanning across eleven medical centres. The "Healthy Bones Program" consists of steps to identify patients at high risk of fractures, then assess and treat them for osteoporosis. The success of this program seems to be related to the utilization of a fully integrated electronic health record. The intervention consisted of a falls reduction program, assessment with DXA, evaluation for secondary causes, as well as a treatment plan. Monitoring occurred on a monthly basis, via reports for "care managers" (FLC) detailing those who needed treatment, and those who received treatment, thereby providing targets, and stimulating further improvements in care.

Study types and patient characteristics

Of the three studies from the United States, there was one 'before and after' analysis [Edwards et al., 2005], one prospective observational study [Dell et al., 2008], and one cross sectional study [Navarro et al., 2011]. All studies included males and females, with Edwards and co-workers (2011) reporting that 75% of subjects were female. Racial background was reported by Navarro et al. (2005) with White subjects representing 64% of the sample. The numbers of subjects varied significantly in each study. Edwards and co-workers (2005) included 203 subjects while in the remaining two studies from the Kaiser Permanente group, Navarro and co-workers included 13,412 subjects seen over a period of one year, and Dell and co-workers studied 620,000 subjects from 2002 to 2006. These large numbers were made possible by an electronically integrated health care system. In the latter two studies, inclusion criteria expanded beyond the patients with minimal trauma fractures to patients who had any risk factor for osteoporosis, including, for example, corticosteroid use or rheumatoid arthritis. All studies included patients with minimal trauma fractures at any site.

Patient identification methods and capture rates

All three studies utilized a fracture liaison co-coordinator. The Kaiser-Permanente model utilized health managers to identify care gaps through electronic lists, thereby identifying all patients in all settings (i.e. inpatients, outpatients, and emergency departments).

Interventions

All studies described a 'type A' FLS, which incorporated patient education, assessment and treatment initiation. All studies assessed and treated subjects on an outpatient basis.

Outcomes

a. Risk factor analysis and pathology testing for secondary causes

Information on the extent of patient assessment was generally limited, with only Edwards and colleagues (2005) reporting specific risk factor assessments. Specifically, 50% of patients had sustained prior fractures. Edwards and colleagues reported pathology testing for secondary causes of osteoporosis only in those with a BMD T-score less than -1.5 SD.

b. BMD testing

Navarro et al (2011) reported osteodensitometry testing and/or initiation of osteoporosis therapy in females of 92% as opposed to 75% in males, in a large cohort of 13,412 subjects. There was no disparity between racial groups. This is in contrast to the racial disparity in health care outcomes in the United States described by others [Wei et al. 2003, Epstein et al. 2010], indicating the significant societal benefits of an integrated electronic health care network.

The same group from Kaiser Permanente demonstrated that the implementation of their FLS resulted in an increase in bone mineral density testing from 21,557 tests in 2002 to 74,770 tests in 2006 [Dell et al., 2008]. This represented a 600% increase in BMD testing for males, and a 220% increase for females. The rate of increase in men was greater than for women, possibly due to the very low rates of testing in men at baseline in 2002 (fig 6).

c. Pharmacological treatment

In the same study [Dell et al., 2008] the number of patients on treatment with specific anti-osteoporosis medications increased from 33,208 in 2002 to 78,058 in 2006 (or from 24% to 60% of at-risk subjects) as shown in Figure 7. Similar to the data on BMD testing, the rate of increase for men was greater than that for women.

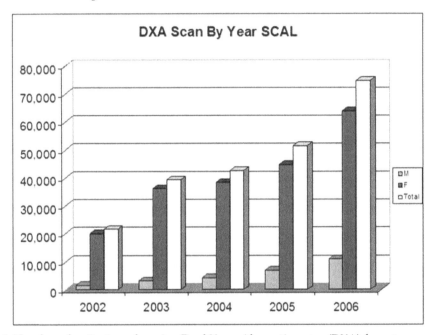

Fig. 6. Number of patients undergoing Dual X-ray Absorptiometry (DXA) for osteoporosis assessment [reproduced from Dell et al., 2008, with permission].

Edwards and co-workers (2005) reported improved treatment rates from 28% at baseline to 70% at six months post-discharge which then declined again to only 25% at twelve months post-discharge. This precipitous decline in adherence at twelve months reflects the need for specific osteoporosis follow-up to reinforce the ongoing need for therapy.

d. Refractures

Dell at el (2008) described the effect of the Healthy Bones Program on hip fracture rates. While there was no concurrent control group, the authors elected to estimate expected rates of hip fracture based on historical data from 1997 – 1999, and then compared these historical data to the actual rate of hip fractures observed in patients cared for by the FLS. Overall, there was a 37.2% relative risk reduction in hip fractures, using data from 2006 (figure 8).

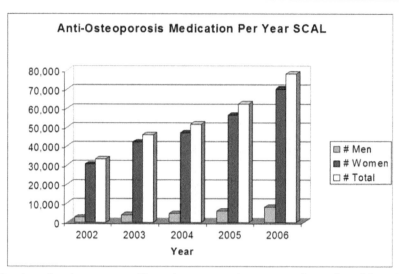

Fig. 7. Number of patients on specific anti-osteoporosis treatment [reproduced from Dell et al.,2008, with permission].

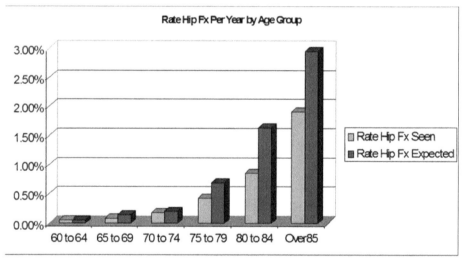

Fig. 8. Age stratified rate of hip fracture seen versus rate of hip fracture expected [reproduced from Dell et al., 2008, with permission].

e. Cost-effectiveness

While there are no formal cost-effectiveness analyses for any of the US studies, one should remember that Kaiser Permanente is a closed health care network which pays for all expenses but also benefits from all savings. The fact that a private provider such as Kaiser Permanente has fully integrated a 'type A' FLS into their health care program strongly suggests that the model is not only cost-effective but actually cost-saving.

5.1.3 'Type A' fracture liaison services in Canada

Study types and patient characteristics

Three 'Type A' FLS have been described in a series of five publications – three randomized controlled trials (RCT) from the same FLS [Majumdar et al., 2007 & Morrish et al., 2009; Majumdar et al., 2011], and one cross-sectional study [Bogoch et al., 2006]. The first two randomized controlled trials compared three different FLS models: firstly a 'type A' versus 'type D' model of care [Majumdar et al., 2007] and secondly a 'type A' versus 'type B' model of care [Morrish et al., 2009] in patients with hip fractures. The third RCT by the same group involved patients with wrist fractures, comparing a 'type A' with 'type C' intervention [Majumdar et al, 2011]. The three services included both males and females, with the proportion of females varying from 65% to 77%. Patient numbers varied significantly in that the randomized controlled trials [Majumdar et al., 2007 & Morrish et al., 2009] had 110 patients in each arm, whilst the trial by Majumdar et al. (2011) had a total of 46 patients. The cross-sectional study evaluated 430 patients. The target population in the RCT's were 50 years of age and over. Between 82% and 95% of patients were white Caucasian. Bogoch and co-workers (2006) included female patients older than 40 years, and male patients over 50 years of age, with a minimal trauma fracture to the hip, wrist, humerus or vertebra.

Patient identification methods and capture rates

All three services utilized a Fracture Liaison Co-coordinator to identify eligible inpatients and outpatients. Bogoch et al. (2006) also engaged the orthopaedic staff in the identification process. There was no indication as to the completeness of identification of eligible patients.

Intervention methods

In all three studies, the FLC coordinated the identification, assessment (clinical risk factors, osteodensitometry, pathology) and treatment of patients with a fragility fracture. In the studies by Majumdar and Morrish it was specified that a letter was sent to the primary care physician once treatment was initiated.

Outcomes

a. Risk factor analysis and pathology testing for secondary causes

Osteoporosis risk factors were evaluated in all studies. A past history of minimal trauma fractures was documented in 37% (Majumdar et al 2007 & Morrish) and 26% (Bogoch). Majumdar and colleagues (2011) was the only trial which stated pathology testing for secondary causes of osteoporosis were performed, although the proportion of positive results was not reported.

b. BMD testing and treatment rates

In the study by Majumdar et al. (2007), 80% of patients in the intervention group underwent BMD testing at six months post-fracture, compared to only 29% in the control group. About 51% of patients in the intervention group were commenced on bisphosphonates at six months, compared to 22% in the control group. A further result reported was "Appropriate Care", which was defined as the proportion of patients commenced on bisphoshponates when the BMD T-score was < -1.5 SD. Appropriate care was achieved in 67% of patients in the intervention group, versus 26% in the control group. The underlying cause of the low rate of appropriate care was not reported.

As an extension of the above trial, patients assigned to the control group ('standard care') were allocated to a new intervention after six months. This new intervention consisted of a BMD scan organised by the FLC ('Type B' intervention) with results being sent to the primary care physician [Morrish et al. 2009]. As a result, the rates of BMD testing, treatment with a bisphosphonate, and "appropriate care" improved compared to usual care ('Type D intervention'), but not to the extent of case management ('Type A' intervention) (fig. 9).

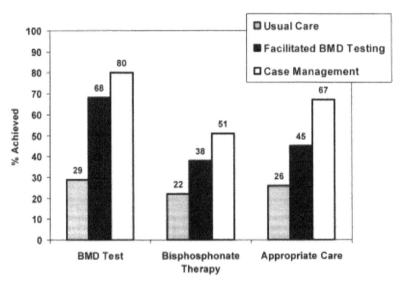

Fig. 9. Comparison of case manager, facilitated BMD testing, and usual care in patients with a hip fracture [reproduced from Morrish et al., with permission].

A further study by Majumdar et al. (2011) which included patients with wrist fractures only, revealed a BMD testing rate of 81% ('type A') versus 52% ('Type C'). The rate of bisphosphonate treatment was better with intensive intervention, at 43% ('type A') versus 12% ('type C').

In the study by Bogoch et al (2006), the proportion of all patients who were previously diagnosed and treated for osteoporosis was 34%, which is higher than expected from the published literature. This study also reported a rate of "appropriate attention" for osteoporosis of 96%, which encompassed referral, diagnosis or treatment of osteoporosis. This unique outcome measure is a good example of the heterogeneity of outcome reporting in various studies, making direct comparison between studies problematic. Reiterating the gender disparity, women (39%) were more likely than men (15%), to have had diagnosis and treatment for osteoporosis prior to their fracture.

c. Re-fractures

Morrish et al. (2009) reported 10 new fractures after a limited follow-up of twelve months. While the authors state that there was no difference in re-fracture rates between groups, they did not specify how many fractures occurred in each arm of the study. Thus, it is likely that the study was underpowered to allow any conclusions on reductions in fracture risk.

d. Cost-effectiveness

Sander and colleagues (2008) performed a cost-effectiveness analysis of the 'type A' model of care described by Bogoch et al. (2006). The FLS was predicted to reduce the annual hip fracture rate from 34 with usual care, to 31, resulting in a cost saving of C$ 49,950. This cost-saving held true assuming at least 350 patients were seen by the FLS over a year. The two limitations of this analysis was firstly, the lack of a control group, resulting in the need to make assumptions in the usual care group based on historical data. Secondly, the cost-saving may not be translated to smaller institutions which have a lower volume of patients seen in the FLS. There was no formal cost-effectiveness evaluation for the RCT by Majumdar et al. (2007) and Morrish et al. (2009), although it was reported that the 'type A' model of care evaluation cost $56 versus $24 for a 'type B' model of care.

5.1.4 'Type A' fracture liaison services in Europe

Study types and patient characteristics

Two cross-sectional studies have described the implementation of a 'Type A' fracture liaison service, one from the United Kingdom [Clunie et al., 2008] and one from France [Boudou et al., 2011]. Clunie and co-workers recruited 2491 male or female patients older than 50 years with a minimal trauma fracture at any site. More than 50% of patients had a hip or wrist fracture. The study by Boudou et al. (2011), evaluated 155 female patients over 50 years of age with wrist, humerus or femur fractures. Racial background was not reported in either study.

Patient identification methods and capture rates

In the study by Clunie et al, (2008), patients were identified in either outpatient or inpatient settings by a FLC. It is unclear as to the proportion of potentially eligible patients who were identified. The study from France also employed a FLC, who utilized an electronic medical record system to identify patients. More that 90% of patients were identified, with only 20% of patients captured for evaluation by the FLS.

Intervention methods

In both studies, patients underwent a complete risk factor assessment, including pathology tests for secondary causes of osteoporosis as well as BMD testing. According to Clunie et al (2008), patients were referred to the Bone clinic when appropriate. Patients more than 75 years of age were assessed for falls risk and referred to the primary care physician. The schema for this service is shown in Figure 10, as another example of a 'Type A' intervention.

Outcomes

a. Risk factor analysis and pathology testing for secondary causes

Patients in both studies underwent risk factor assessment and investigations for secondary causes of osteoporosis. Notably, Clunie et al. (2008) quoted their previous publication relating to the same service, whereby 6% of patients routinely screened for secondary causes of osteoporosis regardless of osteodensitometry results, had a new diagnosis such as hyperthyroidism or primary hyperparathyroidism [Clunie et al., 2005].

b. BMD testing

Clunie and colleagues (2008) reported a high rate (91.2%) of osteodensitometry in those 50-69 years of age, whereas the rate of osteodensitometry was not reported by Boudou and co-workers (2011).

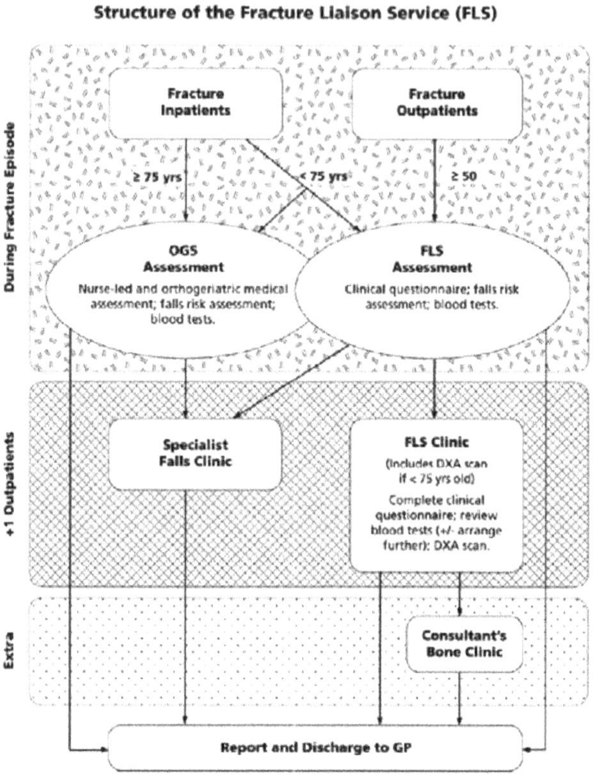

Structure of the Fracture Liaison Service (FLS)

Fig. 10. Structure of 'Type A' fracture liaison service [reproduced from Clunie et al. 2008, with permission].

c. Pharmacological treatment

In the trial by Boudou et al. (2011), approximately 90% of patients initiated treatment prescribed by the FLS, and 80% of these remained on treatment at one year follow-up. After a further follow-up of 27.4 +/- 11.7 months, 68% of patients were persistent with treatment. This trial represents one of the very few studies that report adherence data within the setting of a FLS. Reasons for discontinuation of therapy were adverse events, lack of primary care physician encouragement, and polypharmacy. Clunie and colleagues (2008) did not report treatment rates.

d. Re-fractures

After a mean follow-up period of 27.4 +/-11.7 months, 11.4% had sustained a further fracture [Boudou et al. 2011]. The rate of further fractures was not described by Clunie et al. (2008).

e. Cost-effectiveness

Nil data.

5.2 Appendix B

5.2.1 'Type B' fracture liaison services in Europe

5.2.1.1 United Kingdom

In the United Kingdom, there has been a concerted, collective effort towards re-fracture prevention by attempting to establish fracture liaison services in all hospitals based on the Glasgow FLS model [Mitchell 2011]. The strong advocacy towards re-fracture prevention has been supported and catalysed by patient and professional organisations (e.g. the UK National Osteoporosis Society), the government (through integration into a policy framework and providing financial incentives to health providers who adhere to the guidelines), and pharmaceutical companies (through provision of funding). The publication of the second edition of the 'Blue Book' in 2007 provided comprehensive guidelines to promote high quality care of minimal trauma fracture patients in the UK. Specifically, the 'Blue Book' provides guidelines and standards of care for the peri-operative management of patients with a minimal trauma fracture (particularly hip fractures), as well as guidelines on secondary fracture prevention through fracture liaison services. The third major component of the 'Blue Book' details the importance of contributing to and utilising the National Hip Fracture Database (NHFD) allowing the benchmarking of hip fracture care across the UK, thereby catalysing improvements in clinical care. Critical to the implementation of these guidelines was the multi-disciplinary authorship and the strong endorsement it received from most relevant professional organisations. As a testimony to the success of the program, all 200 hospitals in England, Wales and Northern Ireland have subscribed to the database. In addition, the most recent report from the NHFD in 2010 describes 75% of 36,000 hip fracture patients receiving assessment or treatment for osteoporosis prior to being discharged from hospital.

Study types and patient characteristics

There are four publications describing FLS in the UK, originating from two services. The first two were cross-sectional studies describing the Glasgow FLS, which is the model upon which most FLS in the UK are built [McClellan et al., 2003, 2011]. A case control study of the same service evaluated characteristics of those with re-fractures [Langridge et al., 2007]. The second service based in Royal Manchester Infirmary was described in a 'before and after' analysis [Charalambous et al., 2002]. The Glasgow FLS included 4,671 patients, older than 50 years, who sustained a minimal trauma fracture over an 18 month period. Both male and female patients were included. Approximately 30% of patients sustained wrist fractures, and about 23% had sustained hip fractures. Exclusion criteria included patients with skull or facial fractures, patients with dementia, or those unable to tolerate oral bisphosphonate therapy. The study by Charalambous was limited to only female patients with a minimal trauma fracture to the wrist and hip. The number of patients was also smaller, with 100 pre-intervention and 66 in the intervention phase.

Patient identification methods and capture rates

The Glasgow service utilized a fracture liaison co-coordinator to capture patients from orthopaedic wards, orthopaedic outpatient clinics, as well as the emergency department.

The co-coordinator visited wards regularly, with patient lists maintained by close contact with orthodpaedic staff, and utilizing the hospital information technology systems. Thus, almost 100% of patients were identified; although only 78% attended the service (22% had declined the intervention). Charalambous and colleagues (2002) identified orthopaedic inpatients and outpatients, using a monthly list of patients with new fractures. Instead of a co-coordinator, a protocol was instituted to refer patients for osteoporosis evaluation or direct referral for BMD. No comment was made regarding the proportion of potentially eligible patients identified.

Intervention methods

The Glasgow service provided patient education, together with outpatient assessment, followed by treatment recommendations to the PCP. On the other hand, Charalambous and colleagues did initiate inpatient assessment of those with hip fractures (older than 60 years), with direct referral for BMD, followed by recommendations for further assessment and treatment.

Outcomes

a. Risk factor analysis and pathology screening for secondary causes

Risk factor assessment was performed in both studies while pathology screening for secondary causes of bone loss was described only in the Glasgow service. The results of pathology screening was not reported.

b. BMD testing and treatment

The first set of outcome data for the Glasgow service revealed that 44% of patients underwent BMD testing, compared to 10% in historical controls, and 29% of patients were recommended pharmacotherapy [McLellan et al. 2003]. The most recent outcome data from the Glasgow FLS evaluated the rate of patient capture, assessment, treatment, and cost-effectiveness over 8 years of service provision [McLellan et al. 2011]. A total of 11,096 patients were identified, of whom 8,875 (80%) were assessed. The number of patients who underwent BMD scans was 5,405 (49%). Oral bisphosphonate treatment was recommended in 54%, whilst 1,273 (11%) were on treatment previously. As a testimony to the effectiveness of a close liaison between the FLS and the PCP, the study found that 96% of patients had the recommended treatment initiated in primary care. Treatment persistence was reported as 86% at 12 months.

At Manchester Royal Infirmary the implementation of a protocol was shown to be effective in improving "appropriate osteoporosis management" in female patients [Charalambous et al. 2002]. In this study, "appropriate management" simply entailed initiating a referral to a doctor for evaluation of osteoporosis, or initiation of calcium and vitamin D as per protocol.[1]

Pre-intervention, 22% (11/50) of in-patients with hip fractures and 0% of patients with distal radial fractures received "appropriate management". Post-intervention, the corresponding numbers were 76% and 81%, respectively.

---

[1] This highlights the differences in the definition of 'appropriate care', which appears to be a term of considerable heterogeneity. Thus, a number of studies define 'appropriate care' as a clinical assessment with or without a BMD scan, with or without initiation of treatment. Other definitions refer to receiving osteoporosis treatment in keeping with the local guidelines, based on T-scores.

c. Re-fractures

The South Glasgow service published data from January 2001 to August 2004 with up to 3.5 years follow-up of patients older than 65 years [Langridge et al. 2007]. Of the 2,489 patients seen by the service, 129 had re-fractured (5.2%). About 37% of these patients were taking calcium, vitamin D *and* a bisphosphonate. Unfortunately there was no control group to which these results could have been compared. On the other hand, McLellan et al. (2011) reported a 12% rate of re-fracture over 4 years for the West Glasgow service.

d. Cost-effectiveness

The cost-effectiveness analysis of the Glasgow service was based upon an 8% re-fracture rate at 4 years, although the actual re-fracture rate was reported to be 12% [McLellan et al., 2011]. The cost per Quality Adjusted Life Year (QALY) gained was 5,740 pounds. According to the least favourable efficacy data, fifteen fractures are avoided, at the expense of 84,076 pounds per 1000 patients. According to the most favourable efficacy data, thirty six fractures are avoided and 199,132 pounds saved per 1000 patients. Using a hypothetical cohort of 1000 patients, it was estimated there would be 18 fewer fractures with the fracture liaison service. These results illustrate the effectiveness of a 'type B' intervention in the UK setting.

5.2.1.2 'Type B' fracture liaison services outside the UK

Study types and patient characteristics

There are three cross-sectional studies describing 'type B' models of care in Switzerland [Chevalley et al., 2002], Sweden [Astrand et al., 2006], and the Netherlands [Huntjens et al., 2010]. The study from the Netherlands compared five large FLS within the same health care system. All of these European FLS enrolled both male and female patients 50 years of age or older, who presented with a minimal trauma fractures at any site. The proportion of female patients seen in each service ranged from 70% to 88%, with a mean of 78%. The proportion of patients who sustained wrist fractures varied from 3.6% to 58%, with a mean of 27%. The proportion of patients who sustained hip fractures varied from 1.0% to 45%, with a mean of 13%. The number of patients in each study varied from 238 to 2224. The follow-up period ranged from 12 months to 58 months, with a mean of 43 months. The number of patients seen per centre per month varied from 11 to 47, with a mean of 25. In all studies, dementia and pathological fractures were excluded. In the Swedish study, patients who were out of area and non-English speaking were excluded.

Patient identification methods and capture rates

All seven fracture liaison services (apart from Chevalley and colleagues) utilized a co-coordinator to identify patients from the wards, orthopaedic outpatients, the emergency department or radiology. Two sites from the Netherlands utilized radiology reports alone to identify eligible patients. Three services (two from Netherlands and the Swedish study) incorporated electronic medical record and the co-coordinator to identify patients. The proportion of eligible patients identified, who attended the service was not described.

Intervention methods

In all studies patients underwent osteoporosis assessment and treatment recommendations as outpatients, with components as would be expected from the 'type B' intervention. The details of intervention methods are not described by Huntjens et al. (2010), although Chevalley and colleagues (2002) described a multidisciplinary educational intervention. The extent to which the services educated patients is unclear in the studies from the Netherlands.

Outcomes

a. Risk factor analysis and pathology screening for secondary causes

The assessment of risk factors was described in all seven studies. Six of the seven services reported pathology screening for secondary of osteoporosis (apart from Astrand and co-workers); however the threshold varied between fracture liaison services. For instance, in the Netherlands, two FLS reported performing screening tests for secondary causes of osteoporosis in patients younger than 70 years, with a T-score equal to or less than -3.0 SD, whilst another would do so in any patients with a BMD T-score less than -2.0 SD. A fourth FLS in the Netherlands, investigated only men for secondary causes of osteoporosis.

b. BMD testing

All fracture liaison services performed bone mineral density testing. However, only Chevalley et al. and Astrand et al. reported the actual proportion of patients undergoing BMD testing (63% and 93% respectively).

c. Pharmacological treatment

Treatment outcomes were only reported by Chevalley and colleagues - about 33% of patients were recommended anti-osteoporosis medication, of which 66% were initiated on therapy. Adherence declined to 67%, at six months follow-up.

d. Re-fractures

Nil data

e. Cost-effectiveness

Nil data

5.2.2 'Type B' fracture liaison services in the United States

Study types and patient characteristics

In the two 'before and after' studies from the United States, the study by Johnson et al. (2005) focused on male patients (96% of the study population), while the second report included mainly female patients [Cuddihy et al., 2004]. The study by Johnson et al. analysed outcomes in 126 pre-intervention and 136 post-intervention subjects (mean age: 60 years; 64% white Caucasian). Of note, this study looked at all fracture types, including high trauma fractures. As a result, only 32% of fractures were due to 'minimal trauma'. Cuddihy et al. recruited 96 subjects aged 44yrs or older with a minimal trauma fracture to the wrist (mean age: 68 years).

Patient identification methods and capture rates

Both services utilized fracture liaison co-coordinators, who accessed an electronic database to identify patients, from either orthopaedic clinics or wards. Cuddihy et al. reported 100% identification of potentially eligible patients, made possible by the electronic database.

About 61% of those identified attended the fracture liaison service. Johnson and colleagues did not report the rate of identification of potentially eligible patients.

Intervention methods

As is standard in a 'type B' model of care, patients in both groups were assessed for osteoporosis by performing a BMD scan, followed by a referral to the primary care physician with treatment recommendations.

Outcomes

a. Risk factor analysis and pathology testing for secondary causes

Evaluation of risk factors for osteoporosis was specifically reported by Cuddihy et al. (2004), with 37% (19/51) of women and 50% (4/8) for men sustaining prior fractures. Johnson et al. (2005) reported evaluation of osteoporosis risk factors in only the intervention group who underwent BMD testing. Cuddihy et al. (2004) did not detect any secondary causes for osteoporosis after assessing 32 out of 59 patients, whilst Johnson et al (2005) did not report screening for secondary causes.

b. BMD testing

Osteoporosis assessment increased from 16% at baseline, to 45% at six months, although males had a lower rate of BMD testing compared to females [Cuddihy et al. 2004]. In the study by Johnson et al., the rate of BMD testing changed from 13% (16/126) in the pre-intervention group to 63% (85/136) in the intervention group.

c. Pharmacological treatment

Adherence to osteoporosis specific treatment increased from 9% to 36% at six months [Cuddihy et al., 2004]. In the study by Johnson et al., the proportion of patients recommended specific osteoporosis medications increased from 7% to 19%, which is a surprisingly low number, although the majority of patients had traumatic fractures. At six months following the intervention, only 6% of patients in the pre-intervention group were receiving specific osteoporosis treatment, compared to 13% for the intervention group.

5.2.3 'Type B' fracture liaison services in New Zealand

Study types and patient characteristics

A single 'before and after' study from New Zealand reported on 329 subjects in a pre-intervention group, and 193 subjects in the intervention group, of whom 78% were women. About 69% of patients had sustained a hip fracture [Sidwell et al. 2004].

Patient identification methods and capture rates

Patient identification did not require a fracture liaison nurse, because an *inpatient* protocol was implemented in an ortho-geriatrics ward. Therefore, existing staff were educated to implement the protocol. It is unclear if all potentially eligible patients were captured.

Intervention methods

Staff identified patients with a minimal trauma fracture, assessed them with BMD scan and pathology tests, and sent a report to the primary care physician with treatment recommendations.

Outcomes

a. Risk factor analysis and pathology testing for secondary causes

The evaluation of risk factors for osteoporoisis was not reported, although pathology testing for secondary causes of osteoporosis was performed in 63% of patients.

b. BMD testing

BMD testing increased from 11% (pre-intervention group) to 78% in the intervention group.

c. Pharmacological treatment

At nine months post-fracture, those on calcium or vitamin D increased from 13% to 52%. Bisphosphonates or HRT prescription increased from 10% to 31%.

d. Re-fractures

Nil data.

e. Cost-effectiveness

Nil data.

5.3 Appendix C

5.3.1 'Type C' fracture liaison services in the United States

Study types and patient characteristics

We identified six reports describing a 'type C' intervention in the United States. Three were randomised controlled trials (RCT's) [Gardner et al., 2005; Feldstein et al., 2006 & Solomon et al., 2007], one was a cross-sectional design [Skedros et al., 2004], and two were 'before and after' studies, described in the same article [Harrington et al., 2005]. One study included only female patients [Harrington et al., 2005], whilst the other five studies included both male and female patients. The proportion of females reported in two studies was 78% and 86% [Skedros et al., 2004; Gardner et al., 2005]. Two studies included only patients with hip fractures [Gardner et al., 2005; Harrington et al., 2005], whilst the other studies included patients with minimal trauma fractures at any site. The total number of patients in each study varied from 69 to 1973, with the median number of participants in each study being 283. Most studies recruited patients greater than 50 years of age. Three studies specified exclusion criteria, such as dementia, nursing home residence and previous osteoporosis investigation or treatment [Skedros et al., 2004; Gardner et al., 2005; Feldstein et al., 2006].

Patient identification methods and capture rates

A fracture liaison co-coordinator was critical to the implementation of each service, apart from one [Skedros et al, 2004], in which orthopaedic surgeons were asked to educate and recommend further assessment for osteoporosis. In three studies electronic medical records were employed to help with identification of patients [Harrington et al., 2005; Feldstein et al., 2006; Solomon et al., 2007]. The settings in which the intervention took place varied from exclusively outpatient or inpatient, to mixed settings.

Intervention methods

The methods of intervention did not differ significantly between four of the six studies. Uniquely, one RCT compared three groups, using varying degrees of educational interventions [Feldstein et al. 2006]. This study was a well-powered, randomised controlled trial of female patients only. The three groups were 'usual care' (n=101), electronic reminder to PCP (n=101), and electronic reminder to PCP with educational letter mailed to the patient (n=109). Thus, there was an effective comparison between different 'type C' intervention and no intervention at all. Another randomised controlled study used an educational intervention consisting of a one-on-one interview with a PCP by a *pharmacist,* together with a letter and automated phone call to patients regarding the assessment of their bone health [Solomon et al., 2007].

Outcomes

a. Risk factor analysis and Blood tests for secondary causes

Evaluation of risk factors was reported in only one trial [Harrington et al., 2005]. As expected from an educational intervention, pathology testing was not performed, and a clinical risk factor assessment was not a part of this model.

b. BMD testing and Pharmacological treatment

Five studies reported on the outcome of BMD testing and/or treatment with specific anti-osteoporosis therapies with follow-up periods varying from six months (3 studies) to 18 months. The intervention effect ranged from 14% to 46%, with the control or baseline results ranging from 5% to 19%. The average improvement compared to baseline was 23% across all studies. Of interest, the study by Solomon et al. (2007) failed to detect a clinically significant improvement in BMD testing or treatment (14% in intervention group vs. 10% in control group). This is in stark contrast in to all other studies with similar interventions.

Feldstein and co-workers (2006) reported improved BMD testing rates at six months in the intervention group (20%), compared to 5% in the control group. Treatment rates were 20% and 30% in studies by Feldstein and Skedros respectively.

c. Re-fractures

Solomon et al. reported no difference in re-fracture rates at 10 months follow-up, but the study was not powered for this outcome. No other studies reported on re-fractures.

d. Cost-effectiveness

Nil data.

5.3.2 'Type C' fracture liaison services in Canada

Study types and patient characteristics

We identified five reports on 'Type C' models of care from Canada. The study types include one randomized controlled trial [Majumdar et al., 2008], two prospective controlled trials [Ashe et al., 2004; Majumdar et al., 2004], one 'before and after' analysis [Hawker et al., 2003], and one cluster randomized trial [Cranney et al., 2008]. All studies included both male and female patients, with the proportion of females ranging between 74%-78%. Racial background was described as mostly White in one study [Hawker et al., 2003], and 79% White in the study by Majumdar and co-workers (2004). The numbers of patients in each study varied from 51 to 278, with the mean number of participants per study of 195. Most studies recruited patients above 49 years of age, with a mean age of 67 years. All of the trials apart from one [Hawker et al., 2003] included patients with minimal trauma fractures to the wrist only, although one study included moderate trauma wrist fractures as well [Ashe et al., 2004].

Patient identification methods and capture rates

Three studies utilized fracture liaison co-coordinators [Ashe et al., 2004; Majumdar et al., 2004, Majumdar et al., 2008], whilst one study utilized existing staff [Cranney et al., 2008], and another enlisted the help of the orthopaedic surgeons to identify eligible patients [Hawker et al., 2003]. Patients were identified in the emergency department and orthopaedic clinics.

Intervention methods

Intervention methods for 'type C' services have been described in section 2.5 and all of the Canadian services adhered to this model, with little to no variation between studies.

Outcomes

a. Risk factor analysis

Analysis of osteoporosis risk factors was reported in two studies [Hawker et al., 2003; Majumdar et al., 2008]. Hawker and co-workers reported the rate of prevalent fractures amongst subjects of 20%, whilst Majumdar and co-workers reported a rate of 48%.

b. BMD testing

The rate of BMD testing and/or treatment was reported by Majumdar et al., 2004 & 2008. In the 2004 study, at six months, the intervention group did better than the control group (71% versus 21%). In the 2008 study, 38% of the intervention group versus 11% of the control group underwent BMD testing and / or treatment. The average improvement in the outcome was 38.5%.

The rate of BMD testing was reported in all studies, at three to six months follow-up. The rate of BMD testing in the intervention group ranged from 43% to 92%, and in the control group ranged from 18%-28%. The average improvement in BMD testing was 40%.

c. Pharmacological treatment

Three studies reported the rates of anti-osteoporosis treatment after three to six months follow-up [Hawker et al., 2003; Majumdar et al., 2004 and 2008]. The rate of treatment in the intervention groups ranged from 11% to 40%, compared to 7%-10% in the control groups. The average improvement in treatment rates was 15%. The significant variability in results between studies may be due to factors which are difficult to report such as the details of the explanation of osteoporosis, and rapport between co-coordinator and patients.

d. Re-fractures

Nil data.

e. Cost-effectiveness

Nil data.

5.3.3 'Type C' fracture liaison services in Australia

Study types and patient characteristics

Inderjeeth and colleagues (2010) from Perth, Western Australia, published a 'before and after' study, using a historical control group. There were 200 patients in the pre-intervention group and 194 in the intervention group. The educational intervention targeted patients discharged directly from the emergency department, older than 65 years with a minimal trauma fracture at any site.

Patient identification methods and capture rates

Patient identification occurred by utilizing existing hospital staff (e.g. emergency department clinicians), and primary care physicians were made aware of the need for osteoporosis assessment in these patients. Approximately 34% of eligible patients underwent the intervention.

Outcomes

a. Risk factor analysis and pathology testing for secondary causes

Nil data

b. BMD testing

At 12 months follow-up, the rate of BMD testing was 45% in the intervention group vs. 3% in the pre-intervention group.

c. Pharmacological treatment

Calcium and vitamin D supplementation increased from 12% to 37%. Initiation of osteoporosis specific treatment increased from 6% to 30%.

d. Re-fractures

Nil data.

e. Cost-effectiveness

Nil data.

f. Other outcome measures:

Referral to the bone clinic increased from 4% pre-intervention to 26% with the intervention.

5.4 Appendix D

5.4.1 Description of 'Type D' model of care fracture liaison Services

Study types and patient characteristics

We have identified three publications describing 'type D' interventions, two from Australia [Bliuc et al., 2006; Diamond and Lindenberg et al., 2002] and one from Canada [Bessette et al., 2011]. Two were randomized controlled trials [Bliuc et al. and Bessette et al.] while the third was a cross-sectional analysis [Diamond and Lindenberg, 2002]. In the two Australian studies, 65% of patients were females with an average of 160 subjects in each study. On the other hand, the Canadian study recruited 1314 patients who were all female. Bliuc and colleagues recruited patients over 20 years of age, with one–third sustaining a moderate trauma fracture. Diamond and Lindenberg included patients 45 years or older with minimal trauma fractures. Bessette and co-workers included patients above 49 years of age who sustained a 'minimal trauma' fracture at any site. As an indicator of heterogeneity between studies even of the same 'type', 'minimal trauma' was defined as a fall from a height of one metre or less by Bessette and colleagues. This contrasts with most other studies, define 'minimal trauma' as a fall from standing height or less.

Patient identification methods and capture rates

Diamond and Lindenberg identified patients from a private radiology practice, who had sustained a minimal trauma fracture. No co-ordinator was required for this study. About 64% of eligible patients were contacted. On the other hand, Bliuc and colleagues identified patients from the orthopaedic clinic via a fracture liaison co-ordinator. About 46% of eligible patients received the intervention. Bessette and colleagues identified patients from hospital orthopaedic clinics, as well as from the Quebec Ministry of Health database.

Intervention methods

In the study by Diamond and Lindenberg, patients were asked to fill out a survey about osteoporosis, encouraging them to have their bone health assessed. Bliuc and colleagues randomised patients to receiving either a letter educating patients about osteoporosis risk factors, or a similar letter together with an offer for a free BMD scan. Bessette and colleagues divided their cohort into three groups: i) control group ii) letter to patient group iii) letter to patient together with 15min video.

Outcomes

a. Risk factor analysis and pathology testing for secondary causes

Bliuc and colleagues as well as Bessette and co-workers, reported osteoporosis risk factors extensively in both groups, with well matched baseline characteristics. About 46% (Bliuc et al.) and 24% (Bessette et al.) of patients had a prior fracture. There was no information on risk factors by Diamond and Lindenberg, and neither study reported on testing for secondary causes of osteoporosis. .

b. BMD testing

In the study by Bliuc and colleagues, at six-months follow-up, the rate of BMD testing was 38% in those offered the BMD scan compared to 7% in patients who received a letter only. Female sex was a predictor for having a BMD performed. Diamond and Lindenberg reported a rate of BMD testing of 51% at twelve months. Bessette and co-workers revealed a very small effect of the intervention, with only 15% undergoing BMD testing compared to 12% in the control group.

c. Pharmacological treatment

Diamond and Lindenberg reported that 29% of patients were commenced on specific anti-osteoporosis treatment following the intervention, none of whom were men. This indicates the significant gender disparity often evident in osteoporosis management. Bliuc and colleagues reported treatment rates of 6% (free BMD scan group) and 5% (letter only group), at six months, reflecting the limited effectiveness of a 'type D' intervention. Bessette and colleagues reported a treatment rate of 11% (intervention) versus 8% without the intervention, which is not a clinically significant difference.

d. Re-fractures

Nil data

e. Cost-effectiveness

Nil data

5.5 Appendix E

5.5.1 Description of 'Type E' model of care fracture liaison services

Study types and patient characteristics

We have identified six studies describing 'type E' interventions in the United States [n=3 - Kamel et al., 2000; Jachna et al., 2003; Streeten et al., 2006], Australia [n=2 – Jones et al., 2005; Chong et al., 2008] and the United Kingdom [n=1 – Wallace et al., 2011]. There were five cross-sectional studies and one 'before and after' analysis [Jones et al., 2005]. In the majority of cases patients included were inpatients who had minimal trauma fractures to the hip, with females representing approximately 67% of the subjects. The number of patients in each study varied from 82 to 834, with a median number of patients of 170. At 80 years, the mean age of subjects was significantly greater than in the other intervention models.

Patient identification methods and capture rates

Only one of the studies utilized a fracture liaison co-coordinator [Wallace et al., 2011], whilst two studies had an inpatient protocol for existing staff to use [Jones et al, 2005; Streeten et al., 2006]. One study asked the orthopaedic team to identify eligible patients [Chong et al., 2008].

Intervention methods

Intervention methods varied from an inpatient fracture protocol, to the involvement of an ortho geriatrics team. In one study, the protocol was introduced to all rotating interns, providing guidelines for commencement of anti-resorptive therapy and ortho geriatric consultation [Jones et al., 2005].

Outcomes

a. Risk factor analysis and pathology testing for secondary causes

Two studies reported risk factor analysis [Streeten et al., 2006; Wallace et al., 2011] as well as pathology testing as part of the intervention [Streeten et al., 2006; Jones et al., 2005]. Reflecting an older and sicker cohort than in the other intervention types, Jones and colleagues found that 77% of patients had hypovitaminosis D (i.e., 25-OH-vitamin D level below 50 nmol/L) and 34% of patients had secondary causes for osteoporosis identified.

b. BMD testing

Implementation of a strategy using an inpatient protocol appeared to be more effective in initiating BMD testing compared to a general medical consultation. Such protocols resulted in BMD testing rates of 66% versus 3% in the absence of a protocol [Streeten et al., 2006].

c. Pharmacological treatment according to intervention type

The rate of inpatient bisphosphonate prescription increased from 5% pre-intervention to 24% with and after the intervention (*inpatient protocol*) [Jones et al., 2005]. Wallace and colleagues (2011), showed improved treatment rates of 90.5% for hip fracture patients in a hospital with an ortho-geriatric service as well as a FLS, compared to 60.5% in a hospital with an ortho-geriatrics service only.

Inpatient physician consultation for patients admitted with a minimal trauma fracture to the hip is ineffective in improving osteoporosis care. That is, at discharge only 7% of patients were on bisphosphonates in one study [Jachna et al. 2003], and 5% in another study [Kamel et al. 2000]. It is important to note that these were retrospective chart reviews, and that the consulting physicians were not asked to specifically manage the patients' bone health.

Specific inpatient Endocrinology consultation for osteoporosis has been shown to be partly effective [Streeten et al, 2006] when compared to no consultation, in a study with 84 subjects. The intervention improved calcium and vitamin D commencement (75% vs 3%), and Bisphosphonate commencement (68% vs. 0%). Of those followed-up, 79% vs. 17% were taking calcium or vitamin D, and 65% vs. 0% taking a bisphosphonate (of those contacted). However, the mean follow-up was much longer for the non-intervention group (39 months) compared to the intervention group (18 months).

d. Re-fractures

Nil data.

e. Cost-effectiveness

Nil data.

6. References

Anonymous (1993) Consensus development conference: Diagnosis, prophylaxis and treatment of osteoporosis. *American Journal of Medicine* 941:646-650

Ashe, M.; Khan, K.; Guy, P. & Kruse, K. (2004). Wristwatch-Distal Radial Fracture as a Marker for Osteoporosis Investigation: A Controlled Trial of Patient Education and a Physician Alerting System. *Journal of Hand Therapy*; 17:324-328

Åstrand, J.; Thorngren, KG. & Tägil, M. (2006). One fracture is enough! Experience with a prospective and consecutive osteoporosis screening program with 239 fracture patients. *Acta Orthopaedica*, 77 (1): 3–8

Bessette, L; Davison, KS.; Jean, S.; Roy, S.; Ste-Marie, LG. & Brown, JP. (2011). The impact of two educational interventions on osteoporosis diagnosis and treatment after fragility fracture: a population-based randomized controlled trial. *Osteoporosis International*, 22:2963–2972

Bliuc, D.; Eisman, JA. & Center, JR. (2006). A randomized study of two different information-based interventions on the management of osteoporosis in minimal and moderate trauma fractures. *Osteoporosis International* 17: 1309–1317

Bliuc, D.; Ong, CR.; Eisman, JA. & Center, JR. (2005). Barriers to effective management of osteoporosis in moderate and minimal trauma fractures: a prospective study. *Osteoporosis International,* 16:977–982.

Bogoch, ER.; Elliot-Gibson, V.; Beaton, DE.;, Jamal, SA.; Josse, RG. & Murray TM. (2006). Effective Initiation of Osteoporosis Diagnosis and Treatment for Patients with a Fragility Fracture in an Orthopaedic Environment. *Journal of Bone & Joint Surgery,* 88-A (1):25-34

Boudou, L. ; Gerbay, B. , et al. (2011). Management of osteoporosis in fracture liaison service associated with long-term adherence to treatment. *Osteoporosis International,* 22(7): 2099-2106

Burge, R.; Dawson-Hughes, B.; Solomon, DH., et al (2007). Incidence and economic burden of osteoporosis-related fractures in the United States, 2005-2025. Journal of Bone and Mineral Research, 22:465-475

Center JR, Bliuc D, Nguyen TV, Eisman JA (2007) Risk of subsequent fracture after low-trauma fracture in men and women. JAMA 297:387–394.7. Gallacher S. (2005). Setting up an osteoporosis fracture liaison service: background and potential outcomes. Best Practice and Research Clinical Rheumatology 19(6): 1081-1094.

Charalambous, CP.; Kumar, S.; Tryfonides, M.; Rajkumar, P. & Hirst, P. (2002). Management of osteoporosis in an orthopaedic department: audit improves practice. *International Journal of Clinical Practice,* 56(8):620–621

Chevalley, T.; Hoffmeyer, P.; Bonjour, JP. & Rizzoli, R. (2002). An Osteoporosis Clinical Pathway for the Medical Management of Patients with Low-Trauma Fracture. *Osteoporosis International,* 13:450-5

Chong, C.; Christou, J.; et al. (2008). Description of an orthopedic–geriatric model of care in Australia with 3 years data. *Geriatrics & Gerontology International,* 8(2): 86-92

Clunie, G.; Parkinson, C. & Stephenson, S. (2005). Screening patients with fragility fracture: the occurrence of previously undetected disease, particularly endocrine disease, is significant. ASBMR Abstract M319. Supplement: *Journal of Bone and Mineral Research,* July

Clunie, G. & Stephenson, S. (2008). Implementing and running a fracture liaison service: An integrated clinical service providing a comprehensive bone health assessment at the point of fracture management. *Journal of Orthopaedic Nursing,* 12(3-4): 159-165

Cooper, M.; Palmer, AJ. & Seibel MJ. (2011). Cost-effectiveness of the Concord Hospital Minimal Trauma Fracture Liaison service, a prospective, controlled fracture intervention study. *Osteoporosis International:* Online 29/9/2011

Cranney, A.; Lam, M.; et al. (2008). A multifaceted intervention to improve treatment of osteoporosis in postmenopausal women with wrist fractures: a cluster randomized trial. *Osteoporosis International,* 19(12): 1733-1740

Cuddihy, MT.; Amadio, PC.; Gabriel, SE.; Pankratz, VS.; Kurland, RL. & Melton, LJ III. (2004). A prospective clinical practice intervention to improve osteoporosis management following distal forearm fracture. *Osteoporosis International,* 15:695-700.

Dell, R.; Greene, D., et al. (2008). Osteoporosis Disease Management: The Role of the Orthopaedic Surgeon. *The Journal of Bone and Joint Surgery,* 90(Supplement 4): 188-194

Diamond, T. & Lindenberg, M. (2002) Osteoporosis detection in the community: are patients adequately managed? *Australian Family Physician,* 31:751–752

Edwards, BJ.; Bunta, AD.; Madison, LD.; DeSantis, A.; Ramsey-Goldman, R.; Taft, L.; Wilson, C. & Moinfar, M. (2005). An Osteoporosis and Fracture Intervention Program- OFIP-

increases the diagnosis and treatment for osteoporosis for patients with minimal trauma fractures. *Joint Commission Journal on Quality & Patient Safety*, 31:267-74

Epstein, AJ.; Gray, BH. & Schlesinger, M. (2010). Racial and ethnic differences in the use of high-volume hospitals and surgeons. *Archives of Surgery*, 145:179–186

Feldstein, A.; Elmer, PJ.; Smith, DH.; Herson, M.; Orwoll, E.; Chen, C.; Aickin, M. & Swain MC. (2006). Electronic Medical Record Reminder Improves Osteoporosis Management After a Fracture: A Randomized, Controlled Trial. *Journal of the American Geriatrics Society*, 54(3):450-457

Gallacher, SJ. (2005). Setting up an Osteoporosis Fracture Liaison Service: background and potential outcomes. *Best Practice & Research Clinical Rheumatology*,19(6);1081–1094

Gardner, MJ.; Brophy, RH.; Demetrakopoulos, D.; Koob, J.; Hong, R.; Rana, A.; Lin, JT. & Lane JM. (2005). Interventions to improve osteoporosis treatment following hip fracture. A prospective, randomized trial. *Journal of Bone and Joint Surgery Am.*, 87:3-7

Giangregorio, L.; Papaioannou, A.; Cranny, A.; Zytaruk, N. & Adachi, JD. (2006). Fragility fractures and the osteoporosis care gap: an international phenomenon. *Seminars in Arthritis and Rheumatism*, 35:293-305

Giles, M.; Kallen, J., et al. (2010). A team approach: implementing a model of care for preventing osteoporosis related fractures. *Osteoporosis International. Published online 3/11/2010*; print version: (2011)22:2321-28

Harrington, JT.; Barash, HL.; Day, S. & Lease J. (2005). Redesigning the care of fragility fracture patients to improve osteoporosis management: a health care improvement project. *Arthritis Rheum (Arthritis Care & Research)*, 53:198-204

Hawker, G.; Ridout, R.; Ricupero, M.; Jaglal, S. & Bogoch E. (2003). The impact of a simple fracture clinic intervention in improving the diagnosis and treatment of osteoporosis in fragility fracture patients. *Osteoporosis International*, 14:171-8

Huntjens, K.; van Geel, TACM.; Blonk, MC.; Hegeman JH.; van der Elst, M.; Willems, P.; Geusens, P.; Winkens, B.; Brink, P. & van Helden, SH. (2010). Implementation of osteoporosis guidelines: a survey of five large fracture liaison services in the Netherlands. *Osteoporosis International*, 22(7): 2129-2135

Inderjeeth, CA.; Glennon, DA.; Poland, KE.; Ingram, KV.; Prince, RL.; Van, VR. & Holman CDJ. (2010). A multimodal intervention to improve fragility fracture management in patients presenting to emergency departments. *Medical Journal of Australia*, 193: 149-153

Jachna, CM.; Whittle, J.; Lukert, B.; Graves, L. & Bhargava, T. (2003). Effect of hospitalist consultation on treatment of osteoporosis in hip fracture patients. *Osteoporosis International*, 14:665 - 671

Jaglal, S. B., G. Hawker, et al. (2008). "A demonstration project of a multi-component educational intervention to improve integrated post-fracture osteoporosis care in five rural communities in Ontario, Canada." Osteoporosis International20(2): 265-274.

Johnell, O. & Kanis, JA. (2006). An estimate of the worldwide prevalence and disablility associated with osteoporotic fractures. *Osteoporosis International*, 17:1726-1733

Johnell, O.; Kanis, JA.; Oden, A.; Sernbo, I.; Redlund-Johnell, I.; Petterson, C.; De Laet, C. & Jonsson B. (2004). Fracture risk following an osteoporotic fracture. *Osteoporosis International*, 15: 175–179

Johnson, SL.; Petkov, VI.; Williams, MI.; Via, PS. & Adler, RA. (2005). Improving osteoporosis management in patients with fractures. *Osteoporosis International*, 16:1079-1085

Jones, G.; Warr, S.; Francis, E. & Greenaway, T. (2005). The effect of a fracture protocol on hospital prescriptions after minimal trauma fractured neck of the femur: a retrospective audit. Osteoporosis International, 16:1277-80

Kamel, HK.; Hussain, MS,; Tariq, S.; Perry III, HM. & Morley JE. (2000). Failure to diagnose and treat osteoporosis in elderly patients hospitalized with hip fracture. *American Journal of Medicine*, 109:326-8

Kanis, JA.; Johnell, O.; Oden A. et al. (2000). Long-term risk of osteoporotic fracture in Malmo. *Osteoporosis International*, 11:669–674

Kaufman JD, Bolander ME, Bunta AD, Edwards BJ, Fitzpatrick LA and Simonelli C. Barriers and solutions to osteoporosis care in patients with a hip fracture. J Bone Joint Surg Am. 2003;85:1837-43.

Kuo, I.; Simmons, L.; Bliuc, D.; Eisman, J. & Center, J. (2007). Successful direct intervention for osteoporosis in patients with minimal trauma fractures. *Osteoporosis International*, 18: 1633-1639

Langsetmo, L.; Goltzman, D.; Kovacs, CS.; Adachi, J.; Hanley, DA.; Kreiger, N.; Josse, R.; Papaioannou, A.; Olszynski, WP. & Jamal, SA. (2009). *Journal of Bone and Mineral Research*, 24:1515–1522

Langridge, CR.; McQuillian, C.; Watson WS; Walker, B; Mitchell, L. & Gallacher, SJ. (2007). Refracture following Fracture Liaison Service Assessment Illustrates the Requirement for Integrated Falls and Fracture Services. *Calcified Tissue International*, 81:85–91

Lih, A.; Nandapalan, H.; Kim, M,; Yap, C.; Lee, P.; Ganda, K. & Seibel, MJ. (2011). Targeted intervention reduces refracture rates in patients with incident non-vertebral osteoporotic fractures: a 4-year prospective controlled study. Osteoporosis International, 22: 849-58

Majumdar, SR., et al. (2007). Use of a Case Manager to Improve Osteoporosis Treatment After Hip Fracture. *Archives of Internal Medicine*, 167(19):2110-2115

Majumdar, SR.; Johnson, JA.; et al. (2008). Multifaceted intervention to improve diagnosis and treatment of osteoporosis in patients with recent wrist fracture: a randomized controlled trial. *Canadian Medical Association Journal*, 178(5): 569-575

Majumdar SR, Lier DA, Rowe BH, Russell AS, McAlister FA,Maksymowych WP, Hanley DA, Morrish DW, Johnson JA (2011) Cost-effectiveness of a multifaceted intervention to improve quality of osteoporosis care after wrist fracture.Osteoporos Int. 22:1799-1808.

Majumdar, SR.; Rowe, BH.; Folk, D.; Johnson, JA.; Holroyd, BH.; Morrish, DW.; Maksymowych, WP.; Steiner, IP.; Harley, CH.; Wirzba, BJ.; Hanley, DA.; Blitz, S. & Russell AS. (2004). A controlled trial to increase detection and treatment of osteoporosis in older patients with a wrist fracture. Annals of Internal Medicine, 141:366-373

Majumdar, SR.; Johnson, JA.; Bellerose, D.; McAlister, FA.; Russell, AS.; Hanley, DA.; Garg, S.; Lier, DA.; Maksymowych, WP.; MorrishDW. & Rowe, BH. (2011). Nurse case-manager vs multifaceted intervention to improve quality of osteoporosis care after wrist fracture: randomized controlled pilot study. *Osteoporosis International*, 22:223–230

Marsh D et al, Position Paper: Coordinator-based systems for secondary prevention in fragility fracture patients. Osteoporos Int (2011) 22:2051–2065.

McLellan, AR.; Gallacher, SJ.; Fraser, M. & McQuillian, C. (2003). The fracture liaison service: success of a program for the evaluation and management of patients with osteoporotic fracture. *Osteoporosis International*, 14:1028-34

McLellan, A.; Wolowacz, SE.; Zimovetz, EA.; Beard, SM.; Lock, S.; McCrink, L; Adekunle, F. & Roberts, D. (2011). Fracture liaison services for the evaluation and management of patients with osteoporotic fracture: a cost-effectiveness evaluation based on data collected over 8 years of service provision. *Osteoporosis International*, 22:2083-2098

Mitchell, PJ. (2011). Fracture Liaison Services: the UK experience. *Osteoporosis International*, 22 (Suppl 3):S487–S494

Morrish, DW.; Beaupre, LA., et al. (2009). Facilitated bone mineral density testing versus hospital-based case management to improve osteoporosis treatment for hip fracture patients: Additional results from a randomized trial. *Arthritis & Rheumatism*, 61(2): 209-215

Navarro, RA.; Greene, D., et al. (2011). Minimizing Disparities in Osteoporosis Care of Minorities With an Electronic Medical Record Care Plan." *Clinical Orthopaedics and Related Research*, 469(7): 1931-1935

National Institutes of Health; Research Portfolio Online Reporting Tools. Available from http://report.nih.gov/rcdc/categories/

Nickolls C (2004) Care after an osteoporotic non-vertebral fracture: an audit. Honours Thesis, University of Sydney.

Panneman, MJ.; Lips, P.;,Sen, SS. & Herings, RM. (2004). Undertreatment with anti-osteoporotic drugs after hospitalization for fracture. *Osteoporosis International*, 15:120–124

Sambrook, P. & Cooper, C. (2006). Osteoporosis. *Lancet*, 367:2010-18

Sambrook, P.; Seeman, E.; Phillips, SR. & Ebeling, PR. (2002). Osteoporosis Australia; National Prescribing Service. Preventing osteoporosis: outcomes of the Australian Fracture Prevention Simmit. *Medical Journal of Australia*, 15 (176): Suppl: S1-16

Sander, B.; Elliot-Gibson, V., et al. (2008). A Coordinator Program in Post-Fracture Osteoporosis Management Improves Outcomes and Saves Costs. *The Journal of Bone and Joint Surgery*, 90(6): 1197-1205

Sanders, KM.; Nicholson, GC.; Ugoni, AM.; Pasco, JA.; Seeman, E.& Kotowicz, MA. (1999). Health burden of hip and other fractures in Australia beyond 2000: Projections based on the Geelong Osteoporosis Study. *Medical Journal of Australia*, 170:467-470

Sidwell, AI.; Wilkinson, TJ. & Hanger, HC. (2004). Secondary prevention of fractures in older people: evaluation of a protocol for the investigation and treatment of osteoporosis. *Internal Medicine Journal*, 34:129-132;

Shibli-Rahhal, A.; Vaughan-Sarrazin, MS.; Richardson, K. & Cram, P. (2011). Testing and treatmentfor osteoporosis following hip fracture in an integrated U.S. healthcare delivery system. *Osteoporosis International*, 22:2973–2980

Skedros JG. (2004). The orthopaedic surgeon's role in diagnosing and treating patients with osteoporotic fractures: standing discharge orders may be the solution for timely medical care. *Osteoporosis International*, 15: 405–410

Solomon, DH.; Polinski J.; et al. (2007). Improving Care of Patients At-Risk for Osteoporosis: A Randomized Controlled Trial. *Journal of General Internal Medicine*, 22(3): 362-367

Streeten, EA.; Gandhi, MA.; et al. (2006). The inpatient consultation approach to osteoporosis treatment in patients with a fracture. Is automatic consultation needed? *Bone Joint Surg Am*, 88: 1968-1974

The Burden of Brittle Bones: Epidemiology, Costs & Burden of Osteoporosis in Australia - 2007. *Osteoporosis Australia & International Osteoporosis Foundation*. Available from http://www.osteoporosis.org.au/health-professionals/research-position-papers/

Vaile, J., Sullivan, L., et al. (2007). First Fracture Project: addressing the osteoporosis care gap. *Internal Medicine Journal*, 37(10): 717-720

Wallace, I.; Callachand, F.; et al. (2011). An evaluation of an enhanced fracture liaison service as the optimal model for secondary prevention of osteoporosis. Journal of the *Royal Society of Medicine, Short Reports*, 2(2): 8-8

Wei, GS.; Jackson, JL. & Herbers, JE Jr. (2003). Ethnic disparity in the treatment of women with established low bone mass. *Journal of the American Medical Women's Assocication*, 58:173–177

7

Shared Medical Appointments: Implementing Diabetes SMAs to Improve Care for High Risk Patients and Maximize Provider Expertise

Susan Kirsh, Renée Lawrence, Lauren Stevenson,
Sharon Watts, Kimberley Schaub, David Aron,
Kristina Pascuzzi, Gerald Strauss and Mary Ellen O'Day
Louis Stokes Cleveland Veterans Affairs Medical Center
USA

1. Introduction

Worldwide, the burden of diabetes continues to increase to staggering numbers. A recent report from the International Diabetes Foundation estimated that 366 million people have this chronic condition. Additionally, despite advances in diabetes treatment and prevention over the past 30 years, this number continues to rise. This increase applies to both the developing world and the developed world. For example, in 2010, the US Center for Disease Control fact sheet stated 26 million patients in the United States now have diabetes and 79 million have pre-diabetes. Much of the increase is related to the rising rates of obesity. As the numbers of patients with diabetes increases, so does their associated health care expenditures. Not surprisingly, the challenge of diabetes management is greater in those with mental health conditions, (Frayne et al., 2005) the elderly, and minority populations (www.ahrq.gov, 2011). Overall, diabetes and its complications and the often ineffective approaches to delivery of care lead to demonstrable quality gaps and increased costs. As a result, treatment strategies designed to improve outcomes are needed.

Clearly, healthcare systems have many reasons to systematically address diabetes care delivery specifically and chronic disease management in general. A significant barrier for many healthcare systems is their acute-care orientation; they are not designed for chronic illness care. This is particularly true for the United States. Re-orientation toward chronic disease management would necessitate systematic strategies to address high risk patients and prevention of complications. Specifically, the complexities of patients with chronic conditions in the context of changing demands in healthcare systems, requires the development of new models of care delivery which involve collaboration among professionals from different professional disciplines.

One recognized obstacle to the development and implementation of successful multiprofessional models to chronic care management is the traditional silo approach whereby disciplines act in isolation. Accumulating evidence related to chronic care management supports the importance of integrated, multidisciplinary approaches: team-based interventions in chronic disease are associated with better patient outcomes. There is evidence to support greater involvement of professions other than physicians. For example, the involvement of nurses in assessment, treatment, self-management support and follow-up has been linked to improved professional adherence to guidelines, patient satisfaction, clinical health status, and use of health services (Bodenheimer, 2003; Bodenheimer, Wagner & Grumbach, 2002; Kasper et al., 2002; McAlister, Lawson & Teo, 2001; Singh, 2005).

This chapter focuses on one innovation in care delivery designed to help address care gaps for patients with chronic conditions: shared medical appointments (SMAs). We begin by defining SMAs, describing their conceptual roots, and reviewing the literature on their effectiveness. We then describe our experience with SMAs for diabetes – how they were implemented, adapted, and sustained over a 6-year period at our site in the Cleveland Veterans Health Administration. In an effort to help others implement SMAs for diabetes or other chronic diseases, we provide practical details and present a conceptual framework, Consolidated Framework for Implementation Research (CFIR), to assist others in deciding how transferable this model of care is to other settings.

2. Definition, conceptual roots and current literature on SMAs

2.1 SMA definition

Originally conceptualized by E. Noffsinger in the United States, this type of medical appointment occurs with a group of patients who often have a common chronic condition. The term SMA is used interchangeably with group visit, cluster visit and chronic care clinic in the literature and practice. Multiple patients have an appointment at the same time (typically about 90 minutes in length) with a team of healthcare professionals representing differing professions. During an SMA, participants receive education, participate in group discussion with other patients, and interact with a multiprofessional healthcare team. An individualized medication management and treatment plan are developed through collaborative interaction between the patient and the healthcare team. In addition to physicians (specialists or generalists) or other primary care providers, e.g., nurse practitioners, other healthcare professions are represented such as health psychology, nutrition, clinical pharmacy, and nursing. The appointment incorporates patient education into a problem solving and patient activating environment. While patients and the professional team discuss core education, it is done in such a way as to foster patient and family participation in their own care management and often provides support for others in the session. Patients also receive individual medication management. Within this definition there is room to vary the type of patient populations targeted for participation (e.g., high blood pressure vs. elevated blood sugars) and the types of health professionals on the team. More details will be described in Section 3 and 4.

2.2 Conceptual Roots of SMAs

The broad frameworks and service delivery models proposed to help address existing challenges in health care delivery for treatment and management of chronic conditions include the Chronic Care Model (CCM) of Wagner et al. and the Innovative Care for Chronic Conditions Model of the WHO, among others (Singh, 2005; Wagner, Austin & Von Kroff, 1996). The best characterized and studied model is the Chronic Care Model (Bodenheimer, 2003; Bodenheimer, et al., 2002; Wagner, 2000). A recent systematic review and meta-analysis demonstrated the effectiveness of this model and its components (Coleman et al., 2009). In this model six major elements: delivery system; clinical information systems; healthcare organization; self-management; decision support; and community, are viewed from the perspective of their abilities to support productive interactions between a motivated proactive patient and a prepared proactive *health care team*. Column one of Table 1 summarizes the six components of the CCM and provides a brief description of each as initially set up in our local context.

Chronic Care Model Components	Enhanced Dimensions and Practices for SMAs
1. Self-management support: Provide methods and opportunities for patients to be empowered and prepared to manage their health conditions and health care	Tools and information utilized in group format for teaching self-management
	Health topics covered during patient-led discussion to enhance self-management
	Multi-disciplinary team and continuity of team
	Patient-centered group dynamics
	Peer support (helps with problem solving for self-management)
	Reinforced by team members
	Motivational interviewing
2. Decision support: Enhance and promote evidence-based clinical care that recognizes patient preferences	Embedded guidelines into notes
	Standardized electronic note
	Multi-disciplinary team overlap
3. Delivery system design: Promote proactive delivery of clinical care and support of self-management within the system	Debriefing huddle after each session (Continuous Quality Improvement / Evaluation) and continuity of team
	Registry to review and plan
	Multi-disciplinary team with roles and tasks defined and overlapping
	Individual patient (one-on-one) sessions at end
	Cross-training and spread of care practices back to (other) Primary Care Professionals
4. Community Resources & Policies: Identify and mobilize community-based resources to help meet health care management needs of patients	Significant others invited and encouraged to participate
	Peer support group structure with possibilities for linking outside of group
5. Organizational support: Leadership at all levels provides mechanisms to enhance care and Improvements	Personnel time committed for multi-disciplinary team to participate
	Resources and infrastructure (e.g., designated space and staff, and endorse guidelines)
	Continuous Quality Improvement/Evaluation (feedback and goal-setting)
6. Clinical information systems: Organize and utilize data to promote efficient and effective care	Documentation (consistent with evidence-based guidelines)
	Utilize a diabetes registry, other database for identifying patients

Table 1. Application and Enhancement of the Chronic Care Model to SMAs in the VA Health Care System

SMAs constitute the chronic care model's element of delivery system design and are a form of planned visit. For example, at the heart of SMAs is the notion of patients interacting and helping each other (e.g., patient-centered group dynamics and peer support). At the same time, we incorporate motivational interviewing expertise to help guide those discussions to further support self-management skill development. This type of appointment allows patients to see differing perspectives in problem solving, and productive interactions with other patients and healthcare professionals at one medical appointment.

2.3 Evidence for SMAs

SMAs have been gaining in popularity over the past 10 years, in part based on efficacy similar to or better than usual care (Kirsh et al., 2007; Oandasan, 2004; Weinger 2003; Simpson et al., 2001; Trento et al., 2001; Wagner et al., 2001). Many studies of SMAs have been on patients in managed care in the US or the Veterans Health Administration, in Europe within National Healthcare systems. Most of these SMA studies have demonstrated efficacy and effectiveness in diabetes care with improvements in different intermediate outcome (A1c, blood pressure, cholesterol levels) and recommended diabetes process measures (foot examination rates, eye examination rates, etc. (Martin et al., 2007; Sadur et al., 1999; Trento, 2001; Edelman et al., 2010). One study showed improvement in health status of patients with diabetes as measured by the SF-36 (Wagner et al., 2001). Other outcomes shown to have been improved by participation in diabetes SMAs include patient satisfaction, specialty visits, emergency room visits and patient quality of life. The SMA approach has been applied successfully to the management of other patient populations with chronic diseases including those with hypertension, heart failure, hepatitis C, dyslipidemia and other conditions such as urology visits, bariatric surgery, rheumatoid arthritis and geriatrics.

3. Implementing SMAs for patients with diabetes

While SMAs have been growing in popularity, it isn't always clear how to facilitate them and/or how best to adapt them in different settings. We share our experiences by discussing the implementation process in three phases based on our use of SMAs with diabetes patients in the VA setting: 1) Preparation Phase, 2) Early Implementation Phase, and 3) Sustaining Phase.

3.1 Preparation Stage: Initial ground work and decisions

Initially, the components of SMAs include identification of a targeted population, a healthcare team, administrative support, methods to identify patients and track outcomes, and techniques and processes for conducting the visit.

Figure 1 overviews initial issues to be addressed and decisions to be made and how our site developed them. Thus, we highly recommend them as a starting point for making decisions within your local setting. First, a target population needs to be identified.

Shared Medical Appointments: Implementing Diabetes SMAs to Improve Care for High Risk Patients and
Maximize Provider Expertise

143

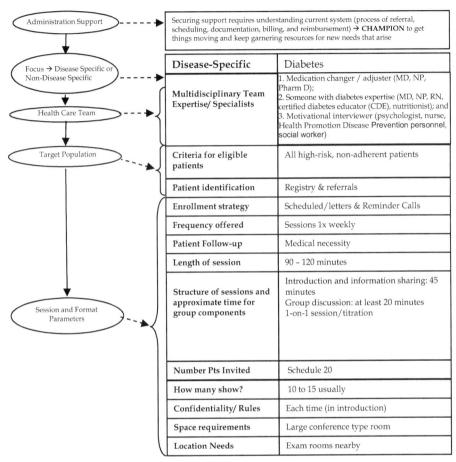

Administration Support	Securing support requires understanding current system (process of referral, scheduling, documentation, billing, and reimbursement) → **CHAMPION** to get things moving and keep garnering resources for new needs that arise
Focus → Disease Specific or Non-Disease Specific	

Disease-Specific	Diabetes
Multidisciplinary Team Expertise/ Specialists	1. Medication changer / adjuster (MD, NP, Pharm D); 2. Someone with diabetes expertise (MD, NP, RN, certified diabetes educator (CDE), nutritionist); and 3. Motivational interviewer (psychologist, nurse, Health Promotion Disease Prevention personnel, social worker)
Criteria for eligible patients	All high-risk, non-adherent patients
Patient identification	Registry & referrals
Enrollment strategy	Scheduled/letters & Reminder Calls
Frequency offered	Sessions 1x weekly
Patient Follow-up	Medical necessity
Length of session	90 – 120 minutes
Structure of sessions and approximate time for group components	Introduction and information sharing: 45 minutes Group discussion: at least 20 minutes 1-on-1 session/titration
Number Pts Invited	Schedule 20
How many show?	10 to 15 usually
Confidentiality/ Rules	Each time (in introduction)
Space requirements	Large conference type room
Location Needs	Exam rooms nearby

Flow diagram labels (left column): Administration Support → Focus → Disease Specific or Non-Disease Specific → Health Care Team → Target Population → Session and Format Parameters

Fig. 1. Developmental Phases and Example of Decisions Made to Help Guide
Implementation of SMAs for Patients with Diabetes

3.1.1 Target population

Identification of patients is a key initial decision. SMAs may be used for patients with well controlled conditions to improve access, or targeted to those with poorly controlled conditions, or a mixture of the two. For example, if the goal of the diabetes oriented SMA is to improve control of chronic illness, remember that patients with poorly controlled blood sugar, blood pressure, proteinuria, or lipids have greatest need to improve and derive the greatest benefit from improvements. They also have poor attendance rate, at times as low as 50%. Depending on goals of the SMA, the targeted population needs to have a pool greater than 500 for a once weekly clinic. This will likely ensure 5-12 patients per clinic for weekly sessions. Starting with once or twice a month SMA sessions may be more manageable in a setting depending on number of patients in need. Among the reasons we chose to focus on diabetes were the desire to meet performance measures, the availability of a clinical diabetes registry (Kern et al., 2008), and interested clinicians. The choice of the target population determines the stakeholders and the members of the team. Of note, in setting up goals for patients, ensure that they are concordant with guidelines in your local setting. For example, the VA/Department of Defense diabetes guidelines provided us with decision support (component of the chronic care model) for our SMA to focus on lowering all patients with A1c levels over 9%. Updated guidelines still utilized during our SMAs are available at www.healthquality.va.gov.

3.1.2 Garnering support

Among the most important early steps are securing buy-in from those staff and administrative sponsors who will be directly involved, rallying stakeholders, and identifying a local champion. It is important to obtain support from all stakeholders -- from administration to patients and their family members because change is always challenging. This is particularly important if change involves a redesign of office practice. We strongly recommend that a physician or other primary care clinician be the champion or the primary champion among a team of champions. A champion of the process is essential to garnering resources for the SMA, both at its inception and in the future. We suggest someone who can leverage support at various levels, and who has a solid understanding of the population and the associated challenges. In our setting, a lead primary care provider is particularly ideal given the fact that SMAs are a change in the format of delivering patient care. We have observed that in our setting, primary provider leaders have been more successful, more quickly, in achieving system redesign regarding direct patient care issues-such as making a case to administration, initiating processes and obtaining current and future resources. Additionally, primary care providers may be in a better position to arrange for outcome data to be made available so that the team can gauge its success. Although our approach flattens the hierarchy with the clinical team, we recognize that the typical bureaucracy may deal more comfortably with a clear hierarchy. Again, it is important to recall that it is the solid core of the team that will keep moving the process forward.

It is also important to remember that the physician or primary care provider does not need to be visible during the entire appointment, does not have to oversee the day-to-day management, or even be the leader of the team once the resources are garnered and team becomes successful in regular SMA visits. The team remains central to the success of the SMAs, but like all changes, needs a liaison with enough status and influence to get support and resources. In our context we are fortunate to have SMAs recognized and prescribed (mandated) as an important management option. Local administration support still is essential and proceeds better if some initial planning and decisions have been made and have been played out to demonstrate feasibility.

Starting with the high-risk patients provided us with the opportunity to obtain initial buy-in from administration and other providers since many recognized that the traditional approaches were not working for our chronic care patients. We found that most of the doubts about starting SMAs came from lack of familiarity and uncertainty about the initial high amount of resources. Locally, we were able to address these by sharing published findings and providing the opportunity for non-team members to observe and participate in a SMA. Once local patients shared their success stories, SMA buy-in was self-perpetuating and providers learned techniques for collaborating with challenging patients. Non SMA providers participating in a few SMAs also provides an opportunity for them to observe motivational interviewing techniques with challenging patients and reinforces the most evidence based approach to care.

Securing provider and staff support helps with informing patients and family members about the new care option. While we use the registry to identify potential patients and also take referral from primary care providers, we recognize that patients and family members may seek reassurance and encouragement from their primary provider. Patients provide a source of buy-in for other patients and family members. Word then travels back to their primary providers, who then are more likely to refer/encourage other patients to participate.

3.1.3 Team members: Main roles and core expertise for each session

After securing leadership support, it is advantageous to focus on deciding who will be part of the team so that other decisions reflect the team working together. The actual size of the team may vary, ranging from 2 members (1 RN and 1 physician or clinical pharmacist or nurse practitioner) to 5 or 6 members. Optimally we recommend three team members but recognize that the composition of the team can also vary and reflect different options for fulfilling expertise requirements, available clinicians and the disease being targeted. For example, a nutritionist may not be available, but a local certified diabetes educator (CDE) has the necessary knowledge of the interface between diabetes and diet. For our SMAs we found that having two or more medication changers at each session was essential for SMA clinics that had more than 12 patients. Again, we recommend at least three total team members be involved at each session (although it does not always need to be the same three people), with each one primarily fulfilling one of the three main roles. Table 2 provides an overview of the roles. The three main roles are further defined by the core or critical expertise that we have found necessary to have present at each session for successful diabetes SMAs. The roles may vary slightly based on the setting or identified disease. We now describe the essential skill sets, not specific health professionals needed since each role can be covered with several different health professionals.

Moderator: The moderator takes main responsibility for facilitating the group session and there are a number of potential staff members who could fill this role. This may be a health psychologist, social worker, or nurse with motivational interviewing experience/group facilitation experience.

The core expertise needed from the moderator is to elicit group discussion and use Motivational Interviewing skills when needed. This technique creates a patient-centered discussion. The moderator helps guide patient generated questions, discussion of challenges and/or educational topics in the group session. It is important to recognize that even though the flow of the discussion is derived from patients and their issues, the moderator and team help ensure that all patients get basic education on physiologic goals, familiarity with medications used to achieve goals, and complications of their disease. The advantage of this context is that the moderator and team build on the discussions so that the information is pertinent to the patient and permits other patients to discuss and make suggestions about common barriers to achieving chronic care management goals.

Role and Core Expertise	Possible Team Members to Fill the Role	Responsibilities
MODERATOR Motivational Interviewer	Psychologist, Pharmacist, Clinical Nurse, Dietician, Certified Diabetes Educator (CDE)	Facilitate discussion related to various aspects of patients' chronic disease
		Answer clinical questions that arise during patient discussion
		Give recommendations to providers as to which order patients should be taken back for their individual physical exam if needed
		Provide, or consult mental health service for smoking cessation classes, weight loss counseling, depression, post traumatic stress disorder (PTSD), insomnia, erectile dysfunction
		Provide, or consult nutrition service for carbohydrate counting
		Provide, or consult pharmacy service for pill box counseling, medication reconciliation (especially new consults), prescription renewals/refills
		Obtain vitals, and assist with check-in process, if necessary
		Assist patients with completion of symptom questionnaire, if indicated
PROVIDER Medication Changer	MD/NP/PA, Clinical Nurse, CDE, Pharmacist	Complete individual patient physical exam if needed, assess functional capacity to engage patient in exercise program

Role and Core Expertise	Possible Team Members to Fill the Role	Responsibilities
		Discuss patients' symptoms, adverse drug reactions, and follow-up on patient response to symptom questionnaire, if needed
		Complete medication reconciliation
		Adjust patient specific pharmacotherapy, if appropriate and as indicated
		Schedule follow-up appointments, as clinically appropriate
		Provide patient option to return to the group for continued discussion or check-out
		Record provider and patient goals for therapy and treatment plan for documentation into the patient's chart (documentation usually occurs during individual patient visits). Partial or complete progress note documentation of the subjective, objective, assessment and plan (SOAP) for each patient.
		Complete take home instruction sheet
CONTENT EXPERT	MD/NP/PA, Clinical Nurse, CDE, Dietician, Pharmacist, Psychologist,	May call patients out for individual consult (e.g., regarding diet), Can help with documentation
		Note that documentation of the assessment and plan can be an individual effort ~or~ a collaborative effort with the team after the clinic visit.
		Understand medical terminology, or have clinical background experience
		Assist with group facilitation

Table 2. Core roles and suggested distribution of responsibilities

Provider: Medication changers in our SMAs include medical doctors (MDs), nurse practitioners (NPs), registered nurses (RNs) with primary provider support, and pharmacists. These team members interact with patients one on one. Titration of medications is completed, if needed. Ideally, this only takes between 5 and 10 minutes for each patient. Consults are placed as needed with a written treatment plan and list of medications for the patient upon check out. If seen in individual rooms for treatment plan, patients may or may not rejoin the group after their individual session. As needed, the provider seeks input from other team members by asking another member in for a quick consult or requesting and relaying information back to patient.

Diabetes Expert (Or Disease Specific Expert): The expert can be a nurse, pharmacist, physician, or nutritionist. We have found that there are several reoccurring themes for patients with diabetes and their families, particularly surrounding food/nutrition related issues (e.g., carbohydrate counting, food preparation, salt intake issues, budget and food). It is critical that at least one member is an expert on the specifics of management of the identified disease.

3.1.4 Session and Format Parameters

In Figure 2 we have summarized our recommended approach for implementing SMAs, but recognize some parameters will be a function of local contextual factors. For example, offering SMAs for patients with diabetes once a week would be ideal to quickly get as many patients as possible involved, however, that may not be feasible given the clinic space and availability of staff.

The visit itself begins with the group format where introductions and information sharing occurs, followed by more open group discussion which also has an educational component. The group discussion facilitates peer support, one of the keys to success in chronic disease management. Arranging chairs in a circular format creates a sharing environment. It is important for the team members to be seen as equal members in the group with the patients and family members, therefore, the group discussion where all team members are sitting rather than standing is recommended.

It is important to stay focused within the SMA visit on chronic illness only to adhere to specified time frames. Recognize that this gets challenging when the patients are part of one's own primary care panel. If need be, and space is a constraint, medication titration and a patient plan can be done in the presence of the whole group or off to the side of the group discussion. We chose not to do so routinely as glucose pattern management for high risk patient with diabetes is complicated to do in front of many other patients. However if clinic is running late, medication titration is often done within the group on the remaining patients.

The last component of the visit is the clinical component (examination if needed and management) where medication titration is done and other issues related to diabetes care are addressed in a one-on-one format with one of the medication changers. Patients may or may not rejoin the group after the individual session.

TIME FRAME	TASKS	MAIN TEAM MEMBER
PREPARATIONS PRIOR TO SESSION		
1 – 2 weeks before	Send Letters of Invitation (At first schedule 10 patients)	CLERK
2 days before	Make reminder phone calls Print note Highlight lab values Assemble handouts	CASE MANAGER CLERK
PREPARATIONS DAY OF SMA SESSION (example start time of 9am):		
8:30am SET UP ROOM	Ensure enough chairs and placed in a Discussion-type format. Put handouts around with pencils	NURSE
8:45 am PATIENTS START ARRIVING	CHECK-IN: Vitals, Download glucose data, Eye and food screening (triage and grabs), Clinical routing slip	NURSE (Screener)
9:00am GROUP SESSION BEGINS	Welcome and privacy reminder. Introductions: ask everyone to introduce self and have patients share their: name, how long had diabetes, whether or not on insulin.	MODERATOR Patients invited via moderator
9:10- 930am GROUP DISCUSSION	Socratic discussion of issues. Begin process by referring to printed notes and asking patients their values and target values. ABCs of Diabetes discussed via questions to engage patients (no lecturing)	MODERATOR and PATIENTS
9:30am START PULLING OUT PATIENTS	INDIVIDUAL SESSIONS: Begin with patients who have time constraints, have hearing problems, are disengaged, are engaging in disruptive behaviors, or have been to previous sessions	PHYSICIAN/MEDICATION CHANGER (Moderator helps identify patients)

Fig. 2. Shared Medical Appointment Schedule

3.1.5 Other considerations

A table for the group is useful for patients to review their health related information and take notes, but is not critical. In the case of people with diabetes, the ability to incorporate home blood glucose monitor readings may add potency to the intervention by informing pharmacological changes, especially for patients on insulin. If feasible it is worth having patients bring their meters to group for review. If the technology is available, we have found that downloading them is helpful for the patient and the team. If your facility uses point-of-care A1c testing, having that available for the session may also be very helpful in titrating pharmacological changes.

3.2 Early implementation

A number of things need to happen early in implementation and include: identifying and contacting patients and their respective family members (or caregivers), mapping out the process during the group session prior to the session itself and identifying the most appropriate guidelines in directing clinical care delivered in the SMA.

Once the criteria have been established, if available, a registry can be used to identify potential participants. Potential patients should be screened for other issues or conditions that would suggest SMAs might not be appropriate. We apply the following exclusions to participation in our diabetes SMAs: an inability to speak English, a diagnosis of dementia or other cognitive impairment, and any behavioral problem which interferes with group participation and discussion.

The letter of invitation is sent about two weeks prior to the SMA session the patient is invited to attend. A reminder phone call is made one or two days prior to the session. Both the letter of invitation and the reminder phone call clarify that significant others are also invited to attend. We should mention that initially we had the team involved in identifying and contacting potential patients, but once the process was established, these steps were handled by one individual on the team (our nurse practitioner who had access to the registry but this could be handled by others who have clerical positions if trained).

Prior to the SMA session, a review of the patient's chart is conducted. Specifically, data is gathered to assess the need for labs prior to the visit and if the patient has been appropriately triaged to the SMA. For example, patients who need insulin initiation are identified and discussed with the designated RN (whose job is to assist patients with insulin starts) prior to the visit, in order to make this process more efficient during the clinic visit. Then during the SMA session, patients are checked in at the site of the group visit, not at the nursing station. This permits meters to be downloaded; blood pressure to be obtained; and foot screening to be conducted, if needed. The patients are given copies of most recent labs, including values for A1c, Ldl-c and Blood Pressure. Additional educational material is provided on hypoglycemia, stress in diabetes, alert identification as well as goal-setting in diabetes.

Our SMAs begin with ground rules, information and reminders about confidentiality. Subsequent to the confidentiality reminder, one must realize that the session introduction is very important to help set the tone. We begin our sessions with introductions of everyone present by going around the room and providing a brief introduction of the clinicians and for the patients including how long s/he has had diabetes and whether they are on insulin. This also helps the care team who may not be familiar with all of the patients at the session. We do not at our site invite the same patients back to each group due to logistical challenges and a desire to provide access to all high-risk patients. Introductions can also be altered to help steer the process of information sharing beyond the basic information. For example, if during prep time you recognize that many of the participants need to start insulin, you could ask patients to share their biggest fear of starting insulin or what was their biggest fear, for those already on insulin. Such alterations help get the discussion moving in the direction that you initially want it to go. It is important to remember to be flexible as the issues the patients want to discuss need to surface and be part of the process.

Typically the group discussion begins with asking an open-ended question to encourage patient participation. The moderator and other team members ensure that relevant educational topics are discussed and that goals are established during the discussion. The topics, and the approach to discussing the topics, are designed to evoke better self-management skills reinforcing the self-management support component of the Chronic Care Model to empower and prepare patients to manage their health conditions and health care. Patients receive educational materials that include target goals for the patient along with his/her own value. Patients set self-management goals around improving diabetes care as well as share perceived confidence in achieving this goal over the ensuing weeks until they return. Additional self-management materials are often provided to patients including pedometers, Blood Pressure Monitors and pill organizers for medication.

An important goal is to get the patients to share and problem-solve with and for each other. The facilitator's role is to keep patients engaged with the group activity to the extent that this is possible. After sufficient discussion (i.e., the topics have been shared and discussed in a patient-driven format), medication adjustment and individualized planning begins by taking patients out individually for the one-on-one session. The other patients remain in the group session and the moderator continues to facilitate relevant discussions. Patients are welcome to return after their one-on-one session to continue to participate in discussion. Typically we start one-on-one sessions with patients who have attended several previous SMAs or have time constraints and/or other commitments (e.g., need to get back to work).

We find it is useful to have a debriefing huddle immediately after SMA session. During the debriefing huddle the health care team discusses the individual and group encounter portion of the patient visit. Additional collaboration happens that may lead to further recommendations for follow up care and/or charting in the medical record. Opinions and consensus occurs during these sessions. In addition, this provides an opportunity for assessing the overall process and goals as well of spread of interprofessional expertise. You may find the debriefing component decreases over time, but it is important to continue debriefing if only for a few minutes. This time may provide an opportunity for interprofessional cross-training and professional development as new evidence-based healthcare practices emerge. This is especially true if trainees of different disciplines are included in this clinical venue. Unintended consequences may arise that may be addressed in the team debriefing session. Further information about how our clinic structure changed with local implementation can be found (Kirsh, Lawrence & Aron, 2008).

3.3 Keys to sustaining SMAs

Sustaining successes for our group has been a result of a continuous quality improvement process, staying alert to unintended consequences and developing supportive tools to track and measure outcomes. Demonstrating value added to clinical care with improved outcomes must be a part of early and ongoing assessment strategies. Improved outcomes may be intermediate outcomes, decreased Emergency Department visits or patient satisfaction with SMAs. It is important to find some measure of improved care to demonstrate value within local systems of care.

3.3.1 Developing supportive tools and environment

We have identified six key ingredients or elements that are associated with successful implementation of SMAs, including improvement of quality of care as evidenced by significant improvement in patient clinical outcomes, high SMA patient and provider satisfaction, and decreased wait times for patients with diabetes. The core keys to success are: 1) multi-professional team development (including continuity of team 2) motivational interviewing 3) nurturing peer support 4) teaching and encouraging self-management 5) a registry for identifying and tracking patients 6) continuous Quality Improvement / evaluation. The keys to success are discussed below and it is important to recognize that they function together to ensure success. Thus, for example, having a highly dynamic group with peer support but without motivational interviewing strategies to focus on what patients' desire as goals is problematic – both are necessary to make improvements in outcomes.

Multi-Professional Team Development (Including Continuity of Team): The more consistent the team members, the more quickly a team can adapt the implementation strategies to their local environment. Deference to expertise, not rank, is an important consideration in fostering teamness; that is the sense of mutual interdependence and supportiveness. An example of this may be to defer to a nurse practitioner about how quickly to titrate insulin since s/he may know how to implement insulin regimens in certain patients. We additionally focus on our successes, which allows for high provider team satisfaction.

Continuity of team need not mean that only the same three people do the session each and every time. What it does mean is that there is continuity in that all team members who rotate or take turns are seen as part of the team and involved with training, updates, debriefing and continuous quality improvement. You may find it helpful to send summaries of the debriefing session to the team member(s) who aren't scheduled for that session, or decide to have a monthly Team Continuity Meeting with all team members to reinforce the common goals and objectives.

Motivational Interviewing: Setting the Tone for Patient-Centered Group Encounters: Healthcare providers and group moderators help promote behavior change in individuals with chronic illness through use of innovative approaches to communication such as motivational interviewing (MI). This approach is particularly useful when patient motivation and adherence are barriers to treatment effectiveness. Given that motivation is often a significant obstacle to behavior change, MI has been used to address many health problems related to lifestyle as well as in the prevention and treatment of many chronic illnesses (Miller, 2004). Although there are many strategies that can be used in the application of this method, MI is not a technique so much as a style for provider-patient communication. MI has been described as a patient-centered counseling style used for eliciting behavior change by helping patients to explore and resolve ambivalence (Miller & Rollnick, 1991; Rollnick & Miller, 1995). Miller (2004) further described it as "a way of being with people, that is also directive in seeking to move the person toward change by selectively evoking and strengthening the patient's own reasons for change" (p. 4). The tenets of Motivational Interviewing acknowledge (Harris, Aldea, & Kirkley, 2006): (a) most people move through a series of steps prior to changing behavior, (b) effective change is self-directed, (c) confrontation and negative messages are ineffective, (d) knowledge alone is insufficient for behavior change, and (e) patient ambivalence about change must be addressed before successful behavior change can be accomplished.

To use this method, the practitioner and the patient work together to address the patient's health care needs, emphasizing a collaborative approach (Miller, 2004). In MI, the practitioner selectively elicits and reinforces positive self-statements, consequently directing the patient to move in the direction of behavior change. However, the patient, not the practitioner, argues for change. To promote positive behavior change, providers must learn to utilize several principles in communicating with patients and these include rolling with resistance, expressing empathy, avoiding arguments, developing discrepancy and supporting self-efficacy (READS). Ambivalence regarding change is considered part of the process. Thus, the central goal in MI is to recognize the discrepancy between the patient's stated goals and his/her present behavior. Eliciting reasons for change from the patient is more powerful than giving the patient prescribed reasons why change is necessary (Miller & Rollnick, 1991; 2002).

Nurturing Peer Support: Peer support is considered an essential component of SMAs and provides an opportunity for participants to share similar life experiences and challenges, offer support and activate one another toward positive behavior change. Among patients dealing with the same chronic illness, sharing experiences with others adjusting to similar medical and/or behavioral regimens has been found to be an effective means of gaining mastery over self-management skills and improving disease outcomes (Heisler & Piette, 2005). Assimilating new knowledge and appraisals through mutual exchange of experiences may occur more effectively when presented by peers with whom the patient identifies and shares common experiences. Group interaction appears to provide emotional support while lessening feelings of isolation and stigmatism that are associated with chronic illness (Weinger, 2003). Peer support also provides an additional social support network that many individuals lack when trying to meet the demands of their illness. Patients are actively involved in decision-making and problem solving in relation to issues raised by others within the group. Moreover, the act of assisting another person can promote a real sense of contribution and certainly increase group cohesiveness (Olsson et al., 2005). Research has shown that patients found meaning and positive reinforcement for their own behavioral goals in seeking also to support other patients' efforts in managing their behavioral goals (Heisler & Piette, 2005).

Promoting peer support in shared medical appointments requires the group moderator to attend to both the content of what is being said and the process of the group (e.g., who is talking, for how long, which patients are disengaged, etc.). Often new moderators interact with patients by either lecturing or engaging in a question/answer session. This interaction sets the norms for the group and will inhibit patients from engaging in discussion with one another. Promoting peer support begins with the initial interaction and can be fostered by the moderator.

In general, the facilitator's job is to find ways to keep the patients talking with one another. Questions/interaction should be aimed at facilitating and promoting peer interaction. Sometimes you have to work harder to get patients interacting, but avoid falling into a lecturing style: ask questions, ask for stories, engage patients you know, rephrase question with another example, and don't feel like you have to fill the silence with information.

Teaching and Encouraging Self-management: The focus of self-management education within our Diabetes SMAs includes an emphasis on self-efficacy and the ABC's of Diabetes (A1c value, Blood pressure [BP] goal, Cholesterol goals, Diet, Eye exam, Foot exam), review of individual lab values and information about Hypoglycemia. This is not meant to take the place of diabetes self-management education but to address those necessary and pertinent topics for safety, and attainment of problem-solving skills in chronic disease care. Patients are encouraged to set a goal to help attain one of the above mentioned values or other health care measures (such as tobacco cessation or weight loss) (Bodenheimer, Lorig, Holman & Grumbach, 2002).

Registry for Identifying and Tracking Patients: The registry is any form of record that identifies actively managed patients in this case with diabetes. Furthermore, the registry can be used to identify patients with A1c, BP, Proteinurias or cholesterol parameters that fall outside the acceptable guideline measure. Our list also provides information on those in need of an eye or foot exam. If there is no current disease specific registry then a generated list of patients fitting the determined population will work.

Continuous Quality Improvement/Evaluation: Measuring the outcomes of the work the team is doing for and with patients is critical. Not only do administrative staff and clinic directors want to see successful improvements in patient measures, but this is critical for the clinical team as well. Often measures are of glycemic targets, blood pressure and cholesterol, which are more difficult to see early results in than process measures such as placing orders for A1c, foot exams and eye exams. Recognize that measures can also be patient satisfaction, care coordination, patient functional status, or number of emergency department visits. Choosing measures at the onset is important to show value to clinical leadership for sustained resources. As mentioned earlier, a key component of success is continuous quality improvement, it is impossible to evaluate progress and make adjustments without measuring aspects of the care provided.

3.3.2 Identifying and addressing challenges

Although we have achieved much success, we have also had several challenges that were met and overcome. The following are several challenges encountered as we have initiated and sustained diabetes SMAs.

Managing Misinformation and Urban Legends: Occasionally patients will want to discuss home remedies for diabetes as if the remedy is scientifically based. This can almost have an infectious effect among group members. They often want to know more about the "cures." Patients have talked about (among other examples) fasting then using honey and vinegar to control blood sugar; sometimes with disastrous outcomes. One way to defuse this type of misinformation is to gently interrupt the discussion, recognize that there are many home remedies that people have tried over centuries, that science is investigating some of these complementary and alternative treatments, but for our discussions we have to stay with what science recommends now, but also realize that other treatment modalities (some based on home remedies) may be included in our treatment options in the future after they have been verified by sound science.

Administrative Hurdles: From an administrative standpoint, pressure to serve patients in a traditional clinic setting may present barriers to changing formats and to allowing staff the initial time needed for developing and adjusting to changes. Emphasis on the long term gains and benefits (increase in patient numbers over time, improved access, cost savings when intermediate outcome measures improve, and high patient satisfaction) must be recognized by administrators in order to persevere through the initial adjustment period. Your champions, are often critical for getting and maintaining administrative support.

Growing Pains: Is important for the team to recognize there is an investment in developing the process for each local setting, with a return, but this must happen over a period of time with those intimately committed and involved helping to refine the process. In our local setting, we met and continue to meet after each shared medical appointment for 10 to 20 minutes to collaborate on patients as well as refine the process and flow (debriefing). Collaboration may mean various health professionals help in ways that are not specific to his/her disciplines. For example, our health psychologist will enter no show notes at the end of the session and our nutritionist will help download glucometers when needed. Flexibility and persistence are necessary and will pay off in the end.

Roles and Cross-Training: The multi/inter- professional nature of SMAs may be uncomfortable until enough cross-training has occurred. The cross-training is critical because it enables more flexible roles to emerge. Being flexible and cross-training help guarantee sustainability, otherwise if you lose one person, the structure of the SMA is lost. If the number of medication changers is limited, other means for facilitating order entry can be considered.

For settings where you are inviting other providers' patients, you may feel hesitant to make recommendations or changes. Our experience is that most non-participating providers appreciate the help and the documentation provided in the individual and collaborative notes. Again, the focus is on diabetes, not the gamut of the patient's other issues.

Clinic Capacity: Clinic capacity depends upon space and available staff. Initially, it is often reasonable to invite fewer patients. This permits the team time to assess acuity, establish flow, and adjust the process of care delivery. Our experience with patients failing to keep this type of appointment ranges from 20 to 50%. At our local site, efforts to reduce the no-show rate have included: reminder phone calls, calling patients who no-show, and scheduling letters. Some sites have also reported use of patient attendance contracts. Adequate patients in clinic can be achieved additionally by overbooking the clinic. If you take this approach, overbook by no more than 40% of the total number of patients desired. Although it makes for a busy clinic if overbooked patients come to clinic, they can usually be accommodated more easily with multiple providers than with one provider. Teamwork is maximized and some patients may opt to be seen and not participate in the group session component due to time constraints.

The group discussion usually occurs in a large group room with individual medication changes occurring in smaller exam rooms. Some clinical sites may be limited by exam rooms and by the number of providers that can make changes to patient medication regimens. Generally, the number of patients per individual making medication changes should be about 6 to 1. Two to four small exam rooms are needed to keep the overall clinic time at 90 to 100 minutes. However, it is important to remember that 'traditional' exam rooms are not usually necessary. It is possible to work quite comfortably if you have access to only one traditional exam room and several private or semi-private spaces. Recall that the focus in the individual patient (one-on-one) session is on medication changes and diabetes-relevant issues; the goal is not to conduct a complete exam.

4. Lessons learned to help guide implementation for others

4.1 An approach to thinking about potential transferability and implementation

Multidisciplinary programs implemented to manage chronic disease are good examples of socially complex interventions that are "described theoretically but implemented subjectively"(Kirsh, Lawrence & Aron, 2009). Contextual characteristics interact in a dynamic way with the program and make the entire process highly individual. Consequently, care must be taken when implementing a model of care developed elsewhere. It is critical to think systematically about the factors involved. One framework that can inform implementation is the Consolidated Framework for Implementation Research (CFIR). The CFIR comprises five major domains (the intervention itself, inner and outer setting, the individuals involved, and the process by which implementation is accomplished.) We have described our implementation of SMAs, but recognize that like many interventions, it needs to be tailored for the specific context into which it is being implemented. The CFIR, interventions can be conceptualized as having components that cannot be altered, the essential and indispensible elements of the intervention, and those that can. The context into which an intervention is implemented is the setting. Generally, the outer setting includes the economic, political, and social context within which an organization resides, and the inner setting includes features of structural, political, and cultural contexts through which the implementation process will proceed, e.g., structural characteristics, networks and communications, culture, climate and readiness. For example, the decision to implement SMAs will depend upon how such visits might be reimbursed. In addition, in some healthcare systems, e.g., US Veterans Health Adminstration, use of group visits has been mandated. How this mandate is put into operational use will vary from facility to facility.

As is true of most system redesign, the unique, local context is the starting point, and existing strengths and limitations need to be carefully considered, utilized, and re-envisioned. The format we found most useful and effective in our local setting includes a multi-professional team working collaboratively to see a group of patients (8-15) with diabetes (and their family members/caregivers) for approximately 90 minutes.

However, the line between the inner and outer setting is somewhat blurry. As to the individuals involved, Greehalgh et al. (2004) describe their significant role as follows: "People are not passive recipients of innovations. Rather (and to a greater or lesser extent in different persons), they seek innovations, experiment with them, evaluate them, find (or fail to find) meaning in them develop feelings about them, challenge them, worry about them, complain about them, 'work around' them, gain experience with them, modify them to fit particular tasks, and try to improve or redesign them-often through dialogue with other uses."(p. 598). Finally, there is the implementation process itself which will vary from program to program and site to site. In our program, the active involvement of internal change agents and local champions was critical.

4.2 Application of SMAs to professional training

Several healthcare professional accrediting bodies have called for integration of multiple professionals working collaboratively, or interprofessionally in care delivery and education. Because the structure and processes of the SMA are designed to promote collaboration, provide multi professional care, and integrate patients' perspectives in the collaboration, it provides a unique opportunity to educate professionals from multiple disciplines. The SMAs provide interprofessional training and collaboration by focusing on the domains of interprofessional competence: communication, teamwork, leadership, knowledge of one's own profession, knowledge of others' professions including each profession's mental models. SMAs also provide trainees an opportunity to understand the provision of care from a systems perspective as well as to appreciate how patients view their illness including the role of barriers in positive outcomes. Role modeling experienced during the SMA team provides education about the complexities of the disease and the knowledge, skills, and attitudes of interprofessionalism. We used this venue for training 3rd and 4th year medical students and Internal Medicine resident physicians. Our initial study involved 3rd and 4th year medical students participating in a four week chronic illness care block in facilities with and without SMAs and found that there was a significant improvement in attitudes toward diabetes among those in the intervention group compared to the control group. There were also greater improvements in recognition of psychosocial impact and seriousness of type 2 diabetes as well as in confidence in the ability to convey logic of clinical recommendations to providers from other disciplines/professions. We have also involved students from other disciplines – psychology, nursing, nutrition and pharmacy.

5. Conclusions and caveats

The patient-centered care in an SMA reinforces the concept that each patient is an individual, with unique life experiences, values, religious and cultural influences and psychological strengths and weaknesses that are taken into account in treatment and discharge planning. Informed and activated patients understand the vital role they play in managing their condition. SMAs provide an opportunity for providers to see and learn things that don't happen during a one-on-one session, providing more insights for helping patients manage their diabetes 365 days a year. This type of appointment allows patient to see differing perspectives in problem solving and productive interactions with other patients and healthcare professionals at one medical appointment. Intermediate outcome measures of aspirin use, annual eye examination, foot examination and patient self-efficacy are all addressed at each visit. Ideally, at the end of each session, a team debriefing occurs where patient issues and clinic processes are reviewed. The SMA promotes collaboration and effectively multiprofessional care while integrating patients; perspectives (Geriatrics Interdisciplinary Advisory Group, 2006; Kirsh, Schaub & Aron, 2009). While implementing a new shared medical appointment, it is prudent to recognize that there will undoubtedly be challenges, but if you are persistent and adhere to the essential phases, core ingredients, and key elements for success, it will be worth the effort for you and your patients.

6. References

Ayoub, W.T., Newman, E.D., Blosky, M.A., Stewart, W.F., and Wood, G.C. (2009). Improving detection and treatment of osteoporosis: Redesigning care using the electronic medical record and shared medical appointments. *Osteoporosis International, 20(1), 37-42.*

Bakitas, M., Lyons, M.D., Hegel, M.T., Balan, S., Brokaw, F.C., Seville, J., Hull, J., Li, Z., Tosteson, T., Byock, I., and Ahles, T.A. (2009). Effects of a palliative care intervention on clinical outcomes in patients with advanced cancer. *JAMA, 302(7), 741-749.*

Yehle, K.S., Sands, L.P., Rhynders, P.A., and Newton, G.D. (2009). The effect of shared medical visits on knowledge and self-care in patients with heart failure: A pilot study. *Heart and Lung: The Journal of Acute and Critical Care, 38(1), 25-33.*

Lorig, K., Sobel, D., Stewart, A., Brown, B., Bandura, A., Ritter, P., Gonzalez, J., Laurent, D., and Halsted, H. (1999). Evidence suggesting that a chronic disease self-management program can improve health status while reducing hospitalization: A randomized trial. *Medical Care, 37(1), 5-14.*

Bodenheimer T. (2003). Interventions to improve chronic illness care: evaluating their effectiveness. *Dis Manag.* 6:63-71.

Bodenheimer, T., Lorig, K., Holman, H. & Grumbach, K. (2002). Patient Self-management of Chronic Disease in Primary Care. *JAMA,* 288:2469-2475.

Bodenheimer T., Wagner E. & Grumbach K. (2002). Improving primary care for patients with chronic illness: the chronic care model. *JAMA.* 288:1775-1779.

Coleman, K., Austin, B. T., Brach, C. & Wagner, E. H. (2009). Evidence on the chronic care model in the new millennium. *Health Aff, 29(1):* 75-85.

Edleman, D., Fredrickson, S. K., Melnuk, S. D., Coffman, C. J., Jefferys, A. S. et al. (2010). Medical clinics versus usual care for patients with both diabetes and hypertension: A randomized trial. *Annals of Internal Medicine, 152(11)*: 689-696.

Frayne, S. M., Halanych, J. H., Miller, D. R., Wang, F., Lin, H. et al. (2005). Disparities in Diabetes Care Impact of Mental Illness *Arch Intern Med.* 165: 2631-2638.

Geriatrics Interdisciplinary Advisory Group. (2006). Interdisciplinary care for older adults with complex needs: American Geriatrics Society position statement. *Journal of American Geriatrics Society.* 54:849-852.

Greenhalgh, T., Robert, G., Macfarlane, F., Bate, P. & Kyriakidou, O. (2004). Diffusion of innovations in service organizations: Systematic review and recommendations. *The Milbank Quarterly, 82(4)*: 581-629.

Harris, R. S., Jr., Aldea, M. A. & Kirkley, D. E. (2006). A motivational interviewing and common factors approach to change in working with alcohol use and abuse in college students. *Professional Psychology Research and Practice, 37* (6): 614-621.

Heisler M. & Piette, J. D. (2005). "I Help You, and You Help Me": Facilitated Telephone Peer Support Among Patients With Diabetes. *The Diabetes Educator*, 31(6): 869 – 879.

Kasper E., Gertoblith G., Hefter G. et al. (2002). A randomized trial of the efficacy of multidisciplinary care in heart failure outpatients at high risk of hospital readmission. *J Am Coll Cardiol.* 39:471-480.

Kern, E. F., Beischel, S., Stalnaker, R., Aron, D. C., Kirsh, S., Watts, S. A. (2008). Building a diabetes registry from the Veterans Health Administration's computerized patient record system. *Diabetes Science and Technology, 2*: 7-14.

Kirsh, S. R, Lawrence, R. & Aron D. C. (2008). Tailoring an intervention to the context and system redesign related to the intervention: A case study of implementing shared medical appointments for diabetes. *Implementation Science*, 3:34.

Kirsh, S. R. & Aron, D. (2008). Integrating the chronic care model and the ACGME competencies: using shared medical appointments to focus on system-based practice. *Quality and Safety in Health Care.* 17:15-19.

Kirsh, S. R., Schaub, K. & Aron, D. C. (2009). Shared medical appointments: A potential venue for education in interprofessional care. *Quality Management in Health Care, 18(3)*: 218-225.

Kirsh S. R., Watts S., Pascuzzi K. et al. (2007). Shared medical appointments based on the chronic care model: a quality improvement project to address the challenges of patients with diabetes with high cardiovascular risk. *Quality Safety in Health Care.* 16:349-353.

Martin, O. J., Wu, W., Taveira, T. H., Eaton, C. B., Sharma, S. C. (2007). Multidisciplinary group behavioral and pharmacologic intervention for cardiac risk reduction in diabetes: A pilot study. *The Diabetes Educator, 33(1)*: 118-127.

McAlister F., Lawson F. & Teo K. (2001). A systematic review of randomized trials of disease management programs in heart failure. *Am J Med.* 110:378-384.

Miller, W. R. (2004). Motivational interviewing in the service of health promotion. Art of Health Promotion in *American Journal of Health Promotion*, 18(3), 1-10.

Miller, W. R. & Rollnick, S. (1991). Motivational interviewing: Preparing people to change addictive behavior. New York: Guilford Press.

Miller, W. R. & Rollnick, S. (1995). What is Motivational Interviewing? *Behavioral and Cognitive Psychotherapy*, 23(4): 325–334.

Miller, W. R., & Rollnick, S. (2002). Motivational interviewing: Preparing people for change (2nd ed.). New York: Guilford Press.

Oandasan, I. (2004). Interdisciplinary Education for Collaborative, Patient-Centred Practice. Research and Findings Report. *Health Canada*. Available from http://www.ferasi.umontreal.ca/eng/07_info/IECPCP_Final_Report.pdf

Olsson, C. A., Boyce, M. F., Toumbourou, J. W. & Sawyer, S. M. (2005). The Role of Peer Support in Facilitating Psychosocial Adjustment to Chronic Illness in Adolescence. *Clinical Child Psychology and Psychiatry*, 10 (1): 78-87.

Sadur, C. N., Moline, N., Michalik, D., Mendlowitz, D., Roller, S. et al. (1999). Diabetes management in a health maintenance organization: efficacy of care management using cluster visits. *Diabetes Care, 22:* 2011-2017.

Simpson G., Rabin D., Schmitt M., Taylor P., Urban S. & Ball J. (2001). Interprofessional health care practice: Recommendations of the National Academies of practice expert panel on health care in the 21st century. *Issues in Interdisciplinary Care.* 3:5-19.

Singh, D. (2005). Transforming Chronic Care: Evidence for Improving Care for People with Long-Term Conditions. Univ. Birmingham Health Services Mgt Ctr, Birmingham, UK.

Trento M., Passera P., Tomalino M. et al. (2001). Group Visits Improve Metabolic Control in Type 2 Diabetes: A 2-year follow-up. *Diabetes Care.* 24:995-1000.

Wagner E. (2000). The role of patient care teams in chronic disease management. *BMJ.* 320: 569-572.

Wagner, E. H., Grothaus, L. C., Sandhu, N., Galvin, M. S., McGregor, M., Artz, K., Coleman, E. A. (2001). Chronic care clinics for diabetes in primary care: A system-wide randomized trial. *Diabetes Care, 24:* 695-700.

Wagner E., Austin B. & Von Korff M. (1996). Organizing care for patients with chronic illness. *Milbank Quarterly.* 74:511-544.

Weinger, K. (2003). Group interventions: Emerging applications for diabetes care. *Diabetes Spectrum,* 16; 86-87.

8

The Effects of Lifestyle Modification on Glycemic Levels and Medication Intake: The Rockford CHIP

Heike S. Englert[1], Hans A. Dieh[2], Roger L. Greenlaw[3] and Steve Aldana[4]
[1]University of Applied Sciences Muenster, Department of Nutritional Sciences,
[2]Lifestyle Medicine Institute, Loma Linda, CA,
[3]Center for Complementary Medicine, SwedishAmerican Health System, Rockford, IL,
[4]Lifestyle Research Group, Mapleton, UT,
[1]Germany
[2,3,4]USA

1. Introduction

The high prevalence of cardiovascular disease (CVD) in the past 50 years has led to intense research, resulting in many improvements in treatment. At the same time, type 2 diabetes, with its concomitant increase in vascular complications, has become a serious, exploding, and costly public health concern (1;2).

Diabetes now affects 285 million adults worldwide and 344 million with pre-diabetes. Of these, 25.8 million diabetics and 79 million pre-diabetics are found in the United States alone (3).

The current cost of diabetes in the US is likely to exceed the $174 billion estimate, which includes 2/3 for direct medical costs and 1/3 for indirect costs, such as disability, work loss, and premature death, but omits the social cost of intangibles (e.g. pain, suffering, lower quality of life) (4-6).

The diabetes epidemic has been accompanied by a similarly drastic increase in obesity. Although the relationship between the two developments is a matter of debate, both are presumably caused by changes in dietary habits and an increasingly sedentary modern lifestyle (7;8). Compelling evidence has shown that lifestyle changes can effectively prevent or delay the occurrence of type 2 diabetes (9-12).

Because individuals at risk for this disease can usually be identified during the pre-diabetic phase of impaired glucose tolerance, early intervention and lifestyle change offer a logical approach to preventing this disease and its devastating vascular complications (13).

Additionally, community-based lifestyle interventions for high risk groups and for the general population are a cost-effective way of curbing the growing burden of the disease (14).

Solidifying the scientific basis for the prevention, treatment and control of this disease and its implementation on a national level, however, remains a difficult challenge (15;16). More research is needed to provide comprehensive and more effective strategies for weight-loss, especially over time (17;18).

Therefore, the objectives of this study were to identify diabetics and those at risk (pre-diabetics) out of the total cohort of 1,517 who selected themselves into an intensive community-based lifestyle intervention program, and to assess its clinical efficacy in effecting medication status as determined and managed by their personal physicians.

2. Methods

CHIP is a 4-week, community-based intensive educational lifestyle intervention program. The project is designed to assess the extent to which a self-selected population can contribute to a shift in coronary risk factors in the community-at-large aiming at primary and secondary prevention.

The participants were recruited from the general population through presentations at service clubs, churches, corporations, as well as through media exposure, billboards, brochures, and healthcare providers.

To be included in the program, participants had to be at least 21 years of age, free of current cancer treatment, at least 3 months post bypass surgery, not afflicted by alcoholism, and able to engage in walking exercises. Eligible and interested participants provided informed consent. All participants were advised to work closely with their personal physicians to monitor clinical changes and to facilitate medication adjustments.

The 40-hour educational intervention with behavioral and skill development content consisted of a carefully crafted 16-session series offered Monday through Thursday for 2 hours over a 4-week period (for details please see Englert et al (19)). Through these almost daily meetings with lectures, clinical Q & A sessions and reading assignments (syllabus, text- and workbooks), the participants became acquainted with some of the extensive epidemiological literature describing the importance of lifestyle factors in the etiology and treatment of chronic circulatory diseases with a focus on a simpler, more *Optimal Diet* used *ad libitum* (20). In addition, several workshops (cooking classes, food-shopping tours, and clinical breakout sessions) were offered during the program to provide the skills needed for adopting a simpler diet. The workshops emphasized the importance of consuming more whole foods, such as fruits and vegetables, legumes and whole-grain products as a way to facilitate lower energy intake with reduced fat ($\leq$20% of total calories), cholesterol ($\leq$50 mg), salt ($\leq$5 gm), and refined sugar, and enhanced fiber content (>30 to 40 gm) (for details please see Englert et al (21)). Furthermore, the CHIP program promoted smoking cessation and recommended a daily exercise program consisting of 30 minutes of walking and general fitness. At the end of the program, participants were encouraged to join the Rockford CHIP Alumni Organization and attend the monthly educational and support meetings for maintenance.

Prior to the educational intervention, all participants underwent blood testing for fasting glucose and lipid levels, and filled out standardized questionnaires on food and tabacco habits and physical activity. The second biometric assessment took place at the conclusion of the 4-

week program. Patients were screened, questionnaires were completed and blood was drawn by the same trained clinical team to assure standardized procedure for quality control.

As part of the "before" and "after" screening, participants were required to complete a lifestyle/nutrition knowledge test and to fill out personal lifestyle evaluation forms, which included a self-reported medical history, socio-economic details, food-frequency diary, stress level, smoking history, and exercise inventory.

The clinical definitions used for fasting glucose levels are set by the American Diabetes Association (22): normal glucose: <100mg/dl; pre-diabetes: 100 to 125 mg/dl; diabetes: >125 mg/dl.

Weekly physical activity was assessed by frequency and duration of exercise during a usual week: *sedentary lifestyle score 0* (no exercise or at the most 2 times/week for 30 minutes or less than 13 min/day); *moderate score 1* (3 to 5 times/week physical activity for 30 minutes or between 13 and 22 min/day); *optimal score 2* (6 to 7 times/week physical activity for 30 minutes or more than 22 min/day) (23).

2.1 Statistical analyses

The following data are from the *consolidation phase* of the Rockford CHIP research project (19). From the fall of 2000 to the fall of 2002, we conducted 5 CHIP programs, with an average enrollment of 300 per program. Out of a total of 1,569 participants, 52 did not meet the graduation criteria, leaving a cohort of 1,517 men and women for this analysis. In the subgroup analysis presented here, we focused on 758 participants with pre-diabetes and type 2 diabetes (21).

Before each lecture, participants signed in at the registration desk. Those who attended fewer than 13 of the 16 meetings or failed to provide complete clinical data sets did not meet the graduation requirements (drop-outs), and their data were not included in this analysis.

Data were entered twice for accuracy and then analyzed using SPSS 13.0. After testing for homogeneity, the 5 datasets were pooled and analyzed. Paired t tests were used to detect before and after changes as continuous variables. McNemar tests were performed for categorical variables and χ^2 –tests for differences in men and women at baseline and after 4 weeks. Analysis of covariance was performed with fasting glucose changes as the dependent variable, and gender, age, and changes in weight (BMI), triglycerides, and physical activity as independent variables.

3. Results

The socio-demographic characteristics of the 758 pre-diabetics and diabetics are presented in Table 1. The gender composition was 432 women and 326 men. The age span ranged from 21 to 81 years. The average age for men was 58 (SD 11) and for women 56 (SD 11). Because no correlation was found between risk improvement and age, data were not age adjusted.

Table 2 depicts the profile of the cohort with reference to diabetes-related risk factors at admission. Of these, 69% were classified as pre-diabetics and 31% as type 2 diabetics, 29% were overweight (BMI between 26 and 30), and 59% were obese (BMI >30). 74% reported a sedentary lifestyle.

	Total (N=758)
Gender	43% men, 57% women
Age (yrs)	58 yrs (men), 56 yrs (women)
Marital status	
married	81%
single	6%
divorced	7%
widowed	6%
Education	
< 12 years	6%
12 years	21%
some college	59%
college or more	14%

Table 1. Socio-demographics: the Rockford CHIP (Illinois, USA)

	Men (N=326)	Women (N=432)	Total (N=758)
Age ≥45 years	91%	89%	90%
Pre-diabetes (Glucose ≥100 to 125 mg/dl)	66%	71%	69%
Diabetes (Glucose >125 mg/dl and/or on hypoglycemic medication)	34%	29%	31%
Overweight (BMI between 26 and 30)	32%	26%	29%
Obese (BMI >30)	57%	61%	59%
Hypertension (SBP ≥130 or DBP ≥ 85mmHg and/or on antihypertensive medication)	87%	79%	83%
Triglycerides (≥250 mg/dl)	20%	15%	17%
LDL Cholesterol (LDL ≥100 mg/dl and/or on hypolipidemic medication)	90%	86%	88%
Sedentary Lifestyle	67%	79%	74%

Table 2. Diabetes related risk factors of pre-diabetics and diabetics at admission: the Rockford CHIP (Illinois, USA)

Figure 1 shows the flow diagram of the total cohort with reference to pre-diabetes and diabetes after the initial screening. Out of the total cohort of 758 participants, 521 (69%) were classified as pre-diabetics and 237 (31%) as type 2 diabetics. Among the latter group, 154 persons were on medication. A significant number of the 83 diabetic subjects not receiving medication were unaware of their condition. The effects of the CHIP lifestyle intervention program on fasting glucose levels in these participants not taking medication with pre-diabetes (n=521) and type 2 diabetes (n=83) can be seen in figure 2. Glucose levels improved significantly in both pre-diabetics and diabetics - the higher the initial glucose, the greater the glucose reduction. In many cases, diabetic glucose levels were brought down into the normal range. Among the pre-diabetics, 47% (25% women and 22% men) were able to lower their glucose below 100mg/dl.

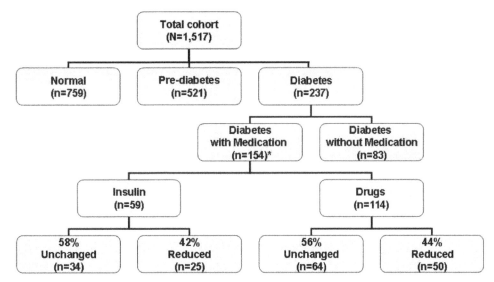

Fig. 1. Flow Diagram according to baseline assessment: the Rockford CHIP (Illinois, USA)

Tables 3 and 4 present the mean changes in fasting glucose in subjects receiving medication (oral hypoglycemics and/or insulin), stratified by gender and medication changes. 44% of those on oral drugs and 42% of those on insulin were advised by their personal physician to reduce their daily medication dosage. In participants whose glucose levels were initially above 125 mg/dl, glucose levels improved on the average between 38 to 49 mg/dl in men and 22 to 27 mg/dl in women. In diabetics with initial levels >125 mg/dl whose medication dosage remained the same, the reductions in glucose levels were equally impressive: the average reduction in men was from 18 mg/dl to 43 mg/dl and in women from 39 to 42 mg/dl. Of those 19 diabetics taking both insulin and drugs, 15 participants were able to reduce their daily doses even so glucose levels dropped by 8 mg/dl and 67 mg/dl in women and men, respectively.

35% of the diabetics were able to reduce their glucose levels below 125 mg/dl. Of these individuals, 10% were even able to reduce them to below 100 mg/dl.

Triglyceride levels in women dropped significantly from 171 mg/dl to 163 mg/dl, and in men from 182mg/dl to 147 mg/dl. LDL levels in women dropped from 122 mg/dl to 112 mg/dl and from 118 mg/dl to 96 mg/dl in men. Moreover average, systolic and diastolic blood pressure was reduced from 140/85 mmHg to 133/79 mmHg in women and 141/85 to 132/80 mmHg in men.

During the 4-week CHIP program, the mean weight reduction was 9 pounds for men and 7 pounds for women. Figure 3 shows that those who needed to lose the most weight lost the most.

	Men (n=57) Means			Women (n=57) Means		
	before	after	change	before	after	change
Glucose (mg/dl)						
drug dosage reduction*						
≤125 (n=12)	108	123	+15	109	118	+9
>125 (n=38)	166	128	-38	175	153	-22
drug dosage unchanged						
≤125 (n=18)	114	109	-5	114	112	-2
>125 (n=46)	178	135	-43	189	150	-39

* reductions: more than 10% of the daily dose

Table 3. Mean changes over 4 weeks in fasting glucose in diabetics on oral drugs by gender (n=114), according to admission levels: the Rockford CHIP (Illinois, USA)

	Men (n=28) Means			Women (n=31) Means		
	before	after	change	before	after	change
Glucose (mg/dl)						
Insulin dosage reductions*						
≤ 125 (n=7)	112	107	-5	114	112	-2
> 125 (n=18)	174	125	-49	178	151	-27
Insulin dosage unchanged						
≤ 125 (n=6)	121	105	-16	110	106	-4
> 125 (n=28)	136	118	-18	131	89	-42

* reductions: more than 10% of the daily dose

Table 4. Mean changes over 4 weeks in fasting glucose in diabetics on insulin by gender (n=59), according to admission levels: the Rockford CHIP (Illinois, USA)

Figure 4 shows significant improvements in physical activity. At the beginning of the intervention, 79% of women and 67% of men reported little or no physical activity, 19% and 28% reported engaging in moderate exercise, and 2% and 5% reported engaging in optimal physical activity. After the 4-week program, only 38% of women and 31% of men reported little or no physical activity, 54% and 58% reported moderate physical activity, and 8% and 12% optimal physical activity.

The Analysis of Covariance for glucose changes in participants with pre-diabetes and type 2 diabetes showed significant results for gender (p≤0.001), BMI (p≤0.001), and triglycerides (p≤0.001) but not for physical activity. Improvements in weight and blood glucose were significantly higher in men than in women. In general, after adjusting for gender, reductions in blood glucose were positively related to weight loss - the higher the weight loss, the greater the improvement in blood glucose.

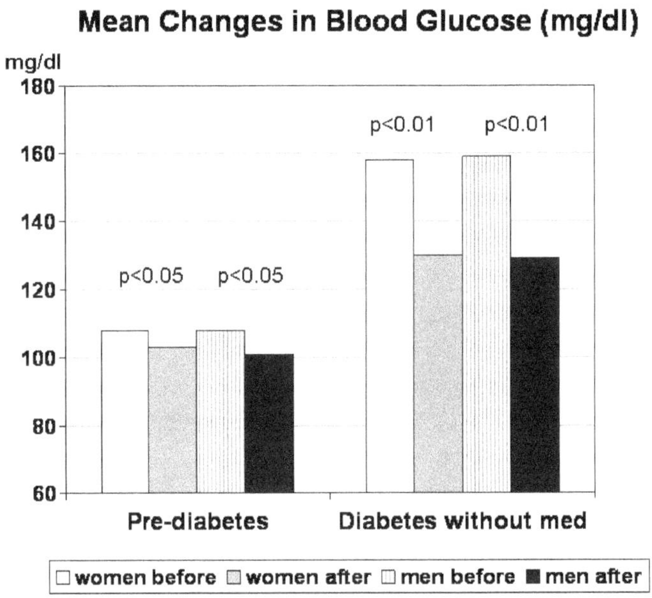

Mean Changes in Blood Glucose (mg/dl)

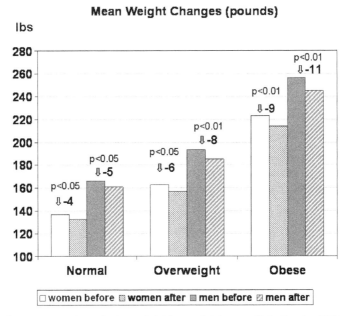

Fig. 2. Mean changes over 4 weeks in fasting glucose in pre-diabetics (n=83) and diabetics (n=521) not on medication: the Rockford CHIP (Illinois, USA)

Mean Weight Changes (pounds)

Fig. 3. Mean changes over 4 weeks in weight (pounds) in pre-diabetics (n=521) and diabetics (n=237): the Rockford CHIP (Illinois, USA)

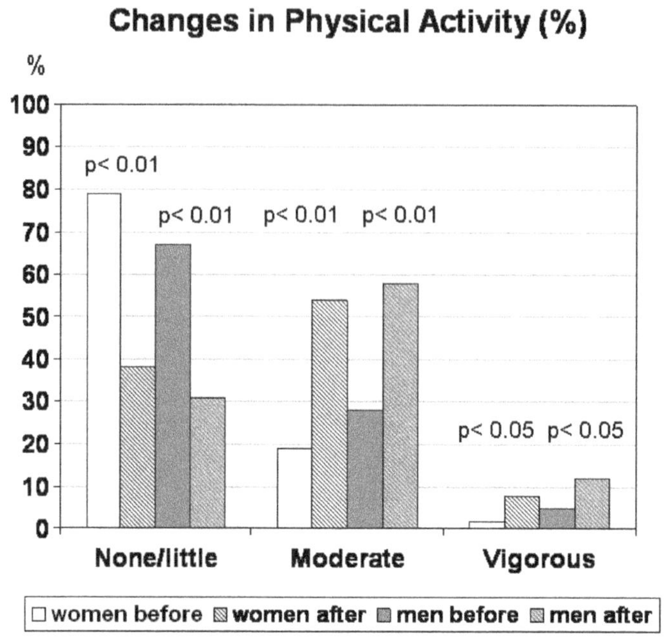

Changes in Physical Activity (%)

Fig. 4. Changes (in %) over 4 weeks in physical activity in pre-diabetics and diabetics (N=758): the Rockford CHIP (Illinois, USA)

4. Discussion

Primary and secondary prevention of type 2 diabetes is the most promising way to alleviate the ever-growing global burden of this disease (24-26). The aim of this community-based CHIP program was thus to translate theoretical knowledge on the subject into well-defined, real-world strategies for screening and treating a population high at risk for type 2 diabetes.

5. Diabetes risk profile

Half of the total cohort of the CHIP consolidation phase (n=1,517) had already or was at risk for diabetes. This sub analysis showed that 35% of the diabetics had never been diagnosed or received diabetes treatment previously. High rates in diabetes related risk factors such as overweight/obesity (88%), hypertension (83%) and LDL-Cholesterol (88%) is most likely an expression of individual lifestyle choices and the interaction with the environment.

6. Effects of CHIP

CHIP led to an improved risk profile in this high risk patient group. Glucose levels in the pre-diabetics and diabetics who were not on medication improved between 5 mg/dl and 30 mg/dl depending on gender and baseline values.

Similar reductions were observed in the 154 participants who were taking diabetes medication. It is noteworthy that these changes in fasting glucose made it possible – under physicians' supervision – to reduce the dose of diabetes medication in approximately 40% of cases. Despite this dosage reduction, the decrease in glucose levels was clinically relevant in the majority of diabetics. Eliminating or reducing the intake of these medications is desirable from both a medical and health economic perspective because of their side effects and costs (27).

7. Critical factors of success of the CHIP program

CHIP focuses mainly on 5 process steps: 1) Identification and enrollment of participants with type 2 diabetes or high at risk. 2) Risk profile assessment (HeartScreen-examination). 3) Behavior change (intense, flexible, culturally sensitive, and individualized 16-lesson curriculum that covers diet, exercise, and behavioral modification). 4) Behavior maintenance (alumni groups and supportive community). 5) Evaluation.

7.1 Lifestyle changes

Diet and exercise: There is little discrepancy about the fact that exercise and weight loss play a vital role in the treatment of pre-diabetes and diabetes. Both have been shown to improve insulin resistance and hyperglycemia (16). A review by Miller & Dustan summarizes data on the effectiveness of physical-activity interventions for treating overweight/obesity and type 2 diabetes. Most of the reported exercise-based interventions have been conducted in clinical settings; and they have often required the use of extensive resources (28). In the CHIP-study we recommended a minimum regimen of 30 min/day of moderate-intensity exercise, such as brisk walking (which harmonizes well the recommendations from the American Diabetes Association (ADA) and also the American Association of Clinical Endocrinologists (AACE). There was a significant improvement in physical activity levels in both men and women. In total, 46% of the participants reported that they had increased their level of physical activity to at least 30 minutes a day, or 210 minutes a week. It is noteworthy that, at the beginning of the program, 74% of participants reported no physical activity at all, while at the end only 35% were physically inactive. Tuomilehto et al observed that achieving a relatively conservative target of at least 210 minutes of exercise per week was associated with a significant reduction in the risk of diabetes, even in subjects without weight loss (9).

Depending on initial weight and gender, the CHIP participants were able to reduce their weight within 4 weeks by up to 5%, which approaches the 7% weight loss goal of the ADA for people with diabetes. Exercise, as an integral part of the CHIP intervention, obviously facilitates loss of excessive weight which contributes to improvements in glycemic control and the need for medication (29). While a BMI >30 has been shown to double the incidence of sudden death, and a moderate increase in BMI can lead to a 4- to 8-fold increase in the risk of diabetes, in males and females, respectively, Mobley and coworkers observed the benefits of weight loss on cardiovascular morbidity and mortality (28). Furthermore, weight reduction has been shown to improve endothelial function and decreased systemic inflammatory reaction (30).

While there is little disagreement about the importance of a sensible and consistent activity program in the prevention and management of diabetes, there is still considerable debate about the most effective therapeutic diet. Several authors and study groups have supported the idea that diets low in carbohydrate content yet relatively high in protein and fat may be more beneficial for pre-diabetics and full blown Type 2 diabetics than high carbohydrate diets since they had been shown to cause hyperglycemia (31-36). Over the years, the ADA gradually reduced their high fat and animal protein recommendations in that they obviously contribute to higher lipid levels thus promoting vascular complications, the very bane of people with diabetes. The ADA also liberalized their once so rigid stand against the intake of sugar and fresh fruits and began to recommend more fresh vegetables and whole grains and more legumes. And yet, while some progress has been made, the current dietary guidelines (recommending the use of meat, poultry, fish and non-rich dairy) are still facilitating an atherogenic diet with up to 7% of the calories consumed coming from saturated fat which also bring along some 200 mg of cholesterol. The current ADA guidelines still reflect the fear of recommending the higher levels of carbohydrate intake, because insufficient attention has been paid to the fundamental difference of how the body handles the digestion and absorption of (1) complex vs. simple carbohydrates (starches vs sugars) and of (2) their unrefined vs refined counterparts (whole grains vs white flour and whole orange vs. orange juice). Unrefined complex carbohydrates with their usually high fiber content become absorbed and digested much more slowly. Thus giving the pancreas more time not to overreact with excessive insulin to reduce the blood glucose levels that usually raise quickly after a slug of sugar, as in a glass of orange juice, where the pancreas has to deal with a highly refined simple carbohydrate totally depleted of any fiber (37).

The CHIP *Optimal Diet* is an *"ad libitum"*, plant-based, very low-fat, low-sugar, high-complex-carbohydrate/low-glycemic, high-fiber regimen with low energy density. In a 22-week clinical trial, Barnard and coworkers were able to show that such a very low-fat plant based, high carbohydrate (70% of calories) diet improved significantly not only the levels of glycemia, but also the levels of lipids and kidney function but clearly exceeded the clinical results of the other intervention diet formulated according to the guidelines of the ADA (38). A recent review concluded that the results from observational and clinical trials demonstrate that low-fat, unrefined plant-based diets are *at least* as effective as more conventional diabetes diets for weight reduction and glycemic control, and that they are significantly more effective in the management of lipid and renal function and in the cost and ease of meal preparation (39).

7.2 Intensive education and curriculum

CHIP is an intensive educational program where participants become aware of the potential benefits of making healthy lifestyle changes and learn how to implement them. The educational curriculum is structured to build progressively and incrementally the concepts of lifestyle medicine. Since habits are best built through daily practice, the program was purposely conducted on an almost every day basis over a period of 4 weeks (40).

7.3 Social support

The group support setting for each of the sessions provided strong social support and may have contributed to the low drop-out rate of 3%.

7.4 Community setting

In the present study we focused on public awareness within the community of Rockford to ensure that individuals high at risk for coronary heart disease and/or diabetes are sensitized. Our experiences show that a successful health management requires an optimal cooperation of health players in the community. Building up a infrastructure of health-facilitators and multiplicators in the community supports the CHIP-philosophy. Effective diabetes lifestyle interventions must target not only the affected individuals, but also families, workplaces, schools etc. Preventing this disease epidemic calls for the identification of culture-sensitive measures that can be applied both to the general population and to high-risk groups. The CHIP strategy is to combine behavior-oriented prevention (e.g. optimal diet, physical activity) with infrastructure-oriented prevention (e.g. supportive community, group support) to promote positive long-term outcomes.

8. Limitations

Self Selection. With its goal of cultural transformation, the CHIP program purposefully aimed at enrolling participants who were probably more motivated and better informed about the need to make healthier lifestyle choices. However, the aim was to build a foundation with motivated people in the community, who, in turn, would become role models in the community-at-large.

Short term results only and lack of control group. It is well known that short-term behavioral changes are subject to decay over time and long-term effectiveness as well as causality cannot be demonstrated without evaluating the program in a randomized controlled trial over an extended period. Moreover, the dimensions to which the CHIP Alumni Association with its refresher courses and monthly meetings can contribute to sustaining these short-term results remain to be subject to further investigation. Even so, the current lack of a randomized control group should not diminish the fact that the vast majority of the subgroup of 758 pre-diabetics and diabetics with multiple risk factors were able to markedly reduce their risk profile in 4 weeks.

9. Conclusion

Diabetes mellitus was very common in this free-living CHIP-cohort with 35% of the individuals being unaware of their condition. The consistently lowered glucose levels in the pre-diabetics and diabetics alike, even in those whose medication dosage had been lowered, suggests that lifestyle changes can be effective in lowering glycemic levels and the need for medication. This lifestyle intervention approach used in a community setting may contribute significantly to reducing the incidence and prevalence of type 2 diabetes at the population level. Until long-term evaluations, however, have been completed, it remains to be seen whether these improvement may **prevent or merely delay** the manifestation on diabetes.

10. Declarations

The study was approved by the IRB of the SwedishAmerican Health System in Rockford, IL, USA.

The study was financially supported by the Swedish American Health System in Rockford, IL, USA.

None of the authors had a conflict of interest.

11. Acknowledgement

We would like to thank the SwedishAmerican Health System for their financial support and the participants for their contribution.

12. References

[1] Nicasio J, El-Atat F, McFarlane SI, LaRosa JH. Cardiovascular disease in diabetes and the cardiometabolic syndrome: focus on minority women. Curr Diab Rep 2005 Jun;5(3):208-13.

[2] AlJaroudi WA, Petersen JL. Obesity, diabetes, and associated risk factors. Curr Treat Options Cardiovasc Med 2006 Feb;8(1):67-78.

[3] Unwin N, Gan D, Whiting D. The IDF Diabetes Atlas: providing evidence, raising awareness and promoting action. Diabetes Res Clin Pract 2010 Jan;87(1):2-3.

[4] Cheng D. Prevalence, predisposition and prevention of type II diabetes. Nutr Metab (Lond) 2005 Oct 18;2:29.

[5] van der Bruggen M HRBGBWBC. Lifestyle Intervention Are Cost-effective in People With Different Levels of Diabetes Risk. Diabets Care 2007;30(1):128-34.

[6] Dall T MSZYMJCYHP. Economic Costs of Diabetes in the US in 2007. Diabtes Care 2008;31(3):596.

[7] Roberts CK, Barnard RJ. Effects of exercise and diet on chronic disease. J Appl Physiol 2005 Jan;98(1):3-30.

[8] Panagiotakos DB, Pitsavos C, Chrysohoou C, Stefanadis C. The epidemiology of Type 2 diabetes mellitus in Greek adults: the ATTICA study. Diabet Med 2005 Nov;22(11):1581-8.

[9] Tuomilehto J, Lindstrom J, Eriksson JG, Valle TT, Hamalainen H, Ilanne-Parikka P, et al. Prevention of type 2 diabetes mellitus by changes in lifestyle among subjects with impaired glucose tolerance. N Engl J Med 2001 May 3;344(18):1343-50.

[10] Lindstrom J, Ilanne-Parikka P, Peltonen M, Aunola S, Eriksson JG, Hemio K, et al. Sustained reduction in the incidence of type 2 diabetes by lifestyle intervention: follow-up of the Finnish Diabetes Prevention Study. Lancet 2006 Nov 11;368(9548):1673-9.

[11] Narayan KM, Kanaya AM, Gregg EW. Lifestyle intervention for the prevention of type 2 diabetes mellitus: putting theory to practice. Treat Endocrinol 2003;2(5):315-20.

[12] Jermendy G. Can type 2 diabetes mellitus be considered preventable? Diabetes Res Clin Pract 2005 Jun;68 Suppl1:S73-S81.

[13] Wylie-Rosett J, Herman WH, Goldberg RB. Lifestyle intervention to prevent diabetes: intensive AND cost effective. Curr Opin Lipidol 2006 Feb;17(1):37-44.

[14] Bantle JP, Wylie-Rosett J, Albright AL, Apovian CM, Clark NG, Franz MJ, et al. Nutrition recommendations and interventions for diabetes: a position statement of the American Diabetes Association. Diabetes Care 2008 Jan;31 Suppl 1:S61-S78.

[15] Bazzano LA, Serdula M, Liu S. Prevention of type 2 diabetes by diet and lifestyle modification. J Am Coll Nutr 2005 Oct;24(5):310-9.

[16] Inzucchi SE, Sherwin RS. The prevention of type 2 diabetes mellitus. Endocrinol Metab Clin North Am 2005 Mar;34(1):199-219, viii.

[17] Wadden TA, Butryn ML, Byrne KJ. Efficacy of lifestyle modification for long-term weight control. Obes Res 2004 Dec;12 Suppl:151S-62S.

[18] Williamson DA, Stewart TM. Behavior and lifestyle: approaches to treatment of obesity. J La State Med Soc 2005 Jan;157 Spec No 1:S50-S55.

[19] Englert HS, Diehl HA, Greenlaw RL. Rationale and design of the Rockford CHIP, a community-based coronary risk reduction program: results of a pilot phase. Prev Med 2004 Apr;38(4):432-41.

[20] Diehl HA. Coronary risk reduction through intensive community-based lifestyle intervention: the Coronary Health Improvement Project (CHIP) experience. Am J Cardiol 1998 Nov 26;82(10B):83T-7T.

[21] Englert HS, Diehl HA, Greenlaw RL. Rationale and design of the Rockford CHIP, a community-based coronary risk reduction program: results of a pilot phase. Prev Med 2007 Feb;44:513-519.

[22] The Expert Committee on the Diagnosis and Classification of Diabetes Mellitus. Position Paper - diagnosis and classification of diabetes mellitus. Diabetes Care 2008;31(1):S55-S59.

[23] Sherwin RS, Anderson RM, Buse JB, Chin MH, Eddy D, Fradkin J, et al. Prevention or delay of type 2 diabetes. Diabetes Care 2004 Jan;27 Suppl 1:S47-S54.

[24] Daskalopoulou SS, Mikhailidis DP, Elisaf M. Prevention and treatment of the metabolic syndrome. Angiology 2004 Nov;55(6):589-612.

[25] Chiasson JL, Brindisi MC, Rabasa-Lhoret R. The prevention of type 2 diabetes: what is the evidence? Minerva Endocrinol 2005 Sep;30(3):179-91.

[26] Laakso M. Prevention of type 2 diabetes. Curr Mol Med 2005 May;5(3):365-74.

[27] Rosenberg DE, Jabbour SA, Goldstein BJ. Insulin resistance, diabetes and cardiovascular risk: approaches to treatment. Diabetes Obes Metab 2005 Nov;7(6):642-53.

[28] Miller YD, Dunstan DW. The effectiveness of physical activity interventions for the treatment of overweight and obesity and type 2 diabetes. J Sci Med Sport 2004 Apr;7(1 Suppl):52-9.

[29] Tonstad S, Butler T, Yan R, Fraser GE. Type of vegetarian diet, body weight, and prevalence of type 2 diabetes. Diabetes Care 2009 May;32(5):791-6.

[30] Mobley CC. Lifestyle interventions for "diabesity": the state of the science. Compend Contin Educ Dent 2004 Mar;25(3):207-2, 214.

[31] Sestoft L, Krarup T, Palmvig B, Meinertz H, Faergeman O. High-carbohydrate, low-fat diet: effect on lipid and carbohydrate metabolism, GIP and insulin secretion in diabetics. Dan Med Bull 1985 Mar;32(1):64-9.

[32] Parker B, Noakes M, Luscombe N, Clifton P. Effect of a high-protein, high-monounsaturated fat weight loss diet on glycemic control and lipid levels in type 2 diabetes. Diabetes Care 2002 Mar;25(3):425-30.

[33] Nielsen JV, Joensson E. Low-carbohydrate diet in type 2 diabetes. Stable improvement of bodyweight and glycemic control during 22 months follow-up. Nutr Metab (Lond) 2006;3:22.

[34] Halton TL, Liu S, Manson JE, Hu FB. Low-carbohydrate-diet score and risk of type 2 diabetes in women. Am J Clin Nutr 2008 Feb;87(2):339-46.

[35] Shai I, Schwarzfuchs D, Henkin Y, Shahar DR, Witkow S, Greenberg I, et al. Weight loss with a low-carbohydrate, Mediterranean, or low-fat diet. N Engl J Med 2008 Jul 17;359(3):229-41.

[36] Sacks FM, Bray GA, Carey VJ, Smith SR, Ryan DH, Anton SD, et al. Comparison of weight-loss diets with different compositions of fat, protein, and carbohydrates. N Engl J Med 2009 Feb 26;360(9):859-73.

[37] American Association of Clinical Endocrinologists: AACE Medical Guidelines fpr Clinical Practice for Developing a Diabetes Mellitus Comprehensive Care Plan. Endocrine Practice 2011March;17(2):1-53.

[38] Barnard ND, Gloede L, Cohen J, Jenkins DJ, Turner-McGrievy G, Green AA, et al. A low-fat vegan diet elicits greater macronutrient changes, but is comparable in adherence and acceptability, compared with a more conventional diabetes diet among individuals with type 2 diabetes. J Am Diet Assoc 2009 Feb;109(2):263-72.

[39] Barnard ND, Katcher HI, Jenkins DJ, Cohen J, Turner-McGrievy G. Vegetarian and vegan diets in type 2 diabetes management. Nutr Rev 2009 May;67(5):255-63.

[40] Boutin-Foster C. In spite of good intentions: patients' perspectives on problematic social support interactions. Health Qual Life Outcomes 2005;3:52.

Section 2

Continuity of Care in Primary Care

9

Palliative Care in General Practice

Imma Cacciapuoti[1], Laura Signorotti[2], Maria Isabella Bonacini[3],
Oreste Capelli[4*], Maria Rolfini[4] and Antonio Brambilla[4]
[1]Dpt. of Mental Health, Modena,
[2]Dpt. of Prevention, Novara,
[3]Pharmacy Department, Derriford Hospital, Plymouth NHS Trust,
[4]The District Primary Care, Emilia-Romagna Region, Bologna,
[1,2,4]Italy
[3]UK

*"You matter because you are you. You matter to the last moment of your life, and we will
do all we can to help you not only to die peacefully, but also to live until you die."*
Dame Cicely Saunders, St. Christopher's Hospice

1. Introduction

The doctor-clown Patch Adams argued that our health care system should not treat the disease, but the patient, in an approach "patient-centered" rather than "disease-centered". Palliative care is a holistic, patient-centered, and culturally sensitive approach to care. According to the Nobel Prize winner Rita Levi Montalcini, "it's better to add life to days, rather then days to life". For those who are dying a good quality of their last days of life is more important rather than prolong unnecessarily the days of the agony. Palliative care focuses on relieving suffering and achieving the best possible quality of life for patients and their family caregivers.

Palliative medicine (from the Latin word "pallium" for mantle, as a synonym of protection) takes care of the patients (and their boundary) rather than the disease(s) that afflicts them.

Palliative care involves not only the patients themselves, but also their families and communities. In practice, palliative care integrates two essential components of care. One is the control of symptoms and pain, the other are the interventions to meet the psychological, social, and spiritual needs of the patient and the family. The palliative care framework calls for varied combinations of these two components to be provided over the full course of the illness, from diagnosis to death, and through the bereavement of family members.

The National Consensus Guidelines for Palliative Care (2011) state the goals of palliative care are to prevent and relieve suffering and to support the best possible quality of life for patients and their families, regardless of the stage of the disease or the need for other therapies.

---

* Corresponding Author

The role of the General Practitioner (GP) is central to community palliative care. Good liaison between the different professionals involved in a patient's care is extremely important for patients in palliative care. In cases where GPs have previously been dissatisfied with palliative services, this may be seen as a barrier to referral when caring for other patients (Bajwah, 2008). With a GP's longitudinal knowledge of patients, and the likelihood that they have shared the journey of the final illness with the patient, it should be beyond dispute that there should be a central role for general practice in palliative care. Physicians must adopt a vision that takes into account the effects that diseases are having not just on patients but also on patients' caregivers and loved ones, a systemic vision. (Emanuel et al, 2011).

The essence of the doctor–patient relationship makes family physicians ideally suited to provide care palliative and end-of-life. Cassell, (1982), has defined that this relationship is the very means to help relieve suffering.

In order to develop the wide term of palliative care, we would like to consider both advance care planning, aid with decision making and clinical care management.

2. Palliative care in general practice: Why is it so important?

> Mr Ralph Smith is a man 74 years old who has suffered from a pulmonary cancer for about 15 months, treated with chemotherapy and radiotherapy on the chest. He lives with his wife (72 y.o.), hemiplegic for an ictus, and a daughter (40 y.o.), who works as a primary teacher. Recently he has developed a metastatic localization in the lumbar spine with increasing pain, severe limitation to movement and urinary retention. The general conditions are quite compromised (Karnofsky Index < 40) with a very poor prognosis (less than 3 months). Ralph refused the antalgic radiotherapy on the lumbar spine proposed by the oncologist. His family doctor proposed him a palliative care program by the Home Palliative Care Team.

Palliative care, with its focus on management of symptoms, psychosocial support, and assistance with decision making, has the potential to improve the quality of care and reduce the use of medical services. However, palliative care has traditionally been delivered late in the course of disease to patients who are hospitalized in specialized inpatient units or as a consultative service for patients with uncontrolled symptoms. Previous studies (Morita et al, 2005; Zimmermann et al, 2008) have suggested that late referrals to palliative care are inadequate to alter the quality and delivery of care provided to patients with cancer. To have a meaningful effect on patients' quality of life and end-of-life care, palliative care services must be provided earlier in the course of the disease (Temel et al, 2010).

To date, evidence supporting a benefit of palliative care is sparse, with most studies having notable methodologic weaknesses, especially with respect to quality-of-life outcomes (Zimmermann et al, 2008). One study showed that Project ENABLE (Educate, Nurture, Advise, Before Life Ends), a telephone-based, psychoeducational program for patients with advanced cancer, significantly improved both quality of life and mood (Bakitas et al, 2009) .

Another recent study (Temel et al, 2010) showed that early outpatient palliative care for patients with advanced cancer can alter the use of health care services, including care at the end-of-life. Early introduction of palliative care led to less aggressive end-of-life care and showed greater documentation of resuscitation preferences in the outpatient electronic medical record, an essential step in clarifying and ensuring respect for patients' wishes about their care at the end-of-life (Walling et al, 2008). Less aggressive end-of-life care did not adversely affect survival.

Given the trends toward aggressive and costly care near the end-of-life among patients with cancer, timely introduction of palliative care may serve to mitigate unnecessary and burdensome personal and societal costs (Emanuel et al, 2002; Earle et al, 2008; Sullivan et al, 2011).

Morrison and Meier (2004) articulate five broad areas of skills that form the core of palliative medicine: physician–patient communication; assessment and treatment of symptoms; psychosocial, spiritual, and bereavement care; coordination of care. This involves defining practice standards, responsibility for educational development and implementation, research in partnership with the academy, and program and systems needs.

In palliative care, the dying is seen as having an important role, complete with tasks and expectations, that is different from the sick role when recovery is expectable (Davies, 2009). The goal is not to prolong or shorten life; rather, the process of dying is to be freed of as much unnecessary suffering as possible. The inevitable dimensions of suffering that accompany dying and death can be soothed by finding meaning and purpose in the life lived and enhancing quality of life and quality of the dying process (Emanuel et al, 2011).

Palliative care is a paradigm of excellence for the generalist. The specific nature of palliative care allows GPs to showcase the strength of a generalist approach. This 'excellence' manifests as a creative tension between evidence-based biomedical care, a patient-centered approach and the more traditional role of 'healer'. GPs think and reflect around patient stories, rather than the abstraction of data to achieve best practice care (Eti & Heidelbaugh, 2011).

Patients repeatedly emphasize the importance of the role of a family physician with whom they have had close ties over the years, and for this role to continue through the palliative stages of life (Emanuel et al, 2007). Physicians must adopt a systemic vision, a vision that takes into account the effects that diseases are having not just on patients but also on patients' caregivers and loved ones (Emanuel et al, 2011). The family physician is also well positioned to address the concerns of the patient's loved ones and assist in coping with grief, as these persons are often patients in the physicians' practice (Lehman & Daneault, 2006).

An in-depth understanding of suffering in those who are seriously ill, and responding to it, is a fundamental role of primary care. Family physicians have the capacity to stay available and involved in care in a way that is reassuring to patients and alleviates patient suffering.

The primary care physicians often must deliver the bad news, discuss the prognosis, and make appropriate referrals. When delivering bad news, it is important to prioritize the key points that the patient should retain. Physicians should assess the patient's emotional state, readiness to engage in the discussion, and level of understanding about the condition. When discussing prognosis, physicians should be sensitive to variations in how much information patients want to know. The challenge for physicians is to communicate prognosis accurately without giving false hope. Physicians also must be aware of how cultural factors may affect end-of-life discussions. Sensitivity to a patient's cultural and individual preferences will help the physician avoid stereotyping and making incorrect assumptions.

Primary care physicians have the opportunity to maintain long-term, trusting relationships with patients and are well positioned to discuss difficult issues such as incurable disease or terminal illness (Ngo-Metzger et al, 2008).

A good primary palliative care is essential, as it allows patients to remain at home as long as possible. It is known that most patients wish to do so and would eventually prefer to die at home among family and friends (Marieke et al, 2007).

A systematic review of studies (Daneaul & Dion, 2004) found that, overall, the majority of the general population as well as patients and caregivers would prefer to die at home, but the findings varied considerably by study, with the percentage of people preferring to die at home ranging from 25% to 100%.

Several studies have repeatedly shown that many terminally ill patients prefer the option of a death at home (Watson, 2008).

However there can be profound shifts in patient and caregiver preference for location of death as the illness progresses. Hinton (1994) found that the preference for a home death changed from 90% initially to 50% as death approached (Higginson & Sen-Gupta, 2000).

Most GPs testify to this being one of the more difficult, but most satisfying, parts of their job. Survey results of different populations vary considerably with regard to preference for home as the location of death (Davies & Higginson, 2004).

Helping patients die with dignity and with minimal distress has been one of the most fundamental aspects of medicine, and over the past 50 years specialistic palliative care services have increasingly worked with general practice to develop more advanced knowledge and skill than ever before.

The European Association of Palliative Care conducted a study, begun in 2003, that evaluated the situation of palliative care through Europe. A report with quantitative and qualitative data was prepared for 43/52 participating countries. In table 1 different organizational models, (Hospital based, Hospice and Home care) in European countries are shown. Iceland is at the first place with a rate of 20 service for million inhabitants, equally distributed as a hospital model or home care assistance.

Different models of service delivery have been developed and implemented throughout the countries of Europe. UK, Germany, Austria and Belgium have a well-developed and extensive network of hospices. Day Centres are a development that is characteristic of the UK with hundreds of these services currently in operation. The number of beds per million inhabitants ranges between 45-75 beds in the most advanced European countries, to only a few beds in others. The model for mobile teams or hospital support teams has been adopted in a number of countries, most notably in France (Centeno, 2007).

Italy and many other countries as Hungary, Bulgaria, Poland, Slovenia, etc. have preferably developed a Home care model based on a multidisciplinary team which include General Practitioners.

Rank	Country	Total Services/ Million Inhabitants	Hospital Support and Unit /Hospice	Home care	First Opioid used
1	Iceland	20,3	50 %	50 %	Morphine
2	United Kingdom	16,0	61 %	39%	Morphine
3	Belgium	11,6	88%	12%	Fentanyl
4	Poland	9,5	36%	64%	Morphine
5	Ireland	8,9	61%	39%	Morphine
6	Luxemburg	8,8	50%	50%	Fentanyl
7	Netherlands	8,5	100%	0%	NA
8	Armenia	8,1	67%	33%	Morphine
9	France	7,8	82%	18%	NA
10	Norway	6,7	97%	3%	Morphine
11	Austria	6,4	67%	33%	Fentanyl
12	Spain	6,0	47%	53%	Fentanyl
13	Bulgaria	5,5	39%	61%	Morphine
14	Switzerland	5,1	63%	37%	NA
15	Finland	5,0	62%	38%	Morphine
16	Hungary	4,3	35%	65%	Morphine
17	Germany	3,9	91%	9%	Morphine
18	Italy	3,8	36%	64%	Fentanyl
19	Israel	3,7	46%	54%	Oxycodone
20	Slovenia	3,6	29%	71%	Morphine
21	Moldova	3,3	15%	85%	Morphine
22	Denmark	3,3	72%	28%	Morphine
23	Cyprus	3,2	50%	50%	Morphine
24	Macedonia	2,9	67%	33%	Morphine
25	Malta	2,6	100%	0%	Morphine

NA: not available

Table 1. Palliative Care Specific Resources in Europe (Modified from EAPC, 2006)

However palliative care is still perceived by most physicians and patients as a waiver to care and a sentence to death. For these main reasons negative myths about palliative care have developed (Table 2).

These often are common barriers to the adoption and effectiveness of palliation in Primary Care. Health Systems should invest in improving the quality of Palliative Home Care to get an assistance really focused on the needs of the patient and his boundary. And it is fundamental to invest on physicians' communication skills.

Negative Myths	Palliative Care (PC) opportunities
PC means that doctors have given up on a patient.	When PC is proposed, it means that the healthcare team has realized that the disease is not curable and that death can't be avoided: PC offers the chance to live out the remaining days as comfortably as they can be, with the care of experts in end-of-life care.
PC means no more treatment.	When a PC team takes over the care of a patient, treatment doesn't automatically stop. Treatment and therapies can continue, but they have a different goal.
PC is only for people with cancer.	PC is offered to anyone with an end-stage of a chronic or terminal illness. Many people who receive PC can have AIDS, heart disease, COPD, multiple sclerosis, muscular dystrophy, and many other fatal illnesses.
PC is only for old people.	Many children are diagnosed with terminal illnesses. They may be born with a birth defect, such as a heart defect, or a disease that will cause them to die as a child or they may develop a terminal illness later on in their childhood.
PC means the patient is very close to death.	When someone is transferred to the PC team, they may die within days or weeks, or they may live for considerably longer. PC isn't offered according to the amount of time left.
In PC the use of narcotics or opioids is a type of euthanasia.	PC is not euthanasia. If the disease cause severe pain, the use of narcotics or opioids is useful to control the pain, but only if patient needs it and only at the dosages he needs it. The goal of PC isn't to help the patient to die, but, on the contrary, to make him as comfortable as possible during the end-of-life period.
PC can be given only in the hospital.	PC services are offered in many communities. Care at end-of-life can be given in a hospital, stand-alone residence, or at home, depending on the resources available.
PC reduce the family role.	One of the benefits of PC is that it's not only for the dying person. The PC team cares for the dying patient and his or her family and friends. The care at the end-of-life isn't just about physical comfort, but it's about emotional and psychological support for everyone who loves and is part of the life of the dying patient.
PC reduce the auto-control of the patient.	PC is a specialty in medicine. A patient in PC is consulted and is part of the team for as long as him or her is able to be (see also the paragraph on ACP).

Table 2. Negative Myths of Palliative Care (PC)

3. Doctor–patient relationship and patient-centered communication

Mrs White Claire, a woman 40 years old, with two adolescent sons, is affected with a breast cancer with multiple liver, bones and brain metastases. Her mother died at 33 for breast cancer. She is currently receiving home care with opioids for bone pain. Her husband, John, requires to their GP a hospice admission for the appearance of a deep venous thrombosis in the right leg. At the admission the leg is edematous but not sore. The hospice doctor says to John that the general conditions are very compromised and the Claire prognosis is very poor (few days). He proposes not him initiate therapy with low molecular weight heparin, but to provide only supportive therapy. John is distressed and confused, he would like to counsel with their family doctor.

The patient–doctor relationship is an important concept in health care, especially in primary care. One of the main competences required to the General Practitioner (GP) in the field of palliative care is to establish a good relationship both with the patient, the family and the other health care professionals engaged in the care process. In order to provide high quality assistance, effective communication between patients and health care providers is an essential element.

The clinicians need establish a therapeutic relationship based on trust and mutual respect with patients who often access a great deal of medical information, come from culturally diverse, have varying levels of social support, and confront the existential and spiritual aspects of dying, all while trying to access complicated health care systems (Foley & Gelband, 2001; Hewitt & Simone, 1999).

The primary care physicians form the backbone of an integrated team by providing an unbiased medical perspective and continuity during a stressful disease course, supporting patients and their families through emotional ups and downs, negotiating or mediating decisions, monitoring for complications, and providing perspective on the illness (Parker et al, 2001).

Despite around the 50-90% of the patients want to be informed about the diagnosis, the prognosis, the medical treatments and the side effects, even though it is a diagnosis of terminal phase, a relevant number of physician tends to hide unpleasant truths. In fact, patients affected by neoplasia with higher probabilities of being cured are usually informed more correctly and completely than patients affected by advanced disease (D'Errico & Valori, 2011).

When a patient and his/her physician enter into end-of-life discussions, each brings individual cultural backgrounds and values, which influence the discussions. Although understanding cultural norms is important, physicians must be careful to avoid stereotyping patients based on their culture (Kagawa- Singer et al, 2001).

The stress of disease and its treatment are often associated with intense negative emotions: sadness, fear, and anger. Though physicians often cannot "fix" the causes of these emotions, empirical studies indicate that providing emotional support ameliorates distress. Patients feel emotionally supported when their doctor shows care for them as a person, by spending enough time with them, allowing them to ask questions, and listening to their concerns (Wenrich et al, 2001).

The physicians should assess how much information to provide using patient-centered communication. After assessing the patient's readiness to receive prognostic information, the physician should focus on communicating the prognosis without giving false hope (Back et al, 2003). Though many clinicians equate honesty about a poor prognosis with destroying hope, healthy coping continually generates hope, even in difficult life situations. Even under situations of severe stress, positive emotions are prominent, and are an integral part of the coping process (Meier et al, 2001).

An American study described patients' hopes for a good death: freedom from pain and other symptoms, clear decision making, preparation for death, having a sense of completion, contributing to others, affirmation of the whole person, being at peace with God, being in the presence of family, being kept clean, and trusting one's physician (Steinhauser et al,

2000). Maintaining hope is essential to patients and their families at the end-of-life (Clayton et al, 2005; Shiozaki et al, 2005).

Retrospective studies (Ptacek et al, 2001; Salander, 2002; Wenrich et al, 2001) identified what patients want when hearing bad news. They prefer to have: bad news discussed in person, and in a private, quiet place; a physician who is able to communicate their diagnosis, prognosis, and treatment options clearly; full attention of the physician; time to ask questions; and to be given informations about how the diagnosis will affect their life (Back et al, 2008).

The Evidence-based recommendations and the best practices on the communication of bad news are summarized in box 1:

• Find a comfortable and private place to talk;
• Ask whether the patient would like to have others present;
• Minimize interruptions;
• Assess the patient's understanding of the situation;
• Let the patient know explicitly that bad news is forthcoming;
• Provide information honestly and in simple language;
• Give time for questions;
• Encourage patient to express emotions and respond empathically;
• Check understanding;
• Arrange a clear follow-up plan.

Box 1. Best practice for communicating bad news (adapted from Back et al, 2008).

The goals of care change as the disease progresses. At each stage, the physician should help the patient create realistic, achievable goals and hopes. Focusing on stage-specific goals and hopes can prevent over- and under-treatment while relieving the patient's psychological distress (Block, 2006).

Breaking bad news, particularly discussing prognosis, requires a combination of disease-specific biomedical knowledge and excellent communication skills (Back & Arnold, 2006).

Therefore, recommendations have been developed to help physicians appropriately deliver bad news, as reported in box 2:

• It is important for physicians to assess the patient's level of understanding about the disease and expectations for the future.
• It is important for the physician to assess how much information the patient wants to know and to tailor the discussion appropriately.
• The primary care physician should remain involved with patient care during the early, middle, and late stages of disease.
• Physicians should avoid phrases and words that can be misconstrued by the patient and lead to negative interpretations such as abandonment and failure.
• During end-of-life communication, physicians should assess and be sensitive to the patient's cultural and individual preferences.

Box 2. How to communicate bad news: recommendations for physicians (adapted from Ngo-Metzger et al, 2008)

Frequently, preparing the caregivers for the patient's death is not a main focus of communication (Rabow et al, 2004). Usually the family of a terminally-ill patient prefers that diagnosis is hidden to its loved one. This behaviour can be seen as a psychological defense system through which the patient's relatives face their own anxiety towards death. That is why the GP should also help the family members to understand what are the advantages of a frankly based relationship and what are the risks of a reticent and not honest relationship (D'Errico & Valori, 2011).

Observational studies (Steinhauser et al, 2001; Hebert et al, 2006) suggest that inadequate information and unpredictable situations might contribute to caregiver uncertainty, which is associated with poorer health outcomes for the caregiver himself. On the contrary, other studies demonstrate that when the caregivers perceive that their questions have been answered, they experience fewer depressive symptoms, fewer economic and other burdens, and improve their satisfaction and quality of life (Valdimarsdottir et al, 2004).

Knowledge about factors that hinder or facilitate the communication between GPs and patients in palliative care is needed in order to improve the quality of the palliative care itself and the life quality of the patients (Slort et al, 2011).

The most frequently reported barriers for GP–patient communication are:

- the GPs' lack of time;
- the patients' ambivalence or unwillingness to know about the prognosis;
- the GPs not talking honestly about the diagnosis or prognosis.

The most frequently reported facilitating factors are:

- the availability of the GPs,
- longstanding GPs–patient relationships,
- GPs showing commitment, being open and allowing any topic to be discussed,
- being honest and friendly,
- listening actively and taking patients seriously,
- taking the initiative to talk about end-of-life issues,
- not withholding information,
- negotiating palliative care options,
- being willing to talk about the diagnosis and prognosis, preparation for death, the patient's psychological, social and spiritual issues and the patient's end-of-life preferences.

In conclusion give dignity, space and attention to the communication are essential steps that need to be undertaken by a GP that recognizes a correct relationship with the patient as one of his main means of care and essential for a better advance care planning.

4. Advance care planning

Advance care planning (ACP) is a process that can support individual autonomy with respect to health care choices throughout the course of a life-threatening illness and at the end-of-life. Advance directives (ADs) are documents enabling capable individuals to plan for care in the case of their own incapacity.

The Institute of Medicine (cited by Emanuel et al, 2011) defines ACP as "not only the preparation of legal documents but also discussions with family members and physicians about what the future may hold for people with serious illnesses, how patients and families want their beliefs and preferences to guide decisions (including decisions should sudden and unexpected critical medical problems arise), and what steps could alleviate concerns related to finances, family matters, spiritual questions, and other issues that trouble seriously ill or dying patients and their families".

As such, ACP is a process not a single event with the goal of learning about both what patients want and what they do not want for themselves in the future.

ACP includes (National Hospice and Palliative Care Organization, 2011):

- Getting information on the types of life-sustaining treatments that are available;
- Deciding what types of treatment one would or would not want should one be diagnosed with a life-limiting illness;
- Sharing personal values with loved ones;
- Completing advance directives to put into writing what types of treatment one would or would not want should one be unable to speak for itself.

A systematic review on the emotional impact of discussions about end-of-life decisions showed that the patients involved experienced positive benefits from the process (Song, 2004). Hypothetical benefits of ACP reported in the literature include increased inclusion of patient preferences for health care, more informed decision making, decreased pain and suffering, reduced costs and use of life-sustaining treatments, and improved patient and family satisfaction with care (Royal College of Physician, guideline 2009).

Another review (Knops et al, 2005) identified three domains of patient concern that are relevant for advance care planning conversations:

- feelings about the disease
- feelings about suffering
- feelings about the circumstances of death.

A literature review (Kaldjian, 2008) reported a list of 6 goals can be used to articulate goal-oriented frameworks to guide decision-making toward the end-of-life and thereby harmonize patients' treatment choices with their values and medical conditions:

1. be cured
2. live longer
3. improve or maintain function/quality of life/ independence
4. be comfortable
5. achieve life goals
6. provide support for family/caregiver.

Discussions about end-of-life care and end-of-life decision-making involve cognitive and particularly affective processes and are often emotionally taxing. How end-of-life discussions are delivered and what is discussed can influence patient's decision-making and affective outcomes.

Although the issue has been increasingly in the public eye, few patients have had these discussions with their physician or family; and, even when they have, decisions may not be documented in the patient's record. Without plans, a crisis situation can escalate quickly, especially if the patient cannot communicate or if the family's preferences conflict with the clinician's ones. In these cases, treatment decisions are not made, they simply happen, usually based on habits that are presumed to reflect what patients generally want.

ACP can be difficult, there may be actual barriers (Lynn et al, 2007):

- Everyone is reluctant to talk about the patient's declining health and approaching death.
- Clinicians find it easier to offer comfort, hope, and medical technology rather than to "let people die."
- Patients and families find it hard to believe that treatments such as resuscitation will not restore health.
- Clinicians and family may not accept the patient's treatment priorities and values.

Recently the Royal College of Physicians, (2009), has release some Evidence-based Guidelines for clinical management, "Advance Care Planning". In box 3 recommendations are reported about the physician approach to ACP:

- Ideally, ACP discussions should be initiated in primary care
- ACP should be offered during routine clinical practice, but never forced upon
- Professionals should initiate ACP discussions with patients using their professional judgement to gauge the appropriate time
- The professional should have adequate knowledge about the disease, treatment and the particular individual to be able to give the patient all the information needed to express their preferences to make the plan
- Individuals should be encouraged to choose who they would wish to be included in the discussion, such as next of kin or future proxy

---

Box 3. When and with whom should I be considering ACP discussions?

In box 4 the recommendations about the better way to conduct a discussion on ACP with the patients are reported:

- ACP discussions need to be skilfully led and should be a process, not a single event or a tick box exercise
- Professionals should ensure that individuals have every opportunity to participate in the discussion by treating reversible illness impacting on decision-making, such as delirium or sensory impairment, and ensuring that the patient is pain-free, fed, not too tired etc
- ACP discussions should not be continued if they are causing the patient excessive distress or anxiety
- Professionals should take account of the following factors which influence attitudes to discussing ACP, and ensure that these factors do not act as artificial barriers: older people, the professional's own personal experience and beliefs, the patient's gender, race, culture, sexual orientation, religion, beliefs and values, the patient's concerns about euthanasia

---

Box 4. Recommendations of the RCP on how to conduct a discussion about ACP with a patient.

Finally in box 5 it is clearly reported that all the carers must be trained in ACP discussions and that it is essential to record the patients statements.

- Health and social care staff should be trained in ACP discussions, especially physician, nursing, social workers and other key workers
- Staff training should be workplace-based, recurrent and led by experts and expert patients
- Physicians should be routinely reminded to offer ACP discussion at an appropriate time to their patients
- ACP should be part of the Quality Outcomes Framework
- Medical records should contain a specific section for advance statements
- A register should be created, which stores details about an individual's ACP document, and should be readily accessible with the individual's permission
- ACP documents should be recorded on the electronic patient record (with the patient's consent)

Box 5. Recommendations for training and implementation of ACP

In general, discussion about advance care planning should focus more on goals of care than on specific treatments, and clinicians should be especially careful to respond to the emotional content of the discussion (Tulsky, 2005).

The underlying principle is that the discussion should move back and forth from preferences to reasons and values to information and back, ensuring that the patient understands the implications of his or her stated preferences and that the doctor understands the patients' values. Although little evidence exists to guide practice, it may be more effective for a physician to make a values-based recommendation, rather than offering a variety of choices without guidance (Back, 2008).

5. The evidence based practice in palliative care

The palliative approach towards the patient in terminal phase requires that all the health carers are able to provide a high quality assistance.

Palliative Medicine, like any other branch of medicine, needs research to switch from a medicine based on opinions to a medicine based on scientific evidence. Clinicians should make decisions for the individual patient not only under their own experience, but also with the guide of the best available evidence. Evidence Based Medicine (EBM), should guide one's clinical decisions based on the efficacy and safety of a particular intervention in a specific population. But only few patients have average characteristics. In Palliative Care the difficulty with guidance about symptom control often is the paucity of evidence of sufficient quality (Bausewein et al, 2011).

Since the primary studies are rare, clinically heterogeneous, with small sampling and often of poor quality, the scientific evidences in palliative care not always can provide elements of "best practice" in order to lead the clinic practice.

The shortage of the research in palliative care is connected to different concurring factors; among them there are:

- A particular observation/intervention setting: for example the patient residence that makes difficult to realize of complex research protocols;
- The limited survival of the patients, with short observation times;
- Subjective experience of the patient during the advanced phases of the illness, that usually make impossible a preliminary intervention, even more complicated to be realized at the end-of-life;
- The multidisciplinary integration often is problematic;
- Techniques and assessment tools are not always comparable between countries.

Anyway, different types of research protocols can be adapted to the specificity and limitations of the palliative medicine in Primary Care:

- Guidelines Implementation and Clinical audit;
- Descriptive surveys, quantitative researches with valued questionnaires and qualitative researches with unstructured interviews;
- Testing of pharmaceuticals and equipment, specific but not invasive;
- Descriptive studies, with the method of the Follow-back survey, using as source of information the caregivers, etc.

5.1 Outcome measurement in palliative care

Outcome measurement has a major role to play in improving the quality, efficiency and availability of palliative care (Bausewein et al, 2011):

- Outcome measurement is a way of measuring changes in a patient's health (which can be attributed to preceding healthcare) over time;
- It can be used to improve the quality of healthcare services;
- Outcome measurement can be used for clinical care, audit and research purposes;
- There is an increasing need for robust outcome measurement in the field of palliative care, but this poses particular challenges and requires special consideration with regard to patients' situations at the end-of-life.

A patient's experience can be related to physical (e.g., symptoms and functional status), psychological (e.g., cognition and emotions), social and cultural (e.g., family and friends, organisational and financial), and spiritual (e.g., beliefs, meaning and religion) domains, which are all interlinked.

Palliative care aims to provide holistic care for patients and families and for this reason an outcome measure should be a complex one and ideally cover several of these domains, as well as aspects of care (NICE, 2011).

Most outcome measures (questionnaire or scales) cover various domains and dimensions, dimensions relate to measurable quantities or particular aspects of a problem: for example, the patient, family and carers, or quality of care, as well as physical (Fig. 1).

A large number of outcome measures have been developed to measure specific physical dimensions, for example, symptoms such as pain, breathlessness or fatigue (Table 3).

Outcome measure	Number of items	Completion time	Notes
Palliative care Outcome Scale (POS)	10 items on physical symptoms emotional, psychological and spiritual needs, provision of information and support	mean time 6.9 min (patients) and 5.7 min (staff)	scores from 0 ('no effect') to 4 ('overwhelming') , staff patient of and carer version; widely used palliative care measure freely available after registration
POS-S Symptom list	10 symptoms 2 questions about the symptom that affected the patient the most and that has improved the most	few minutes	scores from 0 ('no effect') to 4 ('overwhelming'); additional symptom versions available for other conditions (POS-S MS, POS-S renal);
Distress Thermometer	overall distress score 20 symptoms, 5 items on practical problems, 4 on family problems, 5 on emotional problems, 2 on spiritual concerns	median length of time 5 min, with 75% taking no more than 10 min	distress score 0-10; other items yes/no
Edmonton Symptom Assessment Scale (ESAS)	9 symptoms and "other problem"	Approximately 5 min	each symptom with NRS 0-10 developed to measure the most commonly experienced symptoms in cancer patients; freely available
Memorial Symptom Assessment Scale (MSAS)	14 items 7 depression 7 anxiety	2-6 min	developed to assess depression and anxiety for people with physical illness; not freely available
European Organization for Research and Treatment of Cancer - EORTC QLQ-C30	5 functional scales (physical, role, emotional, social, and cognitive), 3 symptom scales(fatigue, nausea, vomiting and pain), a global health status/QoL scale and six single items (dyspnoea, insomnia, appetite loss, constipation, diarrhoea, and financial difficulties)	first assessment 12 min (SD 7.5 min), second assessment 11 min (SD 6.5 min)	not freely available, widely used in cancer research; modular supplement available for a range of malignancies (lung, breast, gastric, brain etc.)

Outcome measure	Number of items	Completion time	Notes
EORTC	pain, physical function (3 items), emotional function (2 items), fatigue (2 items), QoL(1 item), symptoms (6 items)	< 20 min	not freely available, shortened, version of the EORTC QLQ-C30 for palliative care patients

Table 3. Examples of multidimensional outcome measures in palliative care (modified from Bausewein et al, 2011)

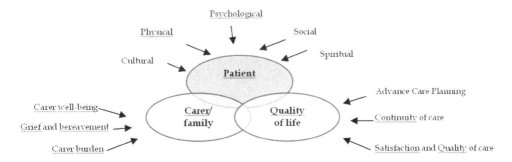

Fig. 1. Domains and dimensions of outocome measures in palliative care
(Bausewein et al, 2011)

Psychological symptoms, such as depression or anxiety, are either measured using separate scales or are included in the symptoms' measures.

5.2 Pain therapy in palliative care

Daniel is a 48 y.o. male, suffering from malignant melanoma with liver metastases, abdominal and thoracic lymph nodes and multiple bone metastases (spinal multidistrict). He is receiving 2 cp of 32 mg hydromorphone/day, oral morphine 50 mg every 4-6 hours (rescue dose), bisphosphonates I.V. every 28 days (in hospital), laxative and anti-emetic therapy. For three days there is an intense nausea due to liver metastases. Daniel is no longer able to take oral therapy. His GP would like to change the oral therapy in a parenteral route. What are the available evidences to support the clinical decision making?

Palliative care is operationalized through effective management of pain and other distressing symptoms, while incorporating psychosocial and spiritual care according to patient and family needs, values, beliefs and culture(s).

Pain is a symptom defined as "An unpleasant sensory and emotional experience associated with actual or potential tissue damage, or described in terms of such damage" (IASP, 1994).

For an adequate estimation of a patient, the Joint Commission Accreditation of healthcare Organization Standard Manual declared in 2002 that the fifth "vital sign" to look for is pain.

Pain has been identified consistently as one of the major problems in end-of-life care.

Chronic pain, present not along in cancer but also in degenerative diseases, neurological disorders, especially in advanced stages and terminal illness, takes on the characteristics of **global pain**, or in other words, of personal suffering, that finds in its etiopathogenesis physical reasons as well as psychological and social causes.

All types of pain (acute, chronic, and cancer pain) are undertreated, and poorly controlled. Adequate pain control can be achieved in most patients at the end-of-life by using a comprehensive approach that includes analgesics, adjuvants, education, support, and monitoring (Emanuel et al, 2011).

Patients should be asked about pain severity, quality, location, and temporal features, such as onset, duration, diurnal variation, or aggravating/relieving factors. They should be actively involved in establishing the goals of palliative pain management, along with family members. It is essential to explain the origin and the type of pain, the initial management plan (including the role of titration), expected adverse effects and how they will be managed, how the pain will be monitored (Emanuel et al, 2011).

5.2.1 Pain classification

Pain is a subjective experience, influenced by cultural factors, specific situations and other psychological variables. The process of pain does not begin with the simple stimulation of the receptors. It is influenced by the personality of the patients, the context in which they live, the cultural level and the experiences of life.

As knowledge about pain has advanced, health care professionals have become increasingly aware of the need to develop a more mechanism-based approach to pain control. Cancer pain is a paradigmatic combination of physical and inflammatory processes, that may result from tissue damage and destruction and/or stimulation of nerves by inflammatory mediators produced by the tumor and by the body in response to tumors, too.

Usually pain can be classified as:

- **Nociceptive pain:** is caused by the activation of nociceptive nerve fibers by physical tissue destruction or by chemical, pressure, or thermal processes; often it is described as sharp and stabbing, while the visceral stimulation derived from the receptors present on the internal organs, (such as the bladder, intestine, stomach, etc...), is poorly localized and may be deaf or cramping.
- **Neuropathic pain:** A new definition was suggested by the IASP Neuropathic Pain Special Interest Group (NeuPSIG, 2008). This group redefines neuropathic pain as "pain caused as a direct consequence of a lesion or condition that affects the somatosensory system". Neuropatic pain is difficult to treat, given the variety of etiologies, mechanical causes and symptoms that characterize it, and its impact on different dimensions of health. The pain is of different intensity, that rarely reaches high levels but causes intense suffering to the patients. It occurs as a continuous pain, throbbing or stabbing, with possible hyperalgesia or hypoalgesia, paresthesia, allodynia.

- **Mixed**: both nociceptive and neuropathic pain are common in illnesses like cancer.

There are several methods to observe pain, based on the patient's ability to define it quantitatively. The measurement of pain is a fundamental tool of the assessment and strategy of pain management for pain control. Routinely using the analgesic scales and keeping records of the results in the patients medical card helps improve the ability of the physician to understand the intensity of pain.

Several instruments are used, some complex, others easier to use in the setting of general practice; the two main categories are:

Intensity scales, such as:

- **Visual Analogical Scale (VAS)** is designed to present to the respondent a rating scale with minimum constraints. Respondents mark the location on the 0-10 centimeters line corresponding to the amount of pain they experienced. VAS data of this type is recorded as the number of millimeters from the left of the line within the range 0-10 centimeters.
- **Numerical Rating Scale (NRS)** is an instrument that requires the rater to assign the rated object that have numerals assigned to them, instruct the patient to choose a number from 0 to 10 that best describes their current pain, 0 would mean 'No pain' and 10 would mean 'Worst possible pain'.
- **Verbal Rating Scales (VRS)** uses specific words to numeric pain describe rather than a scale. In other words, the person in pain describes the intensity of pain, and how they feel.
- **Analogue Chromatic Continuos Scale** is based on gradation of colour along the line (e.g. pale pink to dark red, for the worst pain)

An objective assessment of physical functioning constitutes an important part of the multidimensional assessment of pain. Terminally ill patients may curtail their physical activity because of pain. Physical activity may also be restricted because of fatigue, cachexia, and drowsiness, common in end-stage illness, contributing to rapid deconditioning, with severe impairments in overall functional status.

Multidimensional questionnaires (D'Errico & Valori, 2011) are useful for an overall objective and subjective assessment, but are less used by general practitioners because, if compared with the intensity scales, it means devoting more time to the patients:

- **McGill Pain Questionnaire** can be used to evaluate a person experiencing significant pain, can be used to monitor the pain over time and to determine the effectiveness of any intervention.
- **Memorial Pain Assessment Card**: a scale used to assess 32 physical and psychological symptoms in three different dimensions: intensity, frequency, and distress.
- **Brief Pain Inventory**: provides information on the intensity of pain (the sensory dimension) as well as the degree to which pain interferes with function (the reactive dimension).

5.2.2 Principles of pain control

Pain control is an important aspect of palliative care, in order to improve quality of life. Relief of pain should be seen as part of a comprehensive pattern of care encompassing the physical, psychological, social, and spiritual aspects of suffering. The various components must be addressed simultaneously. Disease progression may necessitate increased dosing of opioids to control pain; this should not be confused with "tolerance." In fact, when a patient with previously well controlled pain develops the need for increasing opioid doses to achieve comfort, advancing illness is almost always the cause (Emanuel et al, 1999).

Flexibility is the key to managing cancer pain. As patients vary in diagnosis, stage of disease, responses to pain and interventions, and personal preferences, so must pain management. The patient should be actively involved in establishing the goals of palliative pain management, along with family members (ICSI Guideline, 2009; NCI, 2009).

The National Cancer Institute (NCI, 2009) emphasizes the patient involvement in 5 recommendations (ABCDE):

* **Ask** about pain regularly. Assess pain and associated symptoms systematically using brief assessment tools. Assessment should include discussion about common symptoms experienced by cancer patients and how each symptom will be treated;
* **Believe** patient and family reports of pain and what relieves the pain (Caveats include patients with significant psychological/existential distress and patients with cognitive impairment);
* **Choose** pain-control options appropriate for the patient, family, and setting;
* **Deliver** interventions in a timely, logical, coordinated fashion;
* **Empower** patients and their families. Enable patients to control their course as much as possible.

There are many barriers to a good pain management in palliative care (NCI, 2009). They include (table 4) discounting a patient's subjective measure of pain, difficulty in assessment of the cognitively impaired, myths believed by both practitioners and patients about opioid therapy and fears of addiction and hastening death.

Problems related to health care professionals	Problems related to patients
Inadequate knowledge of pain management	Reluctance to report pain
Poor assessment of pain	Concern about distracting physicians from treatment of underlying disease
Concern about regulation of controlled substances	Fear that pain means disease is worse
Fear of patient addiction	Reluctance to take pain medications
Concern about side effects of analgesics	Fear of addiction or of being thought of as an addict. This fear may be more pronounced in minority patients.
Concern about patients becoming tolerant to analgesics	Worries about unmanageable side effects such as constipation, nausea, or clouding of thought
	Concern about becoming tolerant to pain medications

Table 4. Barriers to Effective Pain Management (NCI, 2009)

5.2.3 Management of pain

The World Health Organization (WHO, 1996) produced a pain ladder to be used as a guide for prescribing analgesics. The severity of pain, assessed by the scales, is classified as mild, (range VAS 1-4), moderate (VAS 5-6) and severe (VAS 7-10) (figure 2). Different type of analgesics are used, depending on the severity of pain. A telephone survey conducted in 2003 in 15 European countries and Israel, which involved 4,839 patients, showed that there is considerable diversity in the use of analgesics in chronic pain. Countries with greater use of NSAIDs were Poland (71%) and Italy (68%). The weak opioids were used by 36-50% of responders in Sweden, UK and Norway, and only 5-9% in Israel, Denmark and Italy. Strong opioids were almost unused in Italy, Spagna and Switzerland (0-2%), while 12-13% were prescribed in the UK and Ireland (Breivik et al, 2006).

In all three steps it also is possible to use an adjuvant therapy (various drugs, chemotherapy, radiotherapy or/and surgery) to strengthen the action of analgesics (figure 2).

Patients who did not improve their pain should go to the next step of the analgesic ladder.

The consensus statement from the American Pain Society and American Academy of Pain Medicine (1996) states that the undertreatment of pain is unjustified.

For many people experiencing cancer pain that is expected to continue, opioids should be administered on an **"around-the-clock"** basis, rather than given only when pain becomes intense. The "around-the-clock" approach provides a consistent level of the medication in the blood, and this helps to provide a fairly consistent level of pain relief, preventing abrupt peaks and valleys of pain, with the use of short-acting opioids as supplemental agents for Breakthrough pain. Controlled-release formulations can lessen the inconvenience associated with "around-the-clock" administration of short-acting opioids.

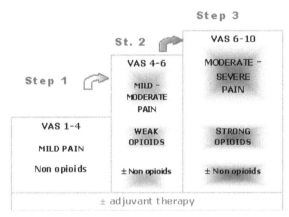

Fig. 2. Pain ladder proposed by WHO (1996).

Recently, the usefulness of step 2 of the WHO ladder has been questioned. Two systematic reviews (McNicol et al, 2004; Maltoni et al, 2005) raised questions about delayed introduction of strong opioids may result in periods of uncontrolled pain. Nowadays, for moderate pain, the recommendation is to consider starting with small doses of a strong opioid. (Pergolizzi et al, 2008).

In table 5, a synopsis of treatment strategies for chronic pain is reported (Emanuel et al, 2011); strong opioids are the reference analgesics for moderate to severe pain both for nociceptive than neuropathic pain.

Type	Nociceptive pain		Neuropathic pain	
	mild	moderate to severe	mild	moderate to severe
Typical Analgesics	Non-opioids $\pm$ weak opioids	Strong opioids	Unuseful (?)	Strong opioids
Adjuvant Analgesics	Acetaminophen (paracetamol) or NSAIDs	Acetaminophen or NSAIDs, Radiotherapy, Surgery	Tricyclic antidepressants Typical and atypical anticonvulsants	

Table 5. Analgesic strategies for Chronic Pain (nociceptive or neuropathic).

5.2.3.1 Non-opioid typical analgesics

The non-opioid analgesics are both typical or adjuvant analgesics. They include nonsteroidal anti-inflammatory drugs (NSAIDs and COXIBs) and acetaminophen, or paracetamol.

NSAIDs and Paracetamol are recommended for use alone or in combination with opioids both as first line therapy (mild pain) or as adjuvant analgesics (moderate to severe pain).

NSAIDs are a group of organic acids with analgesic, antipyretic and anti-inflammatory properties, indicated for rheumatic pain and skeletal muscle inflammation. The effects of NSAIDs are related to inhibition of cyclooxygenase (COX-1 and COX-2) enzyme.

The inhibition of COX-2 determines the analgesic, anti-inflammatory and antipyretic effect typical of **COXIBs**. NSAIDs and COXIBs reduce pain exerting their action primarily at the level of noxious stimuli, which elevate the threshold for activation of nerve endings.

The commonest adverse events with NSAIDs are gastrointestinal (mucosal erosion and bleeding) and renal toxicity.

The analgesic effect of **paracetamol** is expressed at the central level; its mechanism of action is due to inhibition of prostaglandin synthesis in the central nervous system (CNS), but also by the activation of serotonergic pathways descendants. It is administered orally, rectally or intravenously. Oral solutions are absorbed more quickly than traditional tablets and effervescent soluble tablets even better: they contain sodium bicarbonate, the prokinetic action of which promotes gastric emptying and the arrival of the drug in the small intestine that is home to the main absorption.

5.2.3.2 Other adjuvant analgesics

Tricyclic antidepressants (TCAs) may be useful as adjunctive therapy for cancer-related neuropathic pain syndromes. TCAs provide pain relief by independently providing analgesia specific for neuropathic pain, potentiating the effect of opioids, and improving underlying depression and insomnia.

TCAs (amitriptyline, nortriptyline, and desipramine) are also thought to have an inhibitory effect on nociceptive pain , by raising the levels of serotonin and norepinephrine in the CNS by slowing the rate of reuptake by nerve cells. Their analgesic activity seems to be independent from their antidepressant effects. Unfortunately, TCAs also block histaminic, cholinergic, and alpha1-adrenergic receptor sites, and this lack of selectivity is what accounts for the unwanted side effects such as weight gain, dry mouth, constipation, drowsiness, and dizziness.

Several **anticonvulsants** (valproic acid, carbamazepine, gabapentin, pregabalin, clonazepam and others) have a role in the treatment of neuropathic pain. They are thought to inhibit seizures by multiple mechanisms, including functional blockade of voltage-gated sodium channels, functional blockade of voltage-gated calcium channels, direct or indirect enhancement of inhibitory GABAergic neurotransmission, and inhibition of glutamatergic neurotransmission. The effects on neuropathic pain, characterized by neuronal hyperexcitability, are probably mediated by the same molecular mechanisms. Their efficacy is quite variable; antidepressants and anticonvulsants may occasionally be prescribed simultaneously, but it is good clinical practice to introduce only one drug at a time.

5.2.3.3 Opioid analgesics (weaks and strongs)

The most effective analgesics are the opioid analgesics. The opioids include all drugs that interact with opioid receptors in the nervous system. Opioid receptors are a group of G protein-coupled receptors with opioids as ligands. These receptors are the sites of action for the endorphins, compounds that already exist in the body and are chemically related to the opioid drugs that are prescribed for pain. Most opioids undergo biotransformation in the liver and are primarily eliminated by kidneys as a mixture of the parent opioid and their metabolites. Accumulation of active metabolites with analgesic or neurotoxic effects can result in significant toxicity.

WEAK OPIOIDS		
AGONISTS		**PARTIAL AGONISTS**
Codeine Propoxyphene Hydrocodone Dihydrocodeine Tramadol		Buprenorphine
STRONG OPIOIDS		
AGONISTS		**AGONISTS/ANTAGONISTS**
Morphine Oxycodone Hydromorphone Methadone Fentanyl Diamorphine	Oxymorphone Meperidine Levorphanol Sufentanil Alfentanil	Pentazocine Butorphanol Nalbuphine

Table 6. Classification of Opioid Analgesics by Receptor Interactions (modified from Emanuel et al, 2011)

Opioid metabolism knowledge helps in initial selection and titrating the dose in terminally ill patients. On the basis of the interactions with the various CNS receptor subtypes (mu, kappa, and delta) the opioids can be divided into pure agonists, partial agonists, mixed agonists and antagonists (Table 6). The latter two groups are generally not useful in terminal illness, because of partial or total "ceiling effect" (the effect is not dose-dependent) for analgesia and undesired dysesthesia for the activation of K-receptors associated with some agents.

The EAPC survey in 42 European countries (EAPC survey, 2006) showed that the most frequently used opioid (68%) is morphine (see also table 1). Morphine is referred to as the "gold standard" for pain treatment in palliative care, because it is effective, inexpensive and easy-to-holder. In other countries (18%), such as Italy, Spain, Luxemburg, Austria and Belgium, the most widely used opioid was fentanyl, a strong one, but quite expensive and difficult to titrate. Tramadol, a weak opioid, was the first used in 8% of the other countries.

Morphine is the first-choice strong opioid in palliative care, because it is very effective, inexpensive, and easy to titrate. It can administered using many routes including oral, rectal, parenteral, subcutaneous and spinal route. Morphine binds to opioid receptors in the CNS, reducing the perception as well as the emotional response to pain. Alternative opioids have not demonstrated advantages that would make them preferable as first-line drugs for cancer pain. Over the past decade very few new opioids have been developed, but rather new formulations have been made (oral controlled-release formulations, transdermal patches, oral transmucosal devices, buccal adhesive tablets, nasal sprays) to optimise their overall use and to increase usage especially for malignant pain (Janet et al, 2009).

Oxycodone is a strong opioid, used to treat moderate to severe pain. The extended-release form of this medication is for "around-the-clock" treatment of pain. In case of insufficient analgesia and/or intense adverse effects such as sedation, hallucinations and nausea and vomiting a switch from another opioid to oxycodone might be beneficial. Oxycodone is mainly used as controlled-release tablets for chronic pain. The immediate-release solution and tablets are used for acute pain or for BTcP. Parenteral oxycodone is a good alternative when opioids cannot be administered orally (Biancofiore, 2006).

Hydromorphone, is a semi-synthetic morphine derivative that differs slight from morphine in its chemical structure: this makes it 5–10 times more potent and enhances its distribution into the brain making titration of the effects easier. Hydromorphone may be better tolerated than morphine in patients with renal failure (Felden et al, 2011).

Fentanyl is an agonist strong opioid analgesic, effective for the treatment of acute and chronic pain via multiple routes of administration:

- Transdermal fentanyl (Transdermal System – TDS or Patch) releases the opioid for three days, needle-free, easy to use and circumventing barriers to the use of oral analgesics, for example in patients with nausea. The main problem is the dose titration to obtain pain-control: the patch should be introduced only when the pain is under control with an oral opioid.
- Oral transmucosal fentanyl citrate (OTFC), the so-called lollipop, utilizes the rapid uptake through the buccal mucosa to achieve high plasma concentrations rapidly; the OTFC is indicated to treat Break-Through cancer Pain (BTcP).

- The fentanyl buccal tablets (FBT) offer slightly better pharmacokinetics for the same indication, as Fentanyl buccal soluble film (FBSF), a small, bilayered, water-soluble polymer film that adheres to the buccal mucosa and rapidly delivers fentanyl into the systemic circulation.
- The intranasal fentanyl spray (INFS) route is another option to achieve rapid uptake of fentanyl, indicated to treat acute and BTcP relief (Grape et al, 2010).

Despite the current availability of alternatives to morphine, the recommendations of the European Association for Palliative Care (Hanks et al, 2001) on the use of opioids in cancer pain remain still valid. However, most of the recommendations are not based on strong scientific evidence but on the clinical experience of respected authorities from expert committees. Table 7 describes some of the key recommendations.

Grading*	
C	The opioid of first choice for moderate to severe cancer pain is morphine.
C	If patients are unable to take morphine orally the preferred alternative route is subcutaneous There is generally no indication for giving morphine intramuscularly for chronic cancer pain because subcutaneous administration is simpler and less painful.
C	The optimal route of administration of morphine is by mouth. Ideally, two types of formulation are required: normal release (for dose titration) and modified release (for maintenance treatment).
A	Oral transmucosal fentanyl citrate (OTFC) is an effective treatment for 'BTcP' in patients stabilized on regular oral morphine or an alternative step 3 opioid.
A	Hydromorphone or oxycodone, if available in both normal release and modified release formulations for oral administration, are effective alternatives to oral morphine.
B	Transdermal fentanyl is an effective alternative to oral morphine but is best reserved for patients whose opioid requirements are stable.
C	Methadone is an effective alternative, but may be more complicated to use compared with other opioids because of pronounced interindividual differences in its plasma half-life, relative analgesic potency and duration of action.
B	Spinal (epidural or intrathecal) administration of opioid analgesics in combination with local anaesthetics or clonidine should be considered in patients who derive inadequate analgesia or suffer intolerable adverse effects despite the optimal use of systemic opioids and non-opioids.
*The grading system express the robustness of scientific evidence: an A recommendation is sustained by a strong scientific proofs, while a D evidence is mainly based on expert-opinion. Grade B and C express intermediate levels of evidence.	

Table 7. Recommendations about the use of Morphine and alternative opioids in cancer pain (Hanks et al, 2001)

Decision pathway to manage pain in terminally ill patients involves selecting the right opioid at the right dose, frequency, and route, and the prevention and treatment of opioid side effects. Careful opioid titrations with close monitoring of outcomes (eg. pain relief, side effects, physical aid psychosocial functioning) is required to achieve an individualized analgesic response.

• give in adequate dosage
• titrate the dose for each individual patient
• schedule administration according to drug pharmacology
• administer on a strict schedule to prevent pain
• give written instructions for patients on multiple drugs
• give instructions for treatment of Breakthrough pain
• warn of, and give treatment to prevent, adverse effects
• keep the analgesic program as simple as possible
• use the oral route wherever possible
• review and reassess

Box 6. Principles of analgesic administration (modified from Doyle & Woodruff, 2008)

The principles of analgesic administration (particularly for opioid analgesics) in the treatment of chronic pain are summarized in box 6 (Doyle & Woodruff, 2008).

A decision pathway algorithm for opioid therapy (Eti & Heidelbaug, 2011) is reported in Figure 2.

Opioid rotation, especially for patients with cancer, should be considered when opioid side effects are difficult to manage. This approach is based on the clinical observation that intraindividual response varies remarkably from opioid to opioid and that a change to an alternative drug may yield a far better balance between analgesia and side effects. The opioid rotation/switching/ substitution is a strategy that includes:

• changing to a different medication by using the same route of administration, or
• maintaining the current medication, but changing the route of administration, or
• changing both the medication and the route of administration,

because of insufficient pain management, intolerable adverse effects, need for change the administration route and economics.

When opioid rotation is applied in the setting of unacceptable adverse effects, the selection of an alternative opioid is largely empiric. A pure opioid agonist is recommended. Opioid rotation has been shown to be useful in opening the therapeutic window and establishing a more advantageous analgesia/toxicity relation (Vadalouca et al, 2008).

Many patients develop adverse effects such as constipation, nausea, vomiting, urinary retention, pruritus and CNS toxicity (drowsiness, cognitive impairment, confusion, hallucinations, myoclonic jerks and – rarely – opioid-induced hyperalgesia/allodynia). In some cases a reduction in opioid dose may alleviate refractory side-effects. This may be achieved by using a co-analgesic or an alternative approach such as a nerve block or radiotherapy (adjuvant therapy). Other strategies include the continuous use of antiemetics for nausea, laxatives for constipation, antipsychotics for confusion and delirium and psychostimulants for drowsiness. However, since some of the side-effects may be caused by accumulation of toxic metabolites, switching to another opioid agonist and/or another route may allow titration to adequate analgesia without the same disabling effects. This is especially true for symptoms of CNS toxicity like opioid-induced hyperalgesia/allodynia and myoclonic jerks (Jost & Roila, 2010).

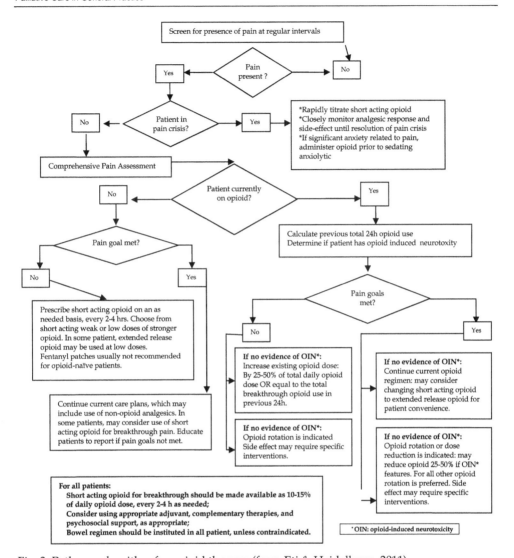

Fig. 3. Pathway algorithm for opioid therapy (from Eti & Heidelbaug, 2011)

Disadvantages of opioid rotation include problems related to inaccurate conversion of the doses, limited availability of certain opioid formulations, drug interactions, and the possibility of increased expense. Weighing the advantages and disadvantages is essential prior to making a decision about opioid rotation selection. This approach requires familiarity with equianalgesic doses of the different opioids (see Table 8).

5.2.4 The Breakthrough (cancer) Pain (BTcP)

Breakthrough (cancer) pain (BTcP) is a common problem in patients with cancer, associated with significant morbidity in this group of patients (Davies, 2006). The original definition of

BTcP was "a transitory exacerbation of pain that occurs on a background of otherwise stable pain in a patient receiving chronic opioid therapy"(Portenoy,1990).

It appears within a few minutes and lasts about 30-45 minutes, distinctly different from the basic pain, with which it shares the location and irradiation.

A newer version has suggested an extension of the definition of BTcP: "a transient exacerbation of pain that occurs either spontaneously, or in relation to a specific predictable

Drug	Oral Route	Parenteral Route	Conversion Ratio to 30mg Oral Morphine (OM)
Morphine sulfate	30mg	10mg	Parenteral morphine is **3 times** as potent as OM
Oxycodone	20mg	NA	Oral Oxycodone is **roughly 1.5 times** more potent than OM
Hydrocodone	20mg	NA	Oral hydrocodone is **roughly 1.5 times** more potent than OM
Hydromorphone	6 mg	1.5 mg	Oral hydromorphone is about **5 times** as potent as OM Parenteral hydromorphone is **20 times** as potent as OM
Fentanyl TDS	NA	12-15 mcg/hr TDS	TDS fentanyl is **approximately 80 times** as potent as OM

Table 8. Opioid Equivalency – Strong Opioid (daily doses)

or unpredictable trigger, despite relatively stable and adequately controlled background pain"(Davies, 2009). The characteristics of pain are:

- High intensity
- Frequent involvement of the same basic site of pain
- Acute clinical manifestation
- Appearance during the day that is repeated with variable frequency

BTcP can place a significant physical, psychological and economic burden on patients. Despite advances in the management of cancer pain, through the application of modern, evidence-based, multimodality management and the availability of new treatment options, recent European surveys have indicated that the diagnosis and treatment of BTcP is still suboptimal. A general lack of consensus on its definition alongside poor recognition and inadequate assessment may often lead to under-treatment and poor patient outcomes (Dickman, 2011).

A task group of the Science Committee of the Association for Palliative Medicine of Great Britain and Ireland (APM, 2009) has produced some up-to-date, evidence-based, practical, clinical guidelines on the management of BTcP in adults. The task group was unable to make recommendations about any individual interventions for the lack of strong evidences; however the group released 12 recommendations about certain generic strategies (Table 9), based on limited evidence (i.e., case series, expert opinion).

Grading*	
D	Patients with pain should be assessed for the presence of BTcP.
D	Patients with BTcP should have this pain specifically assessed.
D	The management of BTcP should be individualized.
D	Consideration should be given to treatment of the underlying cause of the pain.
D	Consideration should be given to avoidance/treatment of the precipitating factors of the pain.
D	Consideration should be given to modification of the background analgesic regimen /"around the clock medication".
D	Modification of the background analgesic regimen has been shown to be a useful approach in managing BTcP, and may involve one or more of the following treatment strategies: • Titration of opioid analgesics. Titrating the opioid can be effective in reducing the intensity and/or frequency of movement-related volitional incident pain (Mercadante et al, 2004). However, his strategy is often limited by the existence/development of dose-dependent adverse effects (e.g., sedation) (Portenoy, 1997). • Switching of opioid analgesics. Switching the opioid and/or the route of administration of the opioid can also be effective in reducing the severity of movement-related volitional incident pain (Kalso et al, 1996; Enting et al, 2002). • Addition of "adjuvant analgesics". Adjuvant analgesics ("co-analgesics") are agents whose primary function is not analgesia, but which provide pain relief in certain circumstances (Lussier & Portenoy, 2004). This strategy can be effective in reducing the impact of specific BTcP syndromes (e.g., antiepileptics for neuropathic pain, anti-spasmodics for visceral pain) (Gannon & Davies, 2006). • Addition of other "adjuvant drugs". Adjuvant drugs are agents whose function is not analgesia, but which provide relief from the adverse effects of analgesic drugs (or the complications of the pain) (Lussier & Portenoy, 2004). This strategy can be effective in allowing titration of the analgesic drugs, which in turn can be effective in reducing the impact of BTcP (e.g., psychostimulants for opioid-related sedation) (Bruera et al, 1992). • Other strategies. In theory, alteration and/or addition of non-opioid analgesic drugs could also lead to improvements in BTcP (e.g., paracetamol, non-steroidal anti-inflammatory drugs) (Gannon & Davies, 2006).
D	Opioids are the "rescue medication" of choice in the management of BTcP episodes.
B	The dose of opioid "rescue medication" should be determined by individual titration.
D	Non-pharmacological methods may be useful in the management of BTcP episodes.

Grading*	
D	Non-opioid analgesics may be useful in the management of BTcP episodes.
D	Interventional techniques may be useful in the management of BTcP.
D	Patients with BTcP should have this pain specifically re-assessed.

*The grading system express the robustness of scientific evidence: an A recommendation is sustained by a strong scientific proofs, while a D evidence is mainly based on expert-opinion. Grade B and C express intermediate levels of evidence.

Table 9. Recommendations for the management of BTcP (Davies et al, 2009)

5.2.5 Constipation and opioid therapy

Side effects are a common and predictable consequence of the opioid therapy; they may either occur acutely and suddenly or as a consequence of a long-term therapy. The most common side effects are constipation, drowsiness, nausea, pruritus and confusion.

Constipation is one of the most common problems experienced by patients in palliative care, particularly those with advanced cancer. The rate of patients with terminal disease affected by constipation varies from 23% to 87% (Librach, 2010; Noguera, 2009; Larkin, 2008; Lagman, 2005), with the highest incidence observed in patients treated with opioids (prevalence 50-95% in several studies: Clark, 2010; Noguera, 2009; Woolery, 2008; Lagman, 2005). Among opioid-treated cancer patients constipation can cause extreme suffering and discomfort. Despite these data, constipation is often undervalued by all the care providers, since it is considered a minor symptom.

Patients' assessement for constipation symptoms should be done at every office visit and a stimulant-based bowel regimen at the beginning of chronic opioid therapy should be routinely initiate. Recommendations (Larkin, 2008; VaDoD, 2010) for the farmacologic treatment of constipation in palliative care patients are listed below:

- Initial bowel regimens should generally consist of a bowel stimulant and a stool softener as well as general measures, such as increased fluid intake, increased dietary fiber, and adequate exercise.
- If inadequate, mild hyperosmotic, saline, and emollient laxatives may be added.
- If possible, reduce or discontinue other drugs that may cause or contribute to constipation.
- Bulk-producing laxatives, such as psyllium and polycarbophil, are not recommended and are relatively contraindicated as they may exacerbate constipation and lead to intestinal obstruction in patients with poor fluid intake.

A revision of clinical guidelines identified only two documents on the management of opioid-induced constipation in palliative care patients (Woolery M, 2008; Librach S. L, 2010); the recommendations are mainly based on expert-opinions:

- Opioids should not be reduced during the treatment of constipation unless it is absolutely necessary (Librach S. L, 2010);
- Switching opioids such as morphine slow-release oral to transdermal fentanyl may decrease constipation (Woolery M, 2008);
- Replace the opioid methadone can lead to a reduction in the consumption of laxatives (Woolery M, 2008);

- Methylnaltrexone is recommended, as an option, to patients treated with opioids that do not respond to usual laxative therapy (Librach S. L, 2010)

Methylnaltrexone (MNTX) is only registered for use in palliative care patients with opioid-induced constipation who did not responde to adequately titrated laxatives, and in whom bowel obstruction has been excluded. MNTX is not a treatment for constipation caused by factors other than opioids. MNTX is an opioid antagonist that, in clinical doses, is unable to cross the blood–brain barrier. Therefore, it can reverse the effect of opioids in the peripheral nervous system and relieve constipation (response of about 50% to laxation after 1 or more doses are given) without reversing the analgesic effect of opioids in CNS (Nerissa & Baumrucker, 2011).

6. Conclusions

Palliative care is a holistic, patient-centered, and culturally sensitive approach to care. To have a meaningful effect on patients' quality of life and end-of-life care, palliative care services should be provided earlier in the course of the disease. However palliative care reach the maximum impact if it can establish a good communication and a respectful relationship with both the patient and his/her carers. Giving dignity, space and attention to the communication are essential steps that need to be undertaken by a doctor that recognizes a correct relationship with the patient as one of his main means of cure and essential for a better Advance Care Planning (ACP).

The essence of the doctor–patient relationship makes family physicians ideally suited to provide home end-of-life care. A good primary palliative care is essential, as it allows patients to remain at home as long as they desire. Many patients want to be informed about their diagnosis, prognosis, treatments and related side effects, even though they are "bad news".

Stimulate and record ACP at an appropriate time is a good clinical practice in palliative care. All the carers should receive an adequate training in ACP discussions with terminally-ill patients. ACP statements should be recorded in medical documents and readily accessible to all the care staff .

The role of Evidence Based Medicine (EBM) in palliative care is limited, since the scientific evidences not always can provide elements of "best practice" in order to lead the clinic practice. However EBM can be useful to handle some situations, such as the treatment of pain and other common symptoms in palliative care. Pain has been identified consistently as one of the major problems in end-of-life care. All types of pain (acute, chronic, and cancer pain) are undertreated and poorly controlled. To obtain effective results in the pain treatment the patient should be fully informed on the origin and type of pain and how it will be monitored; the patient should also be involved in the management plan (including the role of opioid titration) and in the treatment of the expected adverse effects (e.g. the constipation).

7. References

Back L A, Anderson W G, Bunch L, Marr L A, Wallace J A, Yang H B, and Arnold RM, (2008), Communication about cancer near the end-of-life", *Cancer*. Vol. 113(S 7): pp 1897–1910.

Back AL, Arnold RM, Quill TE. (2003), Hope for the best, and prepare for the worst. *Ann Intern Med.*; vol. 138(5): pp 439-443.

Back AL, Arnold RM. (2006), Discussing prognosis: "How much do you want to know?" Talking to patients who are prepared for explicit information, *J Clin Oncol.*, vol. 24(25): pp 4209-4213.

Bajwah, S., Higginson, IJ (2008). General practitioners' use and experiences of palliative care services: a survey in south east England, *BMC Palliative Care*, vol. 7: pp 7-18.

Bakitas M, Lyons KD, Hegel MT, Balan S, Brokaw FC, Seville J,Hull JG, Li Z, Tosteson TD, Byock IR, Ahles TA (2009).: Effects of a palliative care intervention on clinical outcomes in patients with advanced cancer: the Project ENABLE II randomized controlled trial. *JAMA*; vol. 302: pp 741-9.

Bausewein C, Daveson B, Benalia H, Simon ST, Higginson IJ, (2011), Outcome Measurement in Palliative Care:
http://www.eapcnet.eu/LinkClick.aspx?fileticket=-T62WTgTHtU%3d,tabid=1577.

Biancofiore G, (2006), Oxycodone Controlled Release in Cancer Pain Management, Ther Clin Risk Manag. Vol. 2(3): pp 229–234.

Block SD. (2006), Psychological issues in end-of-life care. *J Palliat Med.* Vol. 9(3): pp 751-772.

Breivik H, Collett B, Ventafridda V, Cohen R, Gallacher D, (2006), Survey of chronic pain in Europe: prevalence, impact on daily life, and treatment, *Eur J Pain*; vol. 10(4): pp.287-333.

Cassell EJ. (1982), The nature of suffering and the goals of medicine. *N Engl J Med*; vol. 306: pp 639-45.

Clayton, JM., Butow, PN., Arnold, RM., Tattersall, MH. (2005), Fostering coping and nurturing hope when discussing the future with terminally ill cancer patients and their caregivers; *Cancer*, May 1;vol. 103(9): pp 1965-75.

Coller, JK, Christrup, LL, Somogyi, AA, (2009) Role of active metabolites in the use of opioids, *Eur J Clin Pharmacol* vol. 65: pp 121–139.

D'Errico, Valori, (2011), Manuale sulle cure palliative, per il medico di famiglia e gli operatori sanitari che si dedicano alle cure palliative, *Edicare publishing*, ISBN: 978-88-97137-00-9.

Daneault S., Dion D. (2004) : Suffering of gravely ill patients. *Can Fam Physician*; vol. 50, pp. 1343-1345.

Davies E., Higginson I J., (2004) Palliative care: the solid facts, WHO Regional Office for Europe,:
http://www.euro.who.int/__data/assets/pdf_file/0003/98418/E82931.pdf

Davies, AN., Dickman A, Reid C, Stevens AM, Zeppetella G, (2009) The management of cancer-related Breakthrough pain: recommendations of a task group of the Science Committee of the Association for Palliative Medicine of Great Britain and Ireland. *Eur J Pain.* Vol. 13(4), pp. 331-8.

Dickman A. (2011), Integrated strategies for the successful management of breakthrough cancer pain, *Support Palliat Care.* Vol.5(1): pp 8-14.

Doyle, Woodruff, (2008), The IAHPC Manual of Palliative Care, 2nd Edition, *Published by IAHPC Press* ISBN 0-9758525-1-5.

Earle CC, Landrum MB, Souza JM, Neville BA, Weeks JC, Ayanian JZ. (2008), Aggressiveness of cancer care near the end-of-life: is it a quality-of-care issue? *J Clin Oncol*; vol. 26: pp 3860-6.

Emanuel, LL, von Gunten, CF, Ferris FD. (1999) In The Education for Physicians on End-of-Life Care (EPEC), *American Medical Association.*

Emanuel EJ, Ash A, Yu W, Yu W, Gazelle G, Levinsky NG, Saynina O, McClellan M, Moskowitz M, (2002), Managed care, hospice use, site of death, and medical expenditures in the last year of life, *Arch Intern Med*; vol.162: pp 1722-8.

Emanuel, L., Bennett K, Richardson VE. (2007) The dying role. *J Palliat Med*, Feb; Vol. 10 (1), pp159-68.

Emanuel L, Librach SL, (2011), Palliative care, Core Skills and Clinical Competence, Expert consultant and Print, 2nd Edition, *Elsevier*, ISBN: 978-1-4377-1619-1.

Eti S., Heidelbaugh JJ, (2011), Palliative Care in Primary care: clinics in office practice, *Saunders*, Vol. 38, N° 2, ISSN 0095-4543,ISBN-13:978-1-4557-0497-2.

Felden, C. Walter, S. Harder, R.-D. Treede, H. Kayser, D. Drover, G. Geisslinger, J. Lo¨tsch, (2011), Comparative clinical effects of hydromorphone and morphine: a meta-analysis, British *Journal of Anaesthesia*, vol. 107 (3): pp 319–28.

Foley, KM.; Gelband, H. (2001), Improving Palliative Care for Cancer, Summary and Recommendations. Washington D.C: Institute of Medicine and National Academy Press, Paperback, ISBN-10: 0-309-07563-7; ISBN-13: 978-0-309-07563-3.

Grape S, Schug SA, Lauer S, Schug BS. (2010), Formulations of fentanyl for the management of pain, *Drugs.*; vol. 70(1): pp 57-72.

Hanks GW, de Conno F, Hanks GW, Conno F, Cherny N, Hanna M, Kalso E, McQuay HJ, Mercadante S, Meynadier J, Poulain P, Ripamonti C, Radbruch L, Casas JR, Sawe J, Twycross RG, Ventafridda V; Expert Working Group of the Research Network of the European Association for Palliative Care (2001) Morphine and alternative opioids in cancer pain: the EAPC recommendations. *Br J Cancer.* Vol. 84(5), pp. 587-93.

Hebert, RS., Prigerson, HG., Schulz, R., Arnold, RM.(2006), Preparing caregivers for the death of a loved one: a theoretical framework and suggestions for future research; *J Palliat Med*, vol. 9(5): pp 1164-71.

Hewitt, M, Simone, JV. (1999), Ensuring Quality Cancer Care, Washington D.C, National Academies Press; Institute of Medicine (IOM), Commission on Life Sciences (CLS), Paperback, ISBN-10: 0-309-06480-5, ISBN-13: 978-0-309-06480-4.

Higginson, IJ., Sen-Gupta, GJ (2000), Place of care in advanced cancer: a qualitative systematic literature review of patient preferences *J Palliat Med.* Fall; Vol. 3(3), pp287-300.

Hinton, J, (1994), Can home care maintain an acceptable quality of life for patients with terminal cancer and their relatives? *Palliat Med*; vol. 8: pp 183–96.

Institute for Clinical Systems Improvement, (2009) *Palliative care*, Health Care Guideline http://www.icsi.org/guidelines_and_more/gl_os_prot/other_health_care_conditions/palliative_care/palliative_care_11875.html

International Association for Study of Pain: http://www.iasp-pain.org/ AM/Template.cfm?Section=Pain_Defi...isplay.cfm,ContentID=1728#Pain

Joint Commission Accreditation of healthcare Organization Standard Manual: http://www.jointcommission.org/

Jost L, Roila F, (2010), ESMO Guidelines Working Group, Clinical practice guidelines:" Management of cancer pain: ESMO Clinical Practice", *Annals of Oncology*, vol. 21 (Supplement 5): pp. v257–v260.

Kagawa-Singer M, Blackhall LJ. (2001), Negotiating cross-cultural issues at the end-of-life: "You got to g where he lives." *JAMA*. Vol. 286(23): pp 2993-3001.

Kaldjian LC, Curtis AE, Shinkunas LA, Cannon KT (2008), Goals of care toward the end-of-life: a structured literature review, *Am J Hosp Palliat Care*. Vol. 25(6): pp 501-11.

Knops KM, Srinivasan M, Meyers FJ, (2005), Patient desires: a model for assessment of patient preferences for care of severe or terminal illness". *Palliat Support Care*, vol. 3(4): pp. 289-99:
http://www.caresearch.com.au/caresearch/tabid/2067/Default.aspx

Larkin PJ, Sykes PN, Ellershaw JE, Elsner F, Eugene B, Gootjes JRG, Nabal M, Noguera A, Ripamonti C, Zucco F, Zuurmond WWA, (2008) The European Consensus Group on Constipation in Pallitive Care - The management of constipation in palliative care: clinical practice recomandations - *Palliative Medicine*; vol. 22: pp 796-807.

Lehman, F., Daneault S. (2006), Palliative care: first and foremost the domain of family physicians. *Can Fam Physician*; vol. 52: pp 417-418.

Librach S.L. – Constipation – In Emanuel L.L., Librach S.L. (2011)- Palliative Care Core Skills and Clinical Competencies (2 ed.) - ISBN: 978-1-4377-1619-1USA: *Elsevier Saunders*.

Librach SL, Bouvette M, DeAngelis C, Pereira JL, (2010), The Canadian Consensus Development Group for Constipation in Patients with Advance Progressive Illness - Consensus Recommendations for the Management of Constipation in Patient with Advanced, Progressive Illness - *Journal of Pain and Symptom Management*; vol. 4 (5): pp 761-773.

Lynn J. et al (2007), The Common Sense Guide to Improving Palliative Care, The online edition:
http://www.mywhatever.com/cifwriter/library/commonsense/commonsense301.html.

Maltoni M, et al. (2005) A validation study of the WHO analgesic ladder: a two-step vs three-step strategy. *Support Care Cancer*; vol. 13: pp 888-894.

McNicol E, Strassels S, Goudas L, Lau J, Carr D. (2004) Nonsteroidal anti-inflammatory drugs, alone or combined with opioids, for cancer pain: a systematic review. *J Clin Oncol*. Vol. 22(10): pp 1975-92.

Meier, DE., Back, AL., Morrison, RS. (2001) The inner life of physicians and care of the seriously ill; *JAMA*, vol. 286(23): pp 3007-14.

Morita T, Akechi T, Ikenaga M, Kizawa Y, Kohara H, Mukaiyama T, Nakaho T, Nakashima N, Shima Y, Matsubara T, Uchitomi Y, Late referrals to specialized palliative care service in Japan. J Clin Oncol; vol.23: pp 2637-44.

Morrison, RS, Meier, DE, (2004) Clinical practice: Palliative care *N Engl J Med*, vol. 350(25): pp 2582-2590.

National Consensus Project. Clinical Practice Guidelines for Quality Palliative Care (2011):
http://www.nationalconsensusproject.org/guidelines.html

National Institute for Health and Clinical Excellence (NICE). Quality standard for end of life care for adults (2011):
http://www.nice.org.uk/guidance/qualitystandards/endoflifecare/home.jsp

Nerissa, L., Baumrucker J. (2011) Methylnaltrexone: Treatment for Opioid-Induced Constipation, *AM J Hosp Palliat Care* vol. 28 pp 1 59-61.

Neuropatic Pain Special Interest Group of the International Association for Study of Pain: http://www.neupsig.org/

Ngo-Metzger Quyen, Md, Mph, Kristin J. August, Bs, Malathi Srinivasan, Md, Solomon Liao Md, Frank L. Meyskens (2008), End-of-Life Care: Guidelines for Patient- Centered Communication, *Am Fam Physician*, Jan, vol. 15;77(2), pp167-174.

Parker PA, Baile WF, de Moor C, Lenzi R, Kudelka AP, Cohen L. (2001), Breaking bad news about cancer: patients' preferences for communication. *J Clin Oncol*, vol. 19(7): pp 2049-2056.

Pergolizzi J, Böger RH, Budd K, Dahan A, Erdine S Hans G, Kress HG, Langford R, Likar R, Raffa RB, Sacerdote P., (2008), Opioids and the Management of Chronic Severe Pain in the Elderly: Consensus Statement of an International Expert Panel with Focus on the Six Clinically Most Often Used World Health Organization step III Opioids (Buprenorphine, Fentanyl, Hydromorphone, Methadone, Morphine, Oxycodone), *World Institute of Pain, Pain Practice*, Volume 8, Issue 4, pp 287–313.

Portenoy, RK., Hagen NA (1990), Breakthrough pain: definition, prevalence and characteristics, *Pain*, Vol. 41(3): pp 273-81.

Ptacek, JT,Ptacek, JJ. (2001) Patients' perceptions of receiving bad news about cancer; *J Clin Oncol*, vol. 19(21): pp. 4160-4.

Rabow, MW., Hauser, JM., Adams, J. (2004) Supporting family caregivers at the end-of-life: "they don't know what they don't know"; *JAMA*, vol. 28;291(4): pp 483-91.

Royal College of Physician, (2009), National Guideline:" Advanced Care Planning", Concise Guidance to Good Practice Series, A4 report, 19 pages, CODE: 15119 000(010), ISBN: 9781860163524: http://bookshop.rcplondon.ac.uk/contents/pub267-e5ba7065-2385-49c9-a68e-f64527c15f2a.pdf.

Salander, P.(2002) Bad news from the patient's perspective: an analysis of the written narratives of newly diagnosed cancer patients, *Soc Sci Med* vol. 55(5): pp721-32.

Shiozaki, M., Morita, T.; Hirai, K., Sakaguchi, Y.; Tsuneto, S., Shima Y, (2005), Why are bereaved family members dissatisfied with specialised inpatient palliative care service? A nationwide qualitative study; *Palliat Med*, vol. 19 no. 4 319-327.

Slort W, Schweitzer BPM, Blankenstein AH, Abarshi EA, Riphagen Il, Echteld MA, Aaronson NK, Van der Horst HE and Deliens (2011) L, Perceived barriers and facilitators for general practitioner-patient communication in palliative care: A systematic review, *Palliative Medicine*, vol. 25(6),pp 613–629.

Song MK, (2004), Effects of end-of-life discussions on patients' affective outcomes, *Nurs Outlook*, vol. 52(3): pp 118-25.

Steinhauser, KE., Christakis, NA., Clipp, EC., McNeilly, M., Grambow, S., Parker, J.,Tulsky JA. (2001), Preparing for the end-of-life: preferences of patients, families, physicians, and other care providers; *J Pain Symptom Manage*. Vol. 22(3): pp 727-37.

Steinhauser, KE., Christakis, NA., Clipp, EC., McNeilly, M., McIntyre, L., Tulsky, JA. (2000) Factors considered important at the end-of-life by patients, family, physicians, and other care providers; *JAMA*. p. 2476-82.

Sullivan R, Peppercorn J, Sikora K, Zalcberg J, Meropol NJ, Amir E, Khayat D, Boyle P, Autier P, Tannock IF, Fojo T, Siderov J, Williamson S, Camporesi S, McVie JG,

Purushotham AD, Naredi P, Eggermont A, Brennan MF, Steinberg ML, De Ridder M, McCloskey SA, Verellen D, Roberts T, Storme G, Hicks RJ, Ell PJ, Hirsch BR, Carbone DP, Schulman KA, Catchpole P, Taylor D, Geissler J, Brinker NG, Meltzer D, Kerr D, Aapro M., (2011), Delivering affordable cancer care in high-income countries, *The Lancet Oncology*, Volume 12, Issue 10, Pages 933 – 980.

Temel JS, Greer JA, Muzikansky A, Gallagher ER, Admane S, Jackson VA, Dahlin CM, Blinderman CD, Jacobsen J, Pirl WF, Billings JA, Lynch TJ (2010), Early palliative care for patients with metastatic non-small-cell lung cancer, *N Engl J Med*. 19; vol. 363(8): pp 733-42.

Tulsky, JA. (2005), Beyond advance directives: importance of communication skills at the end-of-life, *JAMA* vol. 294(3): pp 359-65.

VA/DoD (2010) Evidence Based Practice, Clinical Practice Guideline, Management of Opioid Therapy for Chronic pain, Version 2.0, Department of Veterans Affairs, Department of Defense May, 159 p.

Vadalouca, Moka, Argyra, Sikioti, Siafaka, (2008), Opioid rotation in patients with cancer: A review of the current literature, *J Opioid Manag*, Vol.4(4): pp 213-50.

Valdimarsdottir, U.; Helgason, AR.; Furst, CJ.; Adolfsson, J.; Steineck, G. (2004), Awareness of husband's impending death from cancer and long-term anxiety in widowhood: a nationwide follow-up; *Palliat Med*, vol. 18(5): pp 432-43.

Walling A, Lorenz KA, Dy SM, Naeim A, Sanati H, Asch SM, Wenger NS. (2008), Evidence-based recommendations for information and care planning in cancer care. *J Clin Oncol*; vol. 26: pp 3896-902.

Watson, M. Principles of palliative care (2008), *Oxford Journals Medicine InnovAiT*, Volume1 Issue4, Pp. 250-256.

Wenrich, MD., Curtis, JR., Shannon, SE., Carline, JD., Ambrozy, DM., Ramsey, PG. (2001), Communicating with dying patients within the spectrum of medical care from terminal diagnosis to death; *Arch Intern Med*. Vol 161(6) pp 868-74.

Woolery M, Bisanz A, Lyons HF, Gaido L, Yenulevich M, Fulton S, McMillan SC, (2008), Putting evidence into practice: evidence-based interventions for the prevention and management of constipation in patients with cancer - *Clin J Oncol Nurs* vol.12(2): pp 317-37.

Zimmermann C, Riechelmann R, Krzyzanowska M, Rodin G, Tannock I. (2008), Effectiveness of specialized palliative care: a systematic review, *JAMA*; vol. 299: pp 1698-709.

10

Adherence to Long-Term Therapy – A Model of Assessment into Primary Care

Alex Müller
University of Cape Town
South Africa

1. Introduction

Adherence to long-term therapy is a challenge for patients worldwide. In developing countries the focus is placed on adherence to antiretroviral treatment for HIV and antibacterial treatment for TB, while patients and health care providers in developed countries grapple with adherence to treatment of chronic lifestyle diseases such as diabetes. Adherence is a crucial element of successful treatment – some say it is the backbone of any medical treatment. It is therefore of utmost importance for health care providers to assess how adherent their patients are. However, this is often overlooked in routine patient assessments in primary care.

This chapter describes the challenges of adherence with long-term treatments by using the example of antiretroviral treatment for HIV. It introduces the most common adherence measures and describes the experiences of integrating adherence assessment in primary health care settings in Cape Town, South Africa. Even though it focuses on adherence in pediatric patients, the observations and conclusions drawn from this chapter are highly relevant to any age group.

2. Adherence - "Drugs don't work in patients who don't take them"[1]

Chronically ill patients need to take medication for the rest of their life. This requires a lot of discipline and commitment from the patients' part, as well as good education and communication from the health care providers' side. In the past, the term "compliance" was used to characterize the patients' following of health care providers' instructions. As models of patient-physician relationship have changed, so has the definition of "compliance". The new definition challenges the often paternalistic model of decision-making and emphasizes a more equal cooperation between patient and health care provider. The term "compliance" has been replaced with "adherence", to acknowledge the patient's more active participation in the decision-making process and seeing medication-taking behaviour from the patient's perspective: "Adherence is the engaged and accurate participation of an informed patient in

---

[1] Quote by C. EVERETT KOOP, Professor of Pediatrics and Paediatric Surgery, University of Pennsylvania; Surgeon General of the United States 1982 – 1989, quoted in: OSTERBERG and BLASCHKE (2005; p. 487)

a plan of care. It is a broader term than compliance – the extent to which patients follow the instructions of their healthcare providers – and implies understanding, consent, and partnership. Adherence includes entering into and continuing in a program or care plan, attending appointments and tests as scheduled, taking medications as prescribed, modifying lifestyle as needed, and avoiding risk behaviours. It includes adherence to care and adherence to medication, but is usually regarded as more than the sum of its parts."[2]. Osterberg and Blaschke (2005) further elaborate on the difference between compliance and adherence: "The word "adherence" is preferred by many health care providers, because "compliance" suggests that the patient is passively following the doctor's orders and that the treatment plan is not based on a therapeutic alliance or contract established between the patient and the physician." The World Health Organization suggests broadening the definition of the term adherence to "the extent to which a person's behaviour – taking medication, following a diet, and/or executing lifestyle changes, corresponds with agreed recommendations from a health care provider" (WHO 2003; p. 3), according to Berg and Arnsten (2006; p. S79), this behaviour is "individual, complex and dynamic". Table 1 illustrates the various dimensions of adherence, and each dimension's correlate in the patient's behaviour.

Adherence Behaviour	Behavioural Task
Medication-refill adherence	Patient picks up a prescription refill
Medication-interval adherence	Patient takes a medication at the right time of the day
Medication-quantity adherence	Patient takes the right number of pills
Medication-diet adherence	Patient takes medication in accordance with dietary requirements (if specified)

Table 1. Dimensions of adherence

Contrary to this concept, clinical practice often limits the term adherence to the intake of medication and disregards the broader implications of its definition. Adherence is usually reported as the percentage of the prescribed doses actually taken by the patient over a specified period of time, and thus reduced to recommendations that instruct the patient on tablet intake. For these instructions, adherence can vary along a continuum from 0 to 100 percent, sometimes over 100 percent if patients take more than the prescribed amount of medication. Adherence can also be reported as a dichotomous variable, classifying patients into the categories adherent or non-adherent. Since there is no consensual standard for what constitutes adequate adherence, the cut-off value for these categories depends on the patient's condition, the characteristics of the regimen prescribed, on pharmacokinetics of the prescribed medication and on individual research protocols. For HIV infection, an adherence rate greater than 95 percent is considered adequate and necessary for treatment success (Chesney 2003; Paterson et al. 2000). However, common to all these definitions of adherence is the fact that they solely focus on the intake of medication and do not allow for an inclusion of dietary instructions, lifestyle changes or general health behaviour of patients.

In the industrialised world, adherence has been in the focus for medication of chronic diseases such as diabetes and hypertension, or for patients taking immunosuppressants after organ transplantation. In developing countries, HIV infection emerged as a relatively

---

[2] Quote from RABKIN et al. (2005; p. 11)

new chronic illness and the introduction of Highly Active Antiretroviral Therapy (HAART) placed a new emphasis on assessing adherence to HAART. Adherence has a significant impact on all outcome parameters of antiretroviral treatment: on plasma HIV RNA levels, on CD4+ lymphocyte count as well as on survival rates. Bangsberg et al. (2000) demonstrated a strong linear relationship between adherence to HAART and plasma HIV RNA levels, with a 10% decrease in adherence leading to a doubling of HIV RNA plasma levels. Among patients with undetectable HIV RNA load, adherence predicts the time that viral load is kept at undetectable levels (Raboud et al. 2002). Adherence was found to be significantly associated with successful virological outcome (Paterson et al. 2000) and an increase in CD4+ lymphocyte count (Singh et al. 1999). To the same extend that adequate adherence is linked to positive treatment outcomes, non-adherence can result in an increased viral load, emerging drug resistance that limits further treatment options, and, ultimately, in more rapid progression to clinical AIDS and increased mortality (Knobel et al. 2001).

There have been great concerns over whether the infrastructural, socio-economic and political difficulties in the countries of the developing world will allow for demanding and complicated treatment programs resulting in treatment success (Harries et al. 2001). The World Health Organization (WHO) advises that treatment principles in resource-limited settings be the same as for the developed world (WHO 2004); recent initiatives such as the Global Fund To Fight AIDS, Tuberculosis and Malaria (GFATM) and the Presidential Emergency Plan for AIDS Relief (PEPfAR) have provided funding to ensure availability and sustainability of antiretroviral treatment for these countries. Since the number of patients in developing countries is by far greater than in the developed world (UNAIDS 2008), these countries follow a public health approach in providing HAART for adults and children. The choice of antiretroviral drugs is limited, and fixed drug combinations are provided in so-called first- and second-line regimens. The term first-line regimen describes the initial antiretroviral drug combination that a patient starts with. Upon the development of resistance to one or more of the drugs a switch to the second-line regimen, which includes different drugs, is possible. These fixed combinations do not allow the possibility for patient-individualized, "tailor-made" regimens as available in the developed world (WHO 2005). In this way, the cost of antiretroviral drugs is reduced and treatment programs are more affordable and can allow for large amounts of patients. Given this limited choice of treatment options, the imperative of good adherence is of even greater importance in these settings. However, it has been contested whether or not good adherence would be possible.

In a public statement made in 2001, the then chief of the U.S. Agency for International Development (USAID), Andrew Natsios, was quoted to have said that Africans "don't know what Western time is" and thus could not take antiretroviral treatment on the proper schedule. Additionally he reportedly stated that when Africans were asked to take their drugs at a certain time of the day, they "do not know what you are talking about"[3]. This statement, implying that the culture and the general attitude of people living in African countries would render them unable to adhere to antiretroviral treatment, has been strongly condemned by patients, physicians and patients worldwide. In the following years,

---

[3] See ATTARAN et al.: "Dead wrong on AIDS". Published on 15th July 2001 in The Washington Post, United States.

numerous studies from resource-limited settings with HIV-infected adults and children taking HAART have highlighted that adherence is, in fact, rather good (Byakika-Tusiime et al. 2005; Nachega et al. 2004, Vreeman et al. 2008). In the first of two South African studies, Orrell et al. (2003) from Cape Town found that of 278 adults followed over 48 weeks, the median adherence was 94%, and concluded that low socio-economic status was not a barrier to achieving good adherence to antiretroviral triple therapy. In the other South African study Nachega et al. (2004) could show that 97% of HIV-infected adults receiving antiretroviral treatment at a public hospital in Johannesburg had adherence levels of greater than 90 percent. These findings are consistent with a meta-analysis comparing the adherence to antiretroviral treatment in patients from the United States to the adherence in patients from Sub-Saharan Africa, which found that the latter patient group showed higher pooled rates of adherence, and underlined the ability of African patients to adhere to their treatment (Mills et al. 2006).

As lined out above, adherence in resource-limited settings is of even greater importance, yet may also be more difficult to achieve (Gill et al. 2005). In order not to jeopardize the limited options of treatment, virological suppression should be sustained for as long as possible. Emerging studies from various settings in resource-limited countries underline the findings by Mills et al. (2006) and show adherence rates that are as high or even higher than in the developed world (Byakika-Tusiime et al. 2005; Oyugi et al. 2004). In the context of these countries, structural and social inequalities have an unmistakable impact on the health status of patients. A recent report by the WHO Commission on Social Determinants of Health (CSDH 2008) indicates that the quality of urban and rural living conditions such as housing, sanitation and access to clean water are vital contributors to health. This should be borne in mind when comparing the outcomes of antiretroviral treatment in developing countries to outcomes from Europe and North America; it should also be borne in mind that the risk of treatment failure is higher when poorer health statuses exist, regardless of adherence. Since primary care health workers (physicians, nurses, pharmacists and community care workers) are at the forefront of the health care system, they often encounter the patient within her social and economic space. Primary care needs to take the social determinants of health into account, and the same applies to the social determinants of adherence. In order to do this, primary care providers need to know how to assess adherence in their patients.

3. Assessing adherence in primary care

Accurately measuring levels of adherence to medication has importance in clinical trials as well as in clinical practice. For clinical trials, the knowledge of patients actually taking the medication studied is imperative to allow examination of dose-response relationships and treatment efficacy. In clinical practice, the failure of a therapy to provide the desired clinical outcome can be due to either drug failure or poor adherence, and health care providers need information on adherence to make the adequate clinical decision. Most often, it is primary care providers who discuss the importance of adherence with their patients, and on whom it falls to assess whether patients adhere to their treatment plans or not. As with other chronic illnesses, in the case of HAART it is known that adherence levels decrease over time (Howard et al. 2002). The reasons for this are manifold and not difficult to imagine: treatment fatigue, forgetfulness, patients running out of medication, unforeseen circumstances in which medication is not readily available, and, in less resourced countries, medication stock-outs at the point of distribution. Adherence monitoring is necessary to identify patients in need of adherence-improvement interventions before the clinical effects of non-adherence start to show. Measures in clinical settings should be effective, practical and inexpensive, with the aim of identifying poorly adherent patients. This is of even greater importance in resource-limited settings where limited treatment options often do not accommodate for drug changes that become necessary after the development of resistant viral strains due to poor adherence (Gill et al. 2005). Among the variety of available adherence measures, one can differentiate between direct and indirect measures (Farmer 1999). Direct measures of adherence provide proof that the drug has been taken by the patient. There are two ways to achieve this: either by monitoring the drug (or its metabolites) in the patient's body, or by actually supervising the patient taking the drug. The former is called therapeutic drug monitoring, and drug metabolites are usually monitored in blood or urine, although often they can also be traced in other bodily fluids and even hair. This method requires knowledge of the pharmacokinetics of the studied drug and is an invasive procedure. Based on the drug plasma concentration the patient is classified as adherent or non-adherent. Therapeutic drug monitoring is often reserved for clinical trials, where the scientific interest justifies the invasive procedure to obtain the blood/ urine sample. Evidently, it requires a multitude of clinical resources (staff to take the sample and process it in an adequately equipped lab), and the results are not available immediately. On the other hand, directly-observed therapy (DOTS) – the monitoring of the actual intake of the drug by the patient – is relatively inexpensive and requires little to no resources. It is the basis of many successful tuberculosis treatment programs in the developing world. Often, it is carried out in the home of the patients – here, community care workers play a crucial role. While it requires a good infrastructure and availability of care workers (or even relatives) to supervise the patient taking her medication, the resources required from the health care system are minimal.

Indirect measures of adherence can be categorized into subjective (self-reporting by the patient) and objective methods (medication measurement by pill count or estimation of liquid drug formulations, use of electronic monitoring devices and pharmacy prescription record review). These are the most common methods used in primary care settings and will be discussed in detail further on in this chapter.

Each method has advantages and disadvantages that need to be weighed against each other. In general, the accuracy of measures is determined by calculating the sensitivity and specificity of the method with a standard of reference (Ransohoff and Feinstein 1978). For adherence measures, sensitivity denotes the proportion of adherent patients that are correctly identified as adherent. Specificity denotes the proportion of non-adherent patients rightly picked out as non-adherent; high specificity means that as few non-adherent patients as possible should be wrongly identified as adherent. The overall accuracy of the method is calculated by incorporating the proportion of patients that are correctly identified as adherent or non-adherent. However accurate one single measure of adherence may be, it is recommended to use a combination of measures to adjust for possible bias of each single method: "A multi-method approach that combines feasible self-reporting and reasonable objective measures is the current state-of-the-art in measurement of adherence behaviour." (WHO 2003). A further way of validating adherence measures is by determining their correlation with a surrogate marker of adherence. For HIV infection, undetectable HIV RNA plasma levels, indicating that HAART effectively works against the HI virus, serve as surrogate markers for adherence to HAART (Arnsten et al. 2001).

3.1 Patient self-report

Self report is an inexpensive and quick tool to assess adherence at a health care facility or at home. It can be administered by doctors or nurses, counsellors, social workers, clinical psychologists or community care workers. Depending on the relationship of the patient to the interviewer or the administering physician, results can vary in truth and reliability. Self report measures can be structured questionnaires asking about doses that were missed during a specified time before the clinic visit and thus quantifying non-adherence. These questionnaires can be handed out to the patients to be filled out anonymously. For patients with poor literacy or eye-sight, they can be read by the interviewer to assure that the information given is correct. Information on missed doses is used to classify patients or caregivers into adherent and non-adherent groups. Visual Analogue Scales (VAS, see Figure 1) require patients to self-rate their adherence in percent and measure adherence as a continuous variable (Byrne et al. 2002; Giordano et al. 2004). Open interviews can highlight problems around adherence but make it more difficult to quantify adherence rates. A recent meta-analysis of various self-report measures in adult patients with HIV showed that in 85% of all studies reviewed, self-reported adherence was significantly associated with virological outcome (Simoni et al. 2006). There are numerous questionnaires that assess self-reported adherence. Visual Analogue Scales are among the most widely used self-reporting tools. Often abbreviated VAS, they combine the recollection memory with a visual component – patients are asked to rate their adherence on a scale. The scale, ranging from zero to one hundred percent, allows patients to estimate their adherence without forcing them to recollect specific drug intake moments. The visual component makes it suitable for patients who are less literate.

While Visual Analogue Scales ask about drug doses that a patient has actually taken, questionnaires inquire about doses that a patient missed or forgot to take. Different formats of questionnaires span different recollection time intervals. It is common to ask for drug doses that were missed in the previous day, the previous three days, the previous week and the previous month. It is important to note that patients' memories become less accurate the longer the recollection time span is – a very understandable phenomenon, since who would remember forgetting to take medication 3 weeks ago? With the data gained from missed drug dose questionnaires, adherence rates can be calculated. This step might not necessarily be required in clinical practice, but is routinely used to standardise adherence rates in research. Questionnaires that are routinely used in HIV treatment adherence research are the ACTG and PACTG (for adult and paediatric missed drug dose recollection, respectively), developed by the AIDS Clinical Trial Group. These questionnaires are widely available and can serve as a blueprint for tailor-made self-report measures.

An important limitation that needs to be noted for self-reported adherence measures is the inability to objectively confirm the information obtained from the patient. Self-report adherence measures are prone to over-reporting of adherence because patients often feel compelled to answer what they think the health care worker wants to hear. This social desirability (Simoni et al. 2007) can be caused by a lack of faith in the health care worker –

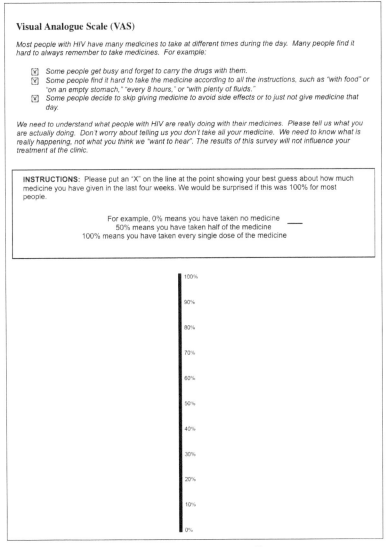

Fig. 1. A Visual Analogue Scale to assess HIV treatment adherence.

patients fear that they would receive inferior treatment for not adhering well enough, or might feel ashamed at their 'failure' (Safren et al. 2006). This is an important issues especially in resource-limited settings where access to health care is limited, patients are less empowered and often depend on the only health care provider in the area. A trustful patient-provider relationship is key to ensuring that patients feel that they can be honest about their adherence behaviour, and it is imperative that health care providers remain non-judgemental and keep encouraging patients to adhere rather than judge or penalise them for not adhering.

3.2 Pill count

For pill count adherence measurement, patients are asked to return their unused medication at each clinic visit. A health care provider or researcher then calculates the percentage of prescribed pills that are absent from the medication container, thus enabling a measurement of adherence as a continuous variable (Steele et al. 2001). Pill count is a relatively quick and easy assessment of adherence, and once a patient has established the routine of returning unused medication, can be completed within a few seconds. For children who receive their medication in liquid form, the pill count concept is also applicable, although slightly more complicated. Upon return of the unused medication syrups, health care workers can measure the amount of liquid returned and calculate an adherence rate based on the amount of liquid the child had initially received. The accuracy of ill count assessment methods depends on the patient's cooperation in returning their unused medication.

3.3 Electronic Monitoring Devices

Electronic Monitoring Devices, also called EMDs are seen as the objective way to measure adherence. They are a relatively new assessment method that uses pressure-sensitive microchips, such as the Medication Event Monitoring System (MEMS), which is implanted in the caps of medication containers (Figure 2). The microchip records time and date of all bottle opening events as presumptive doses taken by the patient; the data is stored in the chip until downloaded onto a computer. MEMS caps allow the examination of patterns of adherence and detailed aspects of medication-taking, such as dose interval adherence, correct timing of dose-taking and prospective adherence assessment over time (Figure 3 shows a sample analysis of data from a MEMS device). In HIV adherence research, MEMS caps are often used as a "gold standard" for adherence assessment in adults, because of a closer correlation with undetectable HIV RNA plasma levels than other single measures (Arnsten et al. 2001). Recently, MEMS caps have also been used to measure the adherence of children who take liquid medication (Müller et al. 2008).

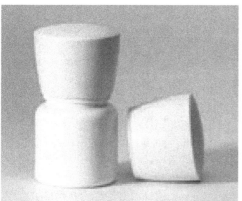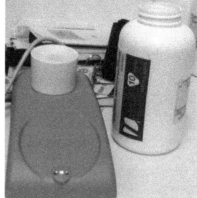

Fig. 2. MEMS container with cap and MEMS terminal to read the microchip

Electronic Monitoring Devices have several advantages over more traditional adherence measures. Most outstanding is their ability to record not only adherence rates, but veritable

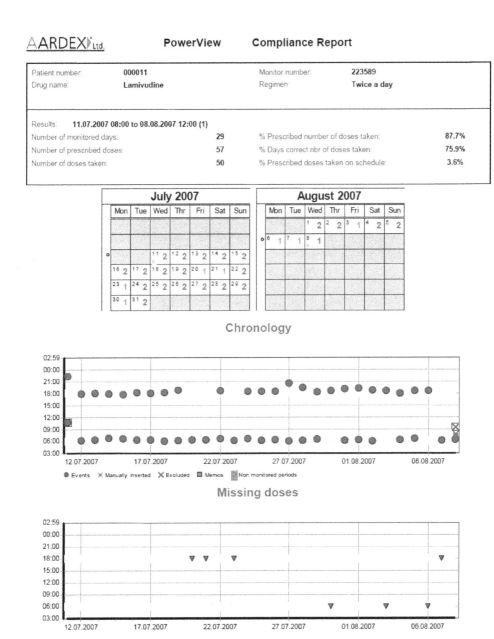

Fig. 3. A report by MEMS, an electronic monitoring device. The report is created with software and shows a) overall adherence statistics, b) drug doses taken by day, c) the chronology (timing) of doses taken and d) missed doses by day

adherence patterns. The microchip records the date and time of every container opening, and health care providers can trace each drug dose in detail. Hence, it is the only adherence measure that can record the exact time of drug dose taking – this is particularly important for drug regimen that depend on constant drug plasma levels, like antiretrovirals against HIV. The detailed report allows the health care worker to analyse together with the patient what the challenges to adherence are – for example if patients struggle more to keep medication times on weekends, or on certain days during the week. Often, these analyses reveal adherence challenges that patients were not aware of before. In this way, adherence assessment with Electronic Monitoring Devices also supports patients to adhere to their drug regimen. Newer electronic devices have evolved even more, and come with build-in timers and alarm clocks that serve as reminders to take drug doses. Another advantage of electronic devices is that they provide the most objective data of all indirect adherence measures. Similar to pill count, health care workers don't rely on information obtained from the patient, but can actually access adherence information directly from the microchip. Unlike pill count, the microchip is also more difficult to tamper with – because it measures medication-taking behaviour over the whole time in-between health facility visits, it cannot be changed or manipulated should patients try to do so before returning it to their health care worker.

3.4 Pharmacy data

Another way of assessing adherence is to record and analyse patient's patterns of obtaining refills and new prescriptions of their medication from pharmacies. Provided that patients either use the same pharmacy, or their records are stored in a central database – or that patients visit a pharmacy affiliated to the primary care facility – records on when patients pick up their renewed prescriptions gives an indication on how much of their previous medication they have taken. The presumption here is that patients who are adherent to their medication will use up all their stock in time for a new prescription (i.e. monthly prescriptions for HIV medication) and failure to adhere will lead to a surplus in medication that is reflected in late pharmacy pick ups. Another assumption is that a patient's adherence to scheduled pharmacy pick-ups is a surrogate marker for her medication adherence.

An adherence rate is calculated in comparing the amount of doses prescribed and the amount of doses obtained from the pharmacy over a specified time period. This method is more applicable for large population-based studies where individual adherence rates are of less importance (Steiner and Prochazka 1997), but it can also be used to get an overview of individual patient's adherences. For HIV treatment adherence, it has been found to be correlated with virological outcome in adults (Grossberg et al. 2004; Low-Beer et al. 2000).

4. Cost comparison of adherence measures - experience from South Africa

In a recent study, a research team from the Desmond Tutu HIV Centre at the University of Cape Town set out to evaluate the cost-effectiveness and feasibility of a range of adherence measures at a paediatric primary care facility (Müller et al. 2010). In a cross-sectional study design, 53 paediatric patients were enrolled to have their adherence monitored by electronic monitoring devices, self-report by Visual Analogue Scale and missed-dose recall, by pharmacy refill data and by pill count (for most children this meant measurement of returned syrups). The feasibility of each measure in a primary care setting was explored by its month-long use through primary care providers, and additionally a cost comparison of all measures was performed. The results highlighted crucial issues in the use of adherence assessment in primary care settings.

The cost comparison of the adherence measures used an ingredients-based methodology in order to most accurately assess the cost of the measures (Drummond et al. 2005). This means measuring the utilization of staff time and measures (the ingredients) required to perform the task, and the cost of each measure. For each adherence measure all tasks performed by staff members over and above standard practice in the absence of adherence measurement were determined. For each task, a research assistant observed the clinic staff using the adherence measures, recording the time taken to perform the task and all consumables and other resources used. The costs of staff time were based on the annual cost of employment of the staff grade performing the task. The costs of other resources were based on their commercial prices with the costs of durable items being depreciated across their expected lifetime. Table 2 shows the costing of each adherence measure. It is quite clear that MEMS, the electronic monitoring device, was considerably more expensive than any of the other measures. This was primarily due to the high initial purchasing cost ($120 per cap; additionally the battery life limits the length of use to 3 years) but also due to high additional expected input from the pharmacist (annual wage $37,341) and pharmacist assistant (annual wage $8,487) in managing the adherence measurement process. All other measures were considerably cheaper, mostly because of the low cost of the required resources, but also because they could easily be carried out by lower qualified health care workers like health counsellors.

Adherence monitoring method	Resources	Annual cost per patient
1. Electronic Monitoring Device	MEMS equipment	$ 46.30
	Staff time	$ 11.53
	Total cost	$ 57.83
2. Pharmacy Refill Data	Staff time	$ 2.58
3. Visual Analogue Scale	Staff time	$ 0.19
4. Missed dose questionnaire	Staff time	$ 0.39

Table 2. Cost comparison of adherence measures

5. Conclusion

Continuous adherence to medication is crucial for therapeutic success for every medical condition. Adherence is always challenging, but even more so for chronic conditions that require patients to take their medication for long periods of time, or even life-long. In the recent 15 years, HIV treatment adherence has become one of the main adherence research areas, and it has added a new perspective on adherence issues, particularly in developing countries with limited resources to spend on health and patient support. Adherence assessment can occur at all levels of the health care system, but most often it is carried out by health care workers in primary care. This is not accidental – it is primary care workers that are most likely to know the patient and her social surroundings, and carry for chronically ill patients in continuous care. Adherence is a team effort and requires constant commitment from patients – but also constant encouragement and support from health care workers. In order to recognise adherence challenges and potential adherence failures, health care workers need to monitor adherence systematically. This chapter has introduced the most common adherence measures in primary care, and highlighted their advantages and disadvantages. Clearly, every patient and every situation requires an individual assessment, and often the best adherence assessment is a combination of more than one measure. Perhaps more than anything else, issues around adherence speak to the challenges of leading a 'normal' life with a chronic illness, and highlight how patients integrate their illness (through their medication) into their daily lives. The implications of poor adherence or even non-adherence are often dire, and health care workers need to support patients by recognising early signs of poor adherence. Often this can be assessed in conversations with patients, but adherence measures provide a crucial tool to quantify and compare adherence in a more structured way.

6. References

Arnsten JH, Demas PA, Farzadegan H, Grant RW, Gourevitch MN, Chang CJ, Buono D, Eckholdt H, Howard Aa, Schoenbaum EE (2001): Antiretroviral therapy adherence and viral suppression in HIV-infected drug users: comparison of self-report and electronic monitoring. *Clinical Infectious Diseases*, 33, 1417-1423

Bangsberg DR, Hecht FM, Charlebois ED, Zolopa AR, Holodniy M, Sheiner L, Bamberger JD, Chesney MA, Moss A (2000): Adherence to protease inhibitors, HIV-1 viral load, and development of drug resistance in an indigent population. *AIDS* 14, 357-366

Berg KM, Arnsten JH (2006): Practical and conceptual challenges in measuring antiretroviral adherence. *J Acquir Immune Defic Syndr* 43 Suppl 1, S79-S87

Byakika-Tusiime J, Oyugi JH, Tumwikirize WA, Katabira ET, Mugyenyi PN, Bangsberg DR (2005): Adherence to HIV antiretroviral therapy in HIV+ Ugandan patients purchasing therapy. *Int J STD AIDS* 16, 38-41

Byrne M, Honig J, Jurgrau A, Heffernan SM, Donahue MC (2002): Achieving adherence with antiretroviral medications for pediatric HIV disease. *AIDS Read* 12, 151-154

Chesney MA, Ickovics J, Hecht FM, Sikipa G, Rabkin J (1999): Adherence: a necessity for successful HIV combination therapy. *AIDS* 13 Suppl A, S271-S278

CSDH: Closing the gap in a generation: health equity through action on the social determinants of health. Final Report of the Commission on Social Determinants of Health. *World Health Organization*, Geneva 2008, p. 62-65

Drummond MF, Sculpher MJ, Torrance GW, O'Brien BJ, Stoddart GL. *Methods for the economic evaluation of health care programmes*. 3rd ed. Oxford: Oxford University Press; 2005.

Farmer KC (1999): Methods for measuring and monitoring medication regimen adherence in clinical trials and clinical practice. *Clin Ther* 21, 1074-1090

Gill CJ, Hamer DH, Simon JL, Thea DM, Sabin LL (2005): No room for complacency about adherence to antiretroviral therapy in sub-Saharan Africa. *AIDS* 19, 1243-1249

Giordano TP, Guzman D, Clark R, Charlebois ED, Bangsberg DR (2004): Measuring adherence to antiretroviral therapy in a diverse population using a visual analogue scale. *HIV Clin Trials* 5, 74-79

Grossberg R, Zhang Y, Gross R (2004): A time-to-prescription-refill measure of antiretroviral adherence predicted changes in viral load in HIV. *J Clin Epidemiol* 57, 1107-1110

Howard AA, Arnsten JH, Lo Y, Vlahov D, Rich JD, Schuman P, Stone VE, Smith DK, Schoenbaum EE, HER Study Group (2002): A prospective study of adherence and viral load in a large multi-center cohort of HIV-infected women. *AIDS* 16, 2175-2182

Knobel H, Guelar A, Carmona A, Espona M, Gonzalez A, Lopez-Colomes JL, Sabalis P, Gimeno JL, Diez A (2001): Virologic outcome and predictors of virologic failure of highly active antiretroviral therapy containing protease inhibitors. *AIDS Patient Care STDS* 15, 193-199

Low-Beer S, Yip B, O'Shaughnessy MV, Hogg RS, Montaner JS (2000): Adherence to triple therapy and viral load response. *J Acquir Immune Defic Syndr* 23, 360-361

Mills EJ, Nachega JB, Buchan I, Orbinski J, Attaran A, Singh S et al. (2006): Adherence to antiretroviral therapy in sub-Saharan Africa and North America: a meta-analysis. *JAMA* 296, 679-690

Müller AD, Bode S, Myer L, Roux P, von Steinbüchel N (2008). Electronic Measurement of Pediatric Adherence in South Africa. *Pediatric Infectious Disease Journal* 27, 257-262

Müller AD, Jaspan HB, Myer L, Hunter A, Harling G, Bekker L-G, Orrell C (2010). Standard Measures are Inadequate to Monitor Pediatric Adherence in a Resource-Limited Setting. *AIDS and Behavior* 15, 422-431

Nachega JB, Stein DM, Lehman DA, Hlatshwayo D, Mothopeng R, Chaisson RE, Karstaedt AS (2004): Adherence to antiretroviral therapy in HIV-infected adults in Soweto, South Africa. *AIDS Res Hum Retroviruses* 20, 1053-1056

Orrell C, Bangsberg DR, Badri M, Wood R (2003): Adherence is not a barrier to successful antiretroviral therapy in South Africa. *AIDS* 17, 1369-1375

Osterberg L, Blaschke T (2005): Adherence to medication. *N Engl J Med* 353, 487-497

Oyugi JH, Byakika-Tusiime J, Charlebois ED, Kityo C, Mugerwa R, Mugyenyi P, Bangsberg DR (2004): Multiple validated measures of adherence indicate high levels of adherence to generic HIV antiretroviral therapy in a resource- limited setting. *J Acquir Immune Defic Syndr* 36, 1100-1102

Paterson DL, Swindells S, Mohr J, Brester M, Vergis EN, Squier C, Wagener MM, Singh N (2000): Adherence to protease inhibitor therapy and outcomes in patients with HIV infection. *Ann Intern Med* 133, 21-30

Raboud JM, Harris M, Rae S, Montaner JS (2002): Impact of adherence on duration of virological suppression among patients receiving combination antiretroviral therapy. *HIV Med* 3, 118-124

Ransohoff DF, Feinstein AR (1978): Problems of spectrum and bias in evaluating the efficacy of diagnostic tests. *N Engl J Med* 299, 926-930

Safren SA, Kumarasamy N, Hosseinipour M, Harwood MM, Hoffman I, McCauley M et al. (2006): Perceptions about the acceptability of assessments of HIV medication adherence in Lilongwe, Malawi and Chennai, India. *AIDS Behav* 10, 443-450

Simoni JM, Montgomery A, Martin E, New M, Demas PA, Rana S (2007): Adherence to antiretroviral therapy for pediatric HIV infection: a qualitative systematic review with recommendations for research and clinical management. *Pediatrics* 119, e1371-e1383

Simoni JM, Kurth AE, Pearson CR, Pantalone DW, Merrill JO, Frick PA (2006): Self-Report Measures of Antiretroviral Therapy Adherence: A Review with Recommendations for HIV Research and Clinical Management. *AIDS and Behavior* 10, 227-245

Singh N, Berman SM, Swindells S, Justis JC, Mohr JA, Squier C, Wagener MM (1999): Adherence of human immunodeficiency virus-infected patients to antiretroviral therapy. *Clin Infect Dis* 29, 824-830

Steele RG, Anderson B, Rindel B, Dreyer ML, Perrin K, Christensen R, Tyc V, Flynn PM (2001): Adherence to antiretroviral therapy among HIV-positive children: examination of the role of caregiver health beliefs. *AIDS Care* 13, 617-629

Steiner JF, Prochazka AV (1997): The assessment of refill compliance using pharmacy records: methods, validity, and applications. *J Clin Epidemiol* 50, 105-116

UNAIDS: Report on the global HIV/AIDS epidemic 2008: executive summary. *Joint United Nations Programme on HIV/AIDS (UNAIDS)*, Geneva 2008.

Vreeman RC, Wiehe SE, Pearce EC, Nyandiko WM (2008): A systematic review of pediatric adherence to antiretroviral therapy in low- and middle-income countries. *Pediatr Infect Dis J* 27, 686-691

WHO: Adherence to Long Term Therapies: Evidence for Action. *World Health Organization*, Geneva 2003

WHO: Antiretroviral treatment of HIV infected in infants and children in resource-limited settings: Towards universal access. *World Health Organization*, Geneva 2005

Section 3

Accountability in Primary Care

Ethics and the Practice of Primary Care Psychiatry

Russell H. Searight
Department of Psychology,
Lake Superior State University,
USA

1. Introduction

1.1 Psychiatric conditions in primary care

In the United States, as in many Western countries, the primary care clinic has become a very common site for diagnosis and treatment of psychiatric conditions. There has been a significant increase in mental health care visits in the primary care sector. In the 1980s, slightly over 40 % of patients receiving mental health care were diagnosed and treated by primary care physicians. Of this patient population, 75% were managed solely by primary care physicians without psychiatric or psychological consultation (Kessler, Demler, Frank, et al., 2005; Wang, Demler, Olfson, et al., 2006). Between the 1980s and 2010, the use of primary medical care for mental health services has increased by over 150%. By 2008, the primary care sector had become the the most common treatment setting for mental health problems in the United States (Cwikel, et al., 2008). For example, 50% of all patients in the U.S. treated for major depressive disorder are managed solely in the primary care sector. These physicians spend a total of 12.1 hours per week--nearly a quarter of their direct patient contact hours--providing mental health services. In the U.S., approximately 20% of psychotherapy sessions are provided by primary care physicians (Himelhoch & Ehrenreich, 2007). In the United Kingdom, mental health counseling is also a major activity among general practitioners. This surge occurred in the context of corresponding increases in the percentage of the general population receiving mental health care—from 12% per year in 1990-92 to 20% by 2000-2001 (Kessler, Demler, Frank, Olfson, et al., 2005).

Even with this level of psychiatric care by primary care providers, there is considerable evidence of a greater need for mental health care among their patients. Psychiatric symptoms are very common in primary care settings. When compared with the general population, primary care patients have elevated levels of psychiatric symptoms. An early large-scale survey of primary care patients found that approximately 20% of them had a current psychiatric condition (Barrett, Barrett, Oxman, & Gerber, 1988) with major depressive and anxiety disorders the most common. An additional 11% were diagnosed with another psychiatric condition. However some of these patients did have depressive symptoms as well. Generalized anxiety disorder was the second most common mental health diagnosis. Of note, when examining the presence of symptoms rather than specific conditions, only 30% of this primary care population was psychiatrically symptom-free with approximately 40% exhibiting mild symptoms (Barrett, et al., 1998).

More recent studies suggest that rates of psychiatric distress in primary care are rising. When examining the prevalence of mental health conditions in primary care patients during the past year, Cwik et al. (2008) found that approximately half of all patients had some type of significant psychiatric symptomatology. Women were more likely (54.8%) than men (44.9%) to be exhibiting significant psychiatric distress. When formal criteria from the Diagnostic and Statistical Manual of Mental Disorders (American Psychiatric Association, 2006) were applied, 26% of men and 34% of women had a mood, anxiety, or eating disorder and/ or somatoform disorder. While mood disorders were the most common with 17.4% of men and 22.2% of women meeting criteria for major depression during the past year, anxiety disorders were a close second with 13.5% of men and 20% of women having at least one of these disorders during the past year (Cswik et al., , 2008; Searight, 2010). With respect to anxiety disorders, among a large sample of primary care patients, 20% of them currently met criteria for at least one anxiety disorder with 8.6% exhibiting posttraumatic stress and 7.6% exhibiting generalized anxiety and finally, 6.8% demonstrated panic disorder (Kroenke, Spitzer, Williams, et al., 2007). Among pediatric patients, the majority of diagnoses of attention deficit hyperactivity disorder are made by pediatricians and family physicians. When examined from the perspective of sheer numbers, the majority of prescriptions for stimulant medication used to treat the condition are also written by primary care physicians (Mayes, Bagwell, Erkulwater, 2009).

1.2 Reasons behind the rise of primary care psychiatry

There are probably multiple reasons for the increase in the practice of primary care mental health in the past three decades. First, there is evidence that the rates of significant psychiatric conditions such as mood and personality disorders are increasing (World Health Organization., 2011). Second, in many universal healthcare systems as well as the in many insurance and/or managed-care plans, primary care physicians are the gatekeepers to specialty care including psychiatry (Bryan & Rudd, 2011).

Third, there has been increased attention to educating primary care physicians about mental health problems. As a result, while they still miss up to half of patients with conditions such as depression and anxiety disorders, their level of competence in assessing these patients has improved. Fourth, the availability of second generation SSRI antidepressants with relatively few side effects have made many physicians more comfortable with treating psychiatric conditions. Efforts by the pharmaceutical companies to educate primary care physicians by providing information about efficient assessment strategies such as patient self-report instruments has made diagnosis somewhat easier (Bryan & Rudd, 2011). Additionally, pharmacotherapy regimens became safer and guidelines for psychotropic medication use have raised non-psychiatric physicians' comfort level with this treatment modality. Because of direct to consumer marketing of psychotropic medications, the general public has become more aware of mental disorders and the availability of treatment. Finally, there continue to be a number of systems barriers to accessing specialty mental health care. In countries such as the U.S., insurance companies have "carved out" specialty mental health services so that access is governed by different procedures than for medical care. In countries such as Canada, with government-funded universal coverage, access to specialty care is often associated with lengthy waiting periods because of the limited number of specialists including psychiatrists and psychologists.

1.3 The role of chronic disease

Another, often unrecognized, factor in the rise of primary care mental health has been the shift from infectious disease to chronic conditions such as Type II diabetes and cardiovascular disease. These conditions are associated with increased levels of psychiatric distress which both directly and indirectly impact theses medical conditions. For example, the presence of major depressive disorder is associated with a three-fold increase in health care non-adherence including issues such as maintaining an appropriate diet and taking medication according to a prescribed schedule (Di Matteo, 2006). The etiology of these common primary care conditions are influenced by lifestyle factors such as physical activity, smoking, alcohol use, and consumption of dietary fat.

1.4 New ethical dilemmas

While psychiatric care has become commonplace in general medicine, a neglected aspect has been the distinctive ethical and professional dilemmas arising when treating patients' mental health problems. As will be discussed below, virtue-based ethical guidelines such as the Hippocratic Oath and formal codes such as the American Medical Association's "Principles of Medical Ethics," do not adequately address common professional and ethical issues arising in providing psychiatric care. For example, while treating colleagues and their families is common for primary care physicians, this practice is strongly discouraged by the American Psychological Association's Ethical Code (Koocher & Keith-Spiegel, 2008).

2. Ethical principles

In much of the western world, there are two prevailing models of medical ethics. The first approach derives from the Hippocratic oath and articulates the virtues of a moral healthcare provider. The second model, principlism, provides a four dimensional framework for analyzing clinical situations. Principlism emphasizes a somewhat detached analysis of ethical dilemmas according to these dimensions.

2.1 Virtue ethics

The first approach, that has a much longer history in biomedicine, is that of virtues. The Hippocratic Oath, a virtue based code, has a long history in medicine. The Oath essentially states what a good physician does ("Whatever houses I may visit, I will come for the benefit of the sick, remaining free of all intentional injustice, of all mischief in particular of sexual relations with both female and male persons, be they free or slaves.").

A contemporary perspective on physician virtues has been described by Pellegrino and Thomasma (1998). These medical ethicists believe that virtues can and should be formally taught to physicians-in-training. Additionally, these virtues typically go beyond the role of physician and encompass what a morally responsible individual would do during the course of their lives. Pellegrino and Mann's virtues include intellectual honesty, benevolence, humility, and therapeutic parsimony. Additional virtues include trust, compassion, prudence, justice, fortitude, temperance, integrity and self-effacement. A key virtue for ethical issues in health care is Prudence – the ability to reason reflectively and respond to concrete life dilemmas in a way that is both technically and morally correct (Pelligrino & Thomasma, 1998).

2.2 Principlism

In contrast, principlism, rather than focusing on the health care provider's character or actions, centers on four abstract dimensions. These dimensions include: respect for autonomy, nonmaleficence, beneficence, and justice.

Respect for autonomy involves a level of self-determination undisturbed by others' control or influence. Autonomy presumes that one is capable of deliberating and/or acting on the basis of their personally-held wishes, plans and values. It has been argued that geunuine autonomy requires that the individual have all relevant knowledge necessary for making a decision about their own welfare. In most parts of the world, the consent form, signed by the patient before any medical procedure is undertaken, is seen as "proof" of autonomous decision-making. .

Nonmaleficence is best summarized by the medical dictum "first, do no harm." Beauchamp and Childress argue that obligations for nonmaleficence are usually more "stringent" than helping or promoting the welfare of another. An example of their perspective is the general acceptance by the medical community of the decision by a competent patient to refuse a life-sustaining treatment such as ventilator support. However, removal of a ventilator from a living patient typically requires a higher level of critical analysis. In the latter situation, Beauchamp and Childress (2009) believe that there is more of a direct causal connection between a harmful outcome stemming from stopping treatment than in failing to initiate therapy.

Beneficence refers to contributing to the welfare of others. In contrast to nonmaleficence, healthcare providers should take positive proactive steps to benefit patients and not just shield them from harm. A current ethical conflict is when providers believe that an intervention, such as childhood immunizations, is in the patient's best interest while the child's parent disagrees because of concerns about side effects. In many instances, the patient's autonomy over-rules the physician's duty to act to protect patient welfare.

Justice refers to fair, equitable, and appropriate treatment in the context of what is owed to an individual. A close corollary is the concept of distributive justice in which there is a fair distribution of rights, responsibilities, and benefits. In the United States, for example, a key public health problem has been that of health disparities. There is ample evidence that people of all ethnic and social backgrounds do not have equal access to healthcare and are not given the same level of treatment. This pattern exists for multiple medical treatments ranging from pain management, to mental health referrals, to coronary artery bypass graft surgery.

One of the most frequent criticisms of principlism is that while it provides a useful and relatively simple framework for analyzing ethical dilemmas in medicine, it does not inherently lead to definite courses of action. A chief reason for this lack of direction is that there is no priority among the four dimensions and at times, principles may be in conflict. For example, providing contraceptive information and care to a 15-year-old girl, raises questions about the patient's autonomy (Is she cognitively and developmentally capable of making well-reasoned decisions?), non-maleficence (Is she aware of and able to appropriately act on any risks associated with contraception such as a greater likelihood of blood clots if she is a smoker ?), beneficence (It is assumed that protection from pregnancy is beneficial to the young woman. Evidence about the adverse effects of teen pregnancy and motherhood would support this view) and justice (Is contraceptive care something that her peers would be able to access as easily?). In this illustration, there is a potential conflict between autonomy and beneficence. Well-meaning parents may assert that their daughter does not have the necessary cognitive capacity or psychosocial maturity to make truly autonomous decisions about either sexual relationships or contraception. From the perspective of beneficence, there is the value that she should be protected from the "harm" of unintended pregnancy associated with sexual activity.

2.3 Ethics in the mental health professions

In the mental health professions, a much more detailed code of ethics has evolved. For example, psychiatry has an annotated set of ethical principles along with those of the American Medical Association (American Medical Association, 2001). Similarly, for psychologists, the American Psychological Association's ethical guidelines for practitioners are much more detailed and explicit than for researchers and teachers. These guidelines examine issues such as confidentiality, competence to practice, conflicts of interest, dual relationships, and duties to protect others from patients who are potentially violent or are otherwise, presenting risks of harm. For example, AMA's psychiatric annotations include specific circumstances in which confidentiality may be breached. In the discussion of dual relationships, the annotations note that psychiatric care is such that "essentially private, highly personal and sometimes intensely emotional material" may arise in the clinical relationship, raising risks of impaired provider objectivity.

The American Psychological Association's (2002) Code of Ethics examines dual relationships in even more detail. In elaborations of APA's guidelines, the distinction between a "personal" and a "psychologist-patient" relationship is described. In the analysis, it is noted that successful personal relationships are oriented toward mutual satisfaction and addressing common needs (Koocher & Keith-Spiegel, 2008). Furthermore, it is noted that agendas in personal relationships are not necessarily associated with attaining specific goals. In contrast, the professional relationship between psychologist and patient is not mutual; it arises to serve the needs of the client with a focus on specific therapeutic goals. Once those goals are attained, termination of the relationship is expected. Socializing and entering into friendships with current, and frequently, with past patients is strongly discouraged. In addition, treating the relatives of patients is also strongly discouraged (Koocher & Keith-Speigel, 2008).

2.4 Mental health ethics and primary care

These examples highlight the inherent ambiguity and complexity of ethical issues that may arise in treating psychiatric conditions in the primary care sector. In essence, the primary care physician becomes the "functional equivalent" of a mental health professional in these clinical encounters. However, ethical dilemmas such as circumstances mandating the breaking of patient confidentiality, responding to third party requests for patients' mental health information (including that of minors), duties to protect third parties and the community-at-large, as well as the boundaries of the physician-patient relationship, do not commonly arise in general medical practice. While mental health professionals typically have had significant didactic coursework as well as supervised clinical training in examining these complex ethical issues, primary care physicians are typically only aware of the more concise, yet general, principles governing general medical practice. The practice of psychiatry by primary care physicians, itself, raises questions about practicing outside the bounds of professional competence. Finally, psychiatric symptoms among primary care patients are often difficult to assess because they are non-specific, based solely on patient report, and frequently co-exist with organic medical conditions. This often leaves the provider with having to diagnose and initiate treatment with a less than optimal diagnostic foundation.

3. Confidentiality

3.1 Mental health content in the medical record

Patients with mental health issues seen in the primary care sector often present with non-specific physical complaints and frequently have comorbid medical illnesses. As a result, medical records may include both information about acute and chronic illnesses, such as hypertension and type II diabetes, but also include psychiatric diagnosis and treatment information. There are a number of situations in which patients' records may be disclosed to third parties including insurance companies, government agencies, attorneys, surrogate medical decision makers, and in the case of minors, parents. Patients, themselves, are often unaware that mental health information may have been documented and may authorize release of their medical record with little reflection on the potential implications. While there is typically little stigma associated with most problems diagnosed and treated in ambulatory primary care, the same cannot be said for mental health issues. Disclosure of mental health information can prevent patients from obtaining health and life insurance, adopting a child, entering the military, and could conceivably have negative effects on current and future employment. Additionally, records of mental health treatment are commonly sought in divorce and child custody legal actions. In these circumstances, the physician should rely on beneficence and non-maleficence by informing the patient of the information in the record and ask if they would still want to share the material with a third party. Without knowledge of the medical record itself and/or its use in these non-medical contexts, the patient cannot make a truly informed, autonomous decision.

When surveyed confidentially, a sample of U.S. general practitioners reported that the issue of external review of records influenced them to misrepresent information in the patient's record, itself. In addition, many of these physicians indicated that they had protected patient privacy by misrepresenting or omitting information on insurance forms. In this survey, 21% of the physicians sampled failed to report illness, such as sexually transmitted diseases, to the local health department (Ullom-Minnich & Kallial, 1993; Roberts, Battaglia, & Epstein, 1999).

3.2 Minors

In both medicine and mental health, issues of informed consent and confidentiality for minors are often areas in which ethics and law conflict. Ethical reasoning is also challenged since the child, rather than their parent or guardian, is the patient whose well-being is entrusted to the physician. Because of cognitive-developmental factors, minors may not be able to engage in the level of reasoning required to make truly informed decisions about their medical or mental health care. Therefore, from Beauchamp and Childress' (2009) perspective, children and some adolescents have inherently diminished autonomy. However, per Pellegrino and Thomasma (1998), the health care provider has a responsibility to establish a trusting relationship and represent the best interests of their young patients.

With a few exceptions, parents generally have legal rights to any information, including medical and mental health records, about their minor children. Additionally, parents and guardians typically have the right to make health care decisions on their child's behalf and can override children's objections or requests. However, there are circumstances in which the physician and parents may differ regarding the child-patient's best interests. Historically, the major controversies arising in primary care around this ethical-legal tension have been those involving sexuality and substance abuse among minors. Many states in the United States have passed laws that include an exception to parental notification so that minors (typically 14, 15, or 16 years old) can seek contraceptive care and also mental health/substance abuse counseling without informing a parent or guardian. These laws, reflecting beneficence, recognize that many minors would be disinclined to seek treatment for these issues if parental notification and disclosure of the material shared with the physician were required. While there are situations in which prescribing contraception may increase risk of adverse outcomes outcomes (birth control pills prescribed to an adolescent who smokes cigarettes), the most pressing issue from the parental perspective is that this risk behavior could potentially be harmful to the minor. If parents are unaware of their child's status with respect to sexual activity or drug use, appropriate parental supervision may not be initiated. In the United Kingdom, persons 16 and older are assumed to have the capacity to provide valid consent (Tan, Passerini, & Stewart, 2007). However, research has suggested that younger adolescents and children of average to above average intelligence may have the cognitive capacity to make these decisions as well.

3.3 Psychotropic medication and children

With respect to psychiatric care, there have been growing concerns about the large number of children and adolescents who are being prescribed psychotropic medications. For example, the majority of prescriptions for stimulant medications are written by primary care physicians such as family physicians and pediatricians rather than by child psychiatrists. Both law and ethics, based on the principle of autonomy, recognize that competent adults, even when exhibiting overt psychiatric symptomatology, can refuse psychotropic medication. This issue has not been explored with respect to children. It is not uncommon for children to express discomfort about taking medications such as methylphenidate because it makes them feel "different" than their peers and implicitly stigmatized. Additionally, while not as common, concerns about difficulty falling asleep, suppressed appetite, and headaches, are also expressed by children taking stimulant medication.

An alternative to consent that has been suggested in working with minors is that of "assent." Assent essentially means that the child has not overtly objected to the treatment recommendations. Their agreement is often inferred from the child's cooperation with parents and the healthcare provider (Tan, Passerini, & Stewart, 2007). When children are raising objections to taking or continuing psychotropic medication, the provider, while attempting to understand and respect the child's reluctance, should also determine the level of risk and treatment urgency involved. There is a corresponding duty of care (beneficence) that should be enacted while maintaining openness to the perspective of the young patient and their family and minimizing coercion.

While focused issues of family planning have often been granted confidentiality with adolescents, this level of confidentiality my not always in the child's best interest when other mental health issues are being addressed (Tan, et al., 2007). First, it is often necessary for parents to monitor the child's behavior and provide the prescribing physician feedback about the patient's behavioral response to stimulant medication. Studies of children with ADHD suggest that they are not accurate self-observers (Searight, Gafford, & Evans, 1998). Additionally, information about the child's performance in school is also critical for assessment as well as for medication management. Optimally, the child should be informed that others will be reporting on their behavior and unless disclosure of information is seen as potentially harmful to the child, the child should be tactfully informed about others' reports of their conduct while being encouraged to offer their own perspective. This open communication policy is particularly important with adolescents since "secret information" about their behavior may seriously damage the provider-patient relationship.

3.4 Child custody issues

Because of their increasing involvement in treating child mental health conditions, primary care providers may become entangled in legal issues in which the confidentiality of a child's psychiatric information may be compromised. Common situations are custody issues in which one parent reports that the child has been either abused or exposed to neglectful supervision while in the other parent's care. The physician may be subpoenaed by the court to provide an opinion about the veracity of these reports—particularly if the disclosures are by the child. Again, forcible disclosures may harm the child's relationship with one or both parents and in some circumstances, could put the child at risk for abuse. This is a situation in which the child's welfare may be best served by refusing to disclose this information on therapeutic grounds.

Among children receiving stimulant treatment for AD/HD, it is not uncommon for separated or divorced parents to disagree about the need for the medication. Again, from an ethical perspective, the physician's first priority is the welfare of the child. In joint custody situations or situations involving a noncustodial parent who disagrees with the treatment being provided by the physician, it is often a useful idea to invite them in for an appointment to discuss the child. Again, in circumstances in which there is joint custody or in which the physician is going to be meeting with a noncustodial parent, they should have written permission from the other parent to initiate and conduct a conference at this time. Finally, in situations in which records about a pediatric patient are requested in a legal context and there is significant judicial pressure to comply, there are several avenues that the physician can employ to benefit patient confidentiality and limit disclosures. First, the provider can send a letter which addresses specific questions raised in a legal context while disclosing minimal amounts of background information. Second, the provider can simply refuse to provide information insisting that disclosure would be harmful to the child. Finally, in a compromise solution, the physician may indicate that they can describe and respond to general questions about a particular mental health condition such as ADHD or childhood mood disorder without specific reference to the patient.

4. Dual relationships

4.1 Providing mental health care to patients who are family friends and colleagues

Mental health education devotes considerable time to the importance of clear roles and professional boundaries. Ethical psychologists would never provide psychotherapy for family or friends. While mental health professionals may have informal conversations with colleagues or office staff about personal and family matters, psychologists and psychiatrists are discouraged from providing professional services to persons with whom they have another relationship—even if their sole contact is as a secretary or receptionist in their large group practice. Primary care physicians, while discouraged from treating friends and family, do not have the same degree of prohibition as psychologists regarding dual relationships. It is not uncommon for physicians to be the personal physician for office staff or even colleagues. Indeed, many physicians either formally or informally provide professional care for family and friends. While treating family members is discouraged; it is not unusual for physicians to treat other physicians that they know, family members of colleagues, as well as employees of their hospital or clinic.

Dual relationships are a particularly challenging issue in smaller communities and rural areas. A survey of general practitioners in Kansas found that nearly half of the physicians practicing in small communities reported having a significant number of patients who were family members, friends, or family members or friends of the physician's staff. Most of the small town physicians surveyed indicated that they had interacted in non-medical roles with patients (Roberts, Battaglia, & Epstein, 1999; Ullom-Minnich & Kallall, 1993).

While there are guidelines established by the American Medical Association for ethical practice, they are not as specific as the American Psychological Association's Ethical Principles in influencing practice or state licensing boards. In addition, the guidelines for non-psychiatric physicians are not nearly as stringent regarding multiple relationships with patients.

The rationale for not providing mental health care to members of one's social network is predicated on the recognition of the intensely emotional and personal nature of the psychotherapeutic relationship. If the provider has another personal or professional relationship with the patient, the patient may be reluctant to disclose concerns such as sexual dysfunction, marital conflicts, substance abuse or suicidal ideation. The rationale is that it would be particularly challenging to maintain appropriate personal-professional boundaries and it would be difficult for this knowledge not to impact the social relationship between physician and patient when they are outside of those roles. Family physicians have been found legally liable when counseling a patient for marital issues and then entering into a sexual relationship with one of the spouses. In these circumstances, it would be difficult not to use the personal information received in counseling to assist in establishing an intimate relationship (Searight & Campbell, 1993). The category of inappropriate dual relationships is one of the most common sources of malpractice litigation and complaints to ethics boards for psychiatrist and psychologists.

4.2 The sick note

A potential for dual relationships and competing priorities occurs when physicians communicate with patients' employers. Often, only medically-authorized absences from work or school prevent loss of pay, a failing grade, or termination of employment. A common term used for a physician provided work excuse is the "sick note." As employment has become scarcer with recent economic downturns, patients are even more likely to request physician documentation of their time off of work to maintain wages and avoid termination. Primary care physicians are well aware of the negative effects of remaining in the sick role for extended periods of time. For example it is relatively well-established that previously employed patients with chronic low back pain are unlikely to ever return to work if they are away from their job for six months or more. Ideally, there would be an interaction between the physician and employer in which work duties could be modified and phased in so as to permit an earlier return to work and reduce the likelihood of the patient being permanently disabled.

From an ethical point of view, the sick note raises both anxiety and frustration for physicians. This is particularly true for sick notes based on psychiatric disability. The subjective nature of mental health complaints and the waxing and waning pattern of symptoms make professional judgment about work-related duties particularly challenging. In addition, healthcare providers tend to have a fairly pronounced work ethic and are likely to be troubled by seemingly physically healthy patients who are seeking their assistance to avoid returning to work. Although paternalistic, a beneficent physician's encouragement to return to work may be guided by a belief that employment would be beneficial to the patient's emotional, and likely, physical health . On the other hand, if the physician views the patient as an autonomous agent who can make decisions about return to work alone, the physician is likely to see their role as simply to document and support the patient's request. However, in addition to their views about the potential longer-range benefits of returning to work, physicians may understandably chafe at supporting unhealthy behavior (nonmaleficence) with a sick note

Finally, many physicians see themselves as inadequately trained to perform evaluations for the workplace. From the perspective of occupational health, a well-documented rationale for sending a patient back to work would include an appreciation of the patient's specific expected duties as well as the environment in which these activities occur. In circumstances where the physician is a contracted Workmen's Compensation provider or company physician, there may be pronounced conflicts of interest between the patient's well-being and that of the physician's employer.

In disability dilemmas involving psychiatric conditions, physicians are encouraged to use objective standards in evaluating the patient's current condition. For example, for major depressive disorder, having the patient complete a standardized rating scale such as the Beck Depression Scale or Hamilton Depression Rating Scale prior to initiating pharmacotherapy and at regular intervals thereafter, can assist the physician by having some objective quantitative standards that are used to assess the patient's current functioning. The Global Assessment of Functioning (GAF) index from the DSM-IV (axis V) provides another useful source of quantitative ratings.

In circumstances in which the patient, workplace representative, and the physician disagree on the patient's ability to return to work, the physician should describe the patient's current level of functioning. If the patient disagrees about their current capacity for work duties, the patient's judgment can also be reported. This approach permits the physician to operate with professional integrity while the patient's perspective is still represented. The final decision would be made by the patient's workplace administrator.

5. Dangerous situations

5.1 Suicidal patients

Approximately half of all individuals in the United States who effect suicide have seen a primary care provider in the past month (Bryan & Rudd, 2011). Among elderly individuals completing suicide, nearly half of had seen their primary care provider in the preceding week. There is considerable evidence that as physical complaints increase, particularly pain, suicide risk increases (Bryan & Rudd, 2011). When patients are actively suicidal and in need of close monitoring, it is often helpful to notify competent adults with whom the patient resides. This is particularly true in situations in which hospitalization does not appear to be imminently indicated but could possibly be required in the near future if the patient continues to deteriorate. In general, primary care patients will agree to allow notification of family members about their status, provided it is done in a sensitive manner. While the disclosure may somewhat diminish their autonomy, the benefits of informing family almost always outweigh any harm from sharing personal information. Finally, if patients are acutely suicidal, yet are refusing hospitalization, the provider is required to do whatever is reasonably necessary to maintain their safety with confidentiality, at least temporarily, a secondary concern.

5.2 Duty to warn/protect

The ethical mandate to protect the public has a long history in the field of public health. The requirement for reporting of sexually transmitted diseases to governmental agencies such as health departments and the use of epidemiological techniques such as contact tracing is well established. In these circumstances, the principal requirement is to notify persons who may have had contact with the infected individual. This general approach has been used for tuberculosis, HIV as well as syphilis and gonorrhea (Sugarman, 2000). The ethical justification in these cases is that the public's well-being outweighs individual confidentiality (Sugarman, 2000).

The involvement of primary care providers in psychiatry has opened up a number of other applications of the duty to warn or protect. Among these, are laws requiring that physicians report suspected child abuse or neglect. Recently, there has also been concern about whether women who are engaging in behavior that places their developing fetus at risk, such as consuming alcohol, should be reported to protective services. Many states have requirements that suspected harm to vulnerable elders is also reported to a state protective services agency-- typically a division of aging. Finally, several states have passed legislation requiring the authorities to be notified if the physician has reason to believe that a patient has sustained injuries associated with partner abuse.

5.3 The basis of the duty to protect in psychiatry

In psychiatry, there is a well-established duty to warn and/or protect. This duty stems from a legal case, Tarasoff versus the Regents of the University of California. In this case, a graduate student at the University of California, Prosenjit Poddar had seen a psychologist at the University clinic. He indicated that he planned to kill a woman who was identifiable as Tatiana Tarasoff. The psychologist notified the campus police but they only held Poddar briefly. Ms. Tarasoff and family were never informed of the threats that had been made. Two months later, Poddar stabbed her to death. Tarasoff's family sued the University. The California Supreme Court concluded that the psychologist had a duty to warn an identifiable intended victim. A subsequent rehearing of the case resulted in a somewhat broader decision termed Tarasoff II. This second decision concluded that there was both a duty to warn as well as a broader duty to protect. In psychiatric case law, mental health providers have been found negligent even in situations in which an intended victim was never formally named. In addition, liability has been imposed in cases in which patients with schizophrenia, months after their last clinical contact, accidentally killed another party in a traffic accident (Searight, 1997).

The concept of the duty to protect has been applied to HIV-positive patients who continue to be sexually active, without informing partners of their status or using condoms. Preventive detention in the form of quarantine has been imposed in some situations of non-adherent patients with serious communicable diseases. This rationale has also been applied to situations in which patients with significant psychiatric and neurological issues such as schizophrenia or seizure disorders were continuing to operate motor vehicles.

Recently, because of the growing aging population, there has been increased concern about harm to others associated with aging drivers. Many older individuals continue to drive despite conditions such as Alzheimer's disease as well as age related medical conditions such as glaucoma. If the physician recommends to the patient that they no longer drive and the patient concurs with agreement that appears to be valid, the physician probably has no further ethical or legal obligation. However, in circumstances in which patients continue to drive despite these impairments, the principle of maleficence indicates an ethical duty to protect the public. A number of jurisdictions have passed laws requiring that physicians report possible impaired drivers to the division of motor vehicles or the government agency which licenses drivers in a particular jurisdiction. These offices in turn should mandate that the patient undergo some type of assessment regarding their driving or forgo their driver's license.

6. Ethical issues in primary care geriatrics

6.1 Capacity for making medical decisions

Another issue that disproportionately impacts elderly primary care patients is decision-making capacity--particularly for health care. Patients refusing treatment for a life-threatening medical condition raise both ethical and legal liability issues. Physicians may be held liable and viewed as failing to act with beneficence for not treating an incompetent patient refusing a procedure in which the absence of the procedure results in death or further disability. However, a physician may be held legally liable and would be seen as violating patient autonomy if they perform a procedure on a competent patient refusing treatment (Searight & Montooth, 2008). Legally a physician's or psychologist's determination of incapacity is usually required before a written advanced directive or durable power of attorney can be acted upon.

In general medical hospitals and occasionally, in outpatient clinics, capacity determinations are often informally conducted. Searight (1992) suggested that the primary care provider, who has known the patient for some time, may be better suited for rendering opinions regarding capacity than a mental health professional. When the patient does not appear cognitively intact or capable of making reasonable decisions, health care providers often turn to the next of kin for decisions

Capacity decisions are heavily focused on patients' ability to make autonomous, well—reasoned judgments (Grisso & Appelbaum, 1988). A four-part framework is often used to conduct these assessments. First, the patient should be able to express a consistent choice. Clinically, this component may involve the patient indicating that they are choosing or refusing a proposed intervention. Patients who repeatedly reverse themselves are often unable to maintain adequate attention or concentration to cognitively process medically-relevant information. The second aspect, demonstrating an understanding of the current situation, is often assessed by asking the patient to describe "in their own words" the recommended medical procedure. Appreciating information refers to the ability to articulate personal consequences of treatment options including no treatment. The ability to actively weigh treatment options is typically a higher standard assessed when patients are refusing an effective treatment and in which the refusal could reasonably result in further disability or death (Grisso & Appelbaum, 1988).

6.2 Physician hastened death

While a source of continuing controversy, physician assisted suicide or euthanasia is legal in several European countries including Switzerland and the Netherlands. In the United States, three states have passed laws permitting some form of physician assisted hastened death. Ruijs and colleagues (2011) note that many of the patients requesting hastened death—particularly those with cancer—are attended by primary care physicians. In the Netherlands in recent years close to 90% of cases of physician assisted suicide were performed by generalist physicians. The majority of their Dutch patients had cancer (Ruijs, et al., 2011). There has been considerable controversy about the criteria that are appropriate for assisting a patient in hastened death.

There is general agreement that patients should be assessed for psychiatric conditions such as major depressive disorder that may be impacting their decision. In addition, appropriate pain control – particularly for patients with cancer-- is an important dimension that should be investigated as part of any hastened death request.

In terminally ill patients, assessment of depression can be an area of ambiguity. A number of the symptoms such as fatigue, sleep difficulty, appetite and weight changes as well as concentration difficulties may not be due to a mood disorder but instead are part of primary illnesses such as cancer or medication to treat the condition.. A further complication is that depression has been construed as either a continuous or a categorical condition. Mood disorders may reflect a continuous set of symptoms as in self-report scales such as the Geriatric Depression Scale in which patients above a particular cutoff score are seen as having a particular level of depressive symptoms ranging from mild to severe. The DSM-IVTR, on the other hand is a categorical system, and views major depressive disorder as a diagnosis when five of nine symptoms are present for two weeks. Research to date on the prevalence of depression among patients requesting PAS has been conflicting. Several studies have indicated that there is a fairly direct relationship between depressive symptoms among cancer patients and a desire for hastened death. However, this finding has not been consistent (Ruijs et al., 2011

7. Professional competence for diagnosing and treating mental health conditions

Because they frequently practice in areas such as rural locations, inner-city settings, and public health clinics, primary care physicians provide a good deal of care to populations that have historically been underserved. These settings often have minimal or inaccessible mental health specialty services. Roberts, Battaglia, and Epstein (1999) point out that in rural communities, there are often significant shortages of qualified mental health professionals, minimal psychiatric inpatient and emergency psychiatric services, and poorly integrated systems of medical and mental health care.

As was noted in the introductory section of this chapter, the prevalence of mental health conditions is very high—it is estimated that half of the U.S. population will meet criteria for a DSM diagnosis at some point in their lives. There are indications that mental health problems are even more prevalent in these underserved populations. While many primary care physicians are professionally comfortable treating mild to moderate mood and anxiety disorders, they often do not believe that they are qualified to treat more severe conditions such as bipolar disorder, schizophrenia, personality disorders, and most childhood mental health conditions. However, patients with these conditions routinely present to primary care providers.

An ethical principle guiding both medical and mental health professionals is that one should not provide services outside the bounds of ones' competence and professional training. This very fundamental issue is in conflict with the clinical needs of many patients seen in primary care and presents a very real dilemma to physicians. Primary care physicians struggle about whether to treat significant psychiatric conditions instead of referring to a mental health professional. The difficulties accessing the mental health system and issues of patient coverage for specialty mental health care are weighed against the possibility of providing suboptimal treatment in the primary care setting. In cases where the physician has referred a patient to a psychiatrist, but the patient must wait multiple months for an appointment, should the primary provider make a "best guess" diagnosis and initiate a similarly tentative treatment? This second issue also arises in countries such as Canada which have universal health care systems. In many of these countries, specialty care is particularly scarce and difficult to access and primary care providers are "stretched" to fill in this gap.

Primary care physicians have varying levels of comfort with mental health issues which is partly dependent on their training and experience. For example, in the United States, behavioral sciences are commonly part of the medical school curriculum as well as the residency training in family medicine, internal medicine, and pediatrics. However in many developing countries, such as Southeast Asia, Africa, Latin America, behavioral science and psychiatry are not taught in much detail, if at all (Searight and Gafford, 2006). As a result, when dealing with psychiatric issues, many physicians will be practicing outside the bounds of their competence. The only instance in which this is ethically permitted in an emergency. Again, the ethical dimensions of prudent judgment and balancing beneficence and non-maleficence, together with open conversations with the patient about this dilemma to optimize their autonomy, may assist the provider in resolving these dilemmas.

8. Conclusion: Ethics and the ambiguity of primary care mental health

Ambiguity and lack of certainty, while present in all areas of medicine and mental health, are particularly prominent in primary care. The majority of patients in this setting are seen for self-limiting conditions that are unlikely to be life-threatening.

Medically unexplained symptoms are very common in primary care. While some of these patients meet psychiatric criteria for somatization disorder, most of them do not meet this formal threshold. However, at the same time, these patients are distressed about their symptoms, certainly functionally impaired, and at risk of receiving unnecessary and possibly harmful test procedures. Finally, they consume a good deal of health resources (Heijmans, olde Hartman, van Weel-Baumgarten et al., 2011).

Kroenke and Mangelsdorf (1989) identified the 14 most common symptom complaints presented in primary care settings over a three year period. These symptoms included headache, fatigue, joint and limb pain, and diarrhea. Of these presenting complaints, only about 15% could be linked to an established "organic" cause. While many of these concerns are likely to be related to life stress, they are typically treated as "medical" conditions. In fact, there is evidence that while most people experience many of these symptoms, those who bring these complaints to physicians have higher levels of anxious and dysphoric mood. As Goldstein (1990) noted, outpatient primary care requires a good deal of intuitive as well as scientific thought:

With uncertainty all around me, I sometimes long for the security that science appears to offer. Unfortunately science can no longer offer the comfort that I need. Positivism has long since given way to probability. Modern science has discarded traditional notions of certainty, but the applied sciences fail to fully absorb the message. An ordered, determinate universe of accurate diagnosis and definitive treatment will always be just beyond my grasp. My patients' fears fall through the cracks of the probabilistic certainty that remains (Goldstein, 1990, page 28).

Given the reality of ambiguity and the blurry boundaries between psychiatric and non-psychiatric conditions with the attendant urgency to "do something" for the primary care patient, the physician genuinely struggles daily with an undercurrent of ethical tension. Making the picture even cloudier is the presence of "subclinical" psychiatric syndromes (Searight, 2010). For example some patients do not meet formal diagnostic criteria for either a mood or anxiety disorder but have symptoms of both conditions (Roy-Byrne, Katon, & Broadhead, et al., 1994). This mixed condition is also associated with a greater number of physical symptoms, disability, and a greater likelihood of developing a major psychiatric disorder (Roy-Byrne, Katon, Broadhead, et al. 1994). There are few clear treatment guidelines for these sub-syndromal conditions.

Another area of ambiguity with ethical implications is assessment of cognitive impairment in the elderly. While primary care is probably one of the most common settings for detection of cognitive deterioration in the elderly, these conditions are often ambiguous as well. Diagnosis is primarily based upon clinical history and mental status testing. Mild cognitive impairment, a "transitional zone" (Olazaren, Torrero, Cruz, et al., 2011) between the cognitive decline associated with normal aging and dementia of Alzheimer's type, raises a number of ethical issues of early diagnosis, and the patient's right to know. While MCI was initially believed to be a relatively benign condition, recent research indicates that about 5 to 10% of these patients per year convert to a dementia diagnosis. After 10 years, 50% of MCI patients will have converted. However, the remaining 50% will have remained at the same level of cognitive functioning and in a few cases have even improved. In a recent study involving 31 months of follow-up of patients with MCI, nearly 60% converted to normal cognitive functioning (Olazaran, et al., 2011). It is highly probable that changes in social circumstances and or the presence of mood or anxiety disorders plays a significant role in many of these patients' baseline level of cognitive impairment. From an ethical perspective, what should the provider say to MCI patients? Should they and their families be informed of the possible outcome? Is the predictive value of MCI so equivocal that the potential harm of informing patients and family members outweighs any benefit from the knowledge gained?

These are the types of "on the ground" ethical dilemmas that shape primary care practice. As Goldstein (1990) notes, primary care dilemmas are complex-both ethically and clinically:

"... to the seasoned clinician, the most interesting variety of knowledge comes not from unilateral action, but from negotiation between the physician and patient, leading to adequate enough agreement to allow them to venture upon a course of therapy. This therapeutic knowledge and its creation are inseparable; the process and product are intertwined. In fact, as the epithet implies, the creation of this knowledge is in itself a therapeutic act. (Goldstein, 1990; p. 26)

9. References

American Medical Association. (2001). Principles of Medical Ethics with Annotations for Psychiatry. Washington DC: Author.

American Psychiatric Association. (2006). The Diagnostic and Statistical Manual of Mental Disorders-IV-TR. Washington DC, American Psychiatric Press.

American Psychological Association (2002). Ethical Principles of Psychologists and Code of Conduct. Washington DC: Author.

Barrett, J. E., Barrett, J.A., Oxman, T.E. & Gerber, P.D. (1988). The prevalence of psychiatric disorders in a primary care practice. Archives of General Psychiatry 45: 1100-1106.

Beauchamp, T.L. & Childress, J.F. (2009). Principles of Biomedical Ethics (Sixth Edition). New York: Oxford.

Bryan, C.J. & Rudd, M.D. (2011). Managing Suicide Risk in Primary Care. New York: Springer

Cwikel, J. Feinson, M & Lerner,Y. (2008). Prevalence and risk factors of threshold and subthreshold psychiatric disorders in primary care. Social Psychiatry and Social Epidemiology 43: 184-191.

Goldstein, J., H. (1990). Desperately seeking science: The creation of knowledge in family practice. Hastings Center Report 20(6). 26-29

Heijmans, M., olde Hartman, T.C., van Weel-Baumgarten, E., Dowrick, C., Lucassen, P. L., & van Weel, C. (2011). Experts' opinions on the management of medically unexplained symptoms in primary care. A qualitative analysis of narrative reviews and scientific editorials. Family Practice, 28, 444-455.

Himelhoch, S. M. Ehrenreich., S. (2007). Psychotherapy by primary care providers: Results of a national survey. Psychosomatics 48(4): 325-330.

Kessler, R.C., Demler, O., Frank, R.G., Olfson, M. et al. (2005). U.S. prevalence and treatment of mental disorders: 1990-2003. New England Journal of Medicine, 352; 2515-2523.

Kroenke, K. & Mangelsdorf, A.D. (1989). Common symptoms in ambulatory care: Incidence, evaluation, therapy, and outcome. American Journal of Medicine, 86, 262-266.

Kroenke, K., Spitzer, R.L., Williams, J.B.W., Monahan, P.O., Lowe, B. (2007). Anxiety disorders in primary care: Prevalence, impairment, comorbidity, and detection. Annals of Internal Medicine, 146, 317-325.

Koocher, G.P. & Keith-Spiegel, P. (2008). Ethics in Psychology and the Mental Health Professions. New York: Oxford,

Mayes, R., Bagwell, C., Erkulwater, J.L (2009). Medicating Children: AD/HD and Pediatric Mental Health. Cambridge MA: Harvard University Press.

Olazaran, J., Torrero, P., Cruz, I. et al. (2011). Mild cognitive impairment and dementia in primary care: the value of medical history. Family Practice, 28, 385-392.

Pellegrino, E. & Thomasma, D. (1998). For the Patient's Good: The Restoration of Beneficence in Health Care. New York: Oxford.

Roberts, L.W., Battaglia, J., & Epstein, R.S. (1999). Frontier ethics: Mental health care needs and ethical dilemmas in rural communities. Psychiatric Services, 50, 497-503.

Roy-Byrne, P., Katon, W., , Brodhead, W., Lepine, J. P., Richard, J., Brantley, P. J., Russo, J., et al. (1994). Subsyndromal (mixed) anxiety and depression in primary care. Journal of General Internal Medicine, 9, 507-512.

Ruijs, C., Kerkhof, A., van de rWal, G., & Onwuteaka-Philipsen, B. (2011). Depression and explicit requests for euthanasia in end-of-life cancer patients in primary care in the Netherlands: A longitudinal, prospective study. Family Practice, 28, 393-399.

Searight, H.R. (1991). Assessing patient competence for medical decision-making. American Family Physician, 45, 751-759.

Searight, H.R. (1997). The Tarasoff Warning and the duty to protect: Implications for family medicine. Journal of Aggression, Maltreatment, & Trauma, 1(2), 153-168

Searight, H.R. (2010). Practicing Psychology in Primary Care. New York and Berlin: Hogrefe and Huber.

Searight, H.R. & Campbell, D.C. (1993). Patient-physician sexual contact: Ethical dilemmas and practical guidelines. Journal of Family Practice, 36, 647-653.

Searight, H.R. & Gafford, J. (2006). Behavioral science education and the international medical graduate. Academic Medicine, 81: 164-170.

Searight, H.R., Gafford, J. & Evans, S. (2005). Attention deficit hyperactivity disorder. In M. Mengel & P. Schwiebert (Eds.), Family Medicine: Ambulatory Care & Prevention (Fourth Edition) (pp. 612-628). New York: McGraw-Hill.

Searight, H.R. & Montooth, A. (2008). Regaining decisional capacity during the hospital course: A narrative case with clinical implications. Archives of Psychiatry and Psychotherapy, 4, 47-55.

Sugarman, J. (2000). Ethics in Primary Care. New York: McGraw-Hill.

Tan, J., PAsserini, G., & Stewart, A. (2007). Consent and confidentiality in clinical work with young people. Clinical Child Psychology and Psychiatry, 12, 191-210.

Ullom-Minnich, P.D. & Kallial, K.J. (1993). Physicians' strategies for safeguarding confidentiality: The influence of practice and community characteristics. Journal of Family Practice, 37, 445-448.

Wang, P.S., Demler, O., Olfson, M., Pincus, H.A., Wells, K.B., Kessler, R.C. (2006). Changing profiles of service sectors used for mental health care in the United States. American Journal of Psychiatry, 163; 1187-1198.

World Health Organization (2011). Mental Health Atlas. Geneva: WHO.

12

Performance Measurement and Optimization of Resource Allocation in a Health Care System

Artie W. Ng[1,*] and Peter P. Yuen[1,2]
[1]*College of Professional & Continuing Education, The Hong Kong Polytechnic University*
[2]*Department of Management and Marketing*
Hong Kong
China

1. Introduction

1.1 Evolution of performance measurement system in health care organizations

While cost control has been a significant concern in public health care, stakeholders increasingly strive for a more balanced approach in assessing performance delivered by the health care service providers. This movement has been driven by health care organizations in the developed nations over the past two decades. For instance, in reviewing performance measurement and management in public health services of UK and Sweden, Ballentine et al. (1998) studied their performance measurement systems under a period of reform for market-based competition and discussed the challenges to striking the balance between cost control in the back office and delivery of quality service at the front. Moreover, Radnor and Lovell (2003) unveiled cases of balanced scorecard implementation in NHS of the UK that provided significant benefits for meeting national targets for better transparency, clarity and accountability for the stakeholders, including the patients and public in general. Their study suggests an effective use of a performance measurement system to enable focus on measuring long-term qualitative targets whereas the traditional financial reporting system could be biased towards short-term measures.

With implementation of a performance measurement system, healthcare practitioners are driven to make improvement on their accountability to stakeholders. An effective performance measurement system is vital for a healthcare organization to deliver cost-effective and quality services (Moullin, 2004). However, the overemphasis on the measurement of cost could have a significant effect on the delivery of performance by a hospital. Studying the hospital cost benchmarking introduced in National Reference Costing Exercise (NRCE), Llewellyn and Northcott (2005) argued that such increasing reliance on hospital cost benchmarking is promoting "averageness" among the hospital making the "average hospitals" cheaper to run and easier to control than the highly differentiated ones. While these hospitals might perform well on certain measures of service improvement in efficiency, they were transformed to comply closely with the "cost accounting average". All

---

* Coordinating Author

in all, these prior studies revealed the imperative of striving for a balanced performance measurement system that embraces delivery of quality services with efficiency.

2. Improving the utilization of health care resources

2.1 Efficiency in using health care resources

Efficiency in the utilization of health care resources is considered to be an important issue not only to developed countries but also to developing economies. With reference to the report by WHO (2010), there could be trillion dollars of wastage in health care spending due to various forms of human related inefficiency, such as misallocation, mismanagement and fragmented administration. It is recommended that countries should attempt to improve the efficiency of their existing health systems so that they can release resources to cover services to people in need. Improvement in efficiency could be achieved through dealing with the incentive issues inherent in the health financing system as to how services are purchased and providers paid. As noted by WHO (2010), "*All countries can look to improve efficiency by taking a more strategic approach when providing or buying health services, e.g. decide which services to purchase based on information on the health needs of the population and link payments to providers on their performance and to information on service costs, quality and impact.*"

2.2 Potential slack in health care organizations

The concept of budgetary slack has been utilized in the prior studies to explain managerial behavioural issues among profitable organizations. However, such managerial accounting concept is also considered relevant to health care organizations that are non-profit in nature with reliance on public funding. For instance, it was documented in a prior management study that slack could enable innovation and improvement in performance and quality among organizations (Bourgeois, 1981). On the other hand, excess slack could cause unnecessary empire building and demote performance in delivery of services to the end users as referenced to agency theory (Tan and Peng, 2003). For healthcare organizations, a prior study further suggests simultaneous improvement in productivity and quality might not be possible even when slack exists (Miller and Adam, 1995). Although slack could enhance efficiency, such resources might not necessarily help improve responses to externalities, such as quality of customer service (Cheng and Kesner, 1997).

2.3 Optimizing the use of health care resources through performance monitoring

Goddard et al. (2000) examined the myopia that could take place within a healthcare organization due to the adoption of indicators that focused heavily on cost control and were short-term in nature. The study extended that such dysfunctional consequences of cost emphasis would not be optimal for quality. It was also pointed out by Van der Stede (2000) about the relationship between budgetary slack creation and managerial short-term orientation on achieving financial targets. With respect to behavioural issues in managing resources, it was examined in another study that incentives are critical to the success of a performance measurement system (Courty and Marschke, 2003). Without an effective performance measurement and control to deal with concerns of the stakeholders, healthcare service provider would have a higher chance of encountering moral hazard in dealing with slack resources (Daniel et al., 2007).

Given the potential inadequacy of resource utilization, resource optimization needs to be considered as an important objective for health care organizations. On one hand a health care organization needs to contain costs while on the other to deliver proper quality services to the end users. Slack resources could be utilized to enhance quality delivery beyond a short timeframe but could also be treated a "buffer" for achieving a certain planned target.

2.4 Performance of health care systems in developing economies

Performance of a health care system could be driven by the emphasis what it aims to measure and monitor. While the developed nations have spent efforts to broaden their measurement of quality, constraint of resources remains as an area of concern. In developing economies of Asia, their rapid economic developments could have provided them with additional resources allocated to their health care systems. For instance, despite China's rapid economic development in the past two decades, the country's expenditures in public health have remained relatively low in comparison with the developed nations. WHO in fact ranked China's health system as 144th out of 190 countries in areas of quality and access, among other developing nations in 2000. In a prior study, it was pointed out that China's health care reform placed emphasis on the utilization of the social medical insurance system in delivery of health care solutions to her citizens; however, its effectiveness has remained debatable (Lee et al., 2007). As shown Figure 1, the mechanism within such a social medical insurance system focuses on procedural compliance with the health care service providers as well as the financial sustainability of the health system. There appears to be extraneous emphasis on quality through a performance measurement system over the service providers (Lee et al., 2007).

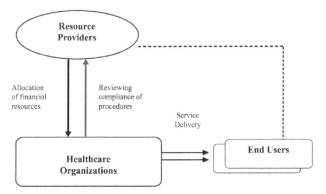

Fig. 1. Resource allocation mechanism (Lee et al. 2007)

Nevertheless, quality performance remains varied in terms of patient satisfaction and outcomes among other developing economies in Asia. In particular, Singapore was ranked 6th in the World Health Organization's ranking of the world's health systems in the year 2000 in terms of overall performance. Hong Kong Special Administrative Region of China (HKSAR) has been ranked as one of the healthiest places in the world reference to life expectancy at birth. The outstanding performance in these two health systems is worth better understanding and a brief review is provided in the following section. The balance between their financial and social sustainability is discussed.

3. Experience of HKSAR and Singapore

3.1 Hong Kong Special Administrative Region (HKSAR)

The Department of Health is HKSAR's agency to execute health care policies and aims to safeguard the health of the community through promotive, preventive, curative and rehabilitative services. In 1991, the government transformed its portfolio of public hospitals into a statutory corporation, the Hospital Authority (HA). The reform denoted an attempt to implement a new management structure for public hospitals and shift the responsibility of operating and managing public hospitals from government bureaucracy to the newly established entity (Cheung, 2002). Major reform measures taken by the HA during the early stage include the organizational restructuring of public hospital systems at both the hospital, region and corporate level with a general management focus; extensive development of information technology and systems; management training and development for staff; the institutionalization of citizens' participation in the management of public hospitals at hospital, regional and corporate levels (Yuen 1991, Yuen 1994, and Yuen and Lieu, 2004).

By 2003, the government further assigned HA with management responsibility of all of the government's primary care general outpatient clinics, which are formerly run by the Department of Health. In assuming responsibility of the clinics, the HA also assumed responsibility for the health of the entire population (Caulfield and Liu, 2006). Under a unified corporate governance structure, HA currently manages 41 hospitals/institutions, 48 Specialist Out-patient Clinics (SOPCs) and 74 General Out-patient Clinics (GOPCs), which are organized into seven regional clusters.

Through this delegation of public health services to HA, the delivery of patient care has been modelled on a cross-functional team approach. Improvement has been observed in the quality of care in public hospital; however, spending has gone up considerably as well. The nature of the mechanisms for accountability for HA and the resulting incentives continued to be mainly driven by the assessment of government officials. HKSAR's Health, Welfare and Food Bureau is responsible for a wide range of health related policy matters, including review of health care delivery and financing systems, development of primary care services, prevention of communicable and non-communicable diseases, as well as provision of hospital services (Yuen and Lieu, 2004).

Direct public funding is provided through an annual subvention mechanism and budgetary control and continues to be the major source of funding for in-patient services. Such funding is however not driven completely by the actual occurrence of services. HA has been receiving its budget directly from the government and serving but also taking the roles of both purchaser and supplier of health services. The dual role of the HA would cause implications about patients' rights and its accountability to the patients. Incentives for performance of the HA were not linked to market exposure (Yip and Hsiao, 2003). As money does not follow patients, there is limited incentive for better service or competition (Yuen & Lieu, 2004).

Although it was expected that the quality of care in public hospital would be improved further after the establishment of the HA, a closer inspection of available evidence revealed that while the physical environment and medical facilities of public hospitals were generally acceptable patients were dissatisfied with the waiting and queuing time in public hospital and clinics.[1] Previous study by Yuen (2004) also indicated that there remained ample room for improvement regarding the quality of care and the attitude of staff in public hospitals. For instance, it was observed that the corporate disclosures by HA revealed that its performance indicators had been focused on the financial aspects of performance with relatively less on the quality ones (Yuen and Ng, 2009). While there is alleged cost efficiency in HKSAR's health care system, the concern about overall quality remains.

In recent years, HKSAR has introduced mechanisms to enhance the resource allocation of funding to its health care system through a performance-driven approach.[2] It was announced by HA's Chief Executive, Shane Solomon, towards end of 2008 that a new internal resource allocation system would be used to renew HA's internal budget allocation system for improved transparency and fairness. The new funding model called "Pay-for-Performance" would link resources with workload while rewarding quality and providing incentive for efficiency. Resource allocation would be driven by a case-mix approach to evaluate the number and complexity of patients treated.

3.2 Singapore

Health care services in Singapore are largely the responsibility of Singapore's Ministry of Health. Singapore has developed a universal healthcare system with emphasis on affordability achieved through compulsory savings and price controls as well as a strong public-private partnership. In fact, its private sector currently plays a significant role in delivery of health care services. Besides its high ranking by the World Health Organization in 2000 for its overall balanced performance, Singapore is among the countries that have attained the lowest infant mortality rate in the world and high life expectancies from birth. Public hospitals in Singapore went through a plan of restructure in the 1990s and were re-organized as government-owned corporations rather than as typical public hospitals in other countries. Unlike the HKSAR's mechanism to form a single, mega health care service organization, Singapore established two major healthcare groups that oversees the operations of restructured hospital: SingHealth and the National Healthcare Group (NHG). In addition, the health care system contains a smaller group affiliated with the National University of Singapore called the National University Health System (NUHS).[3]

With respect to health care financing, Singapore has adopted a system that makes use of a combination of compulsory savings from payroll deductions, a nationalized catastrophic

---

[1] The increase in demand was found not accompanied by increases in resources under an inflexible cost structure. Such constraint in resources can be reflected in the waiting time of public hospital services is long in Hong Kong. The average waiting time for urgent cases to get a first appointment at the Special Out-Patient Clinic (SOPC) was 92 days while 101 days for non-urgent cases. The waiting time of SOPC had been on an increasing trend started from 1999 onwards. The waiting time then varied from 5 to 30 weeks (Soloman, 2006). It was considered relatively long when compared to the OECD average of 2 to 3 months (Hurst and Siciliani, 2003).

[2] Source: http://www.info.gov.hk/gia/general/200811/19/P200811190266.htm

[3] Source: http://www.moh.gov.sg/content/moh_web/home.html

health insurance plan and government subsidies. The deductions from payroll are shared jointly by both employers and employees. To obtain further protection, Singaporeans would purchase supplemental private health insurance on services not covered by the government's schemes. Moreover, the government would actively regulate the supply and prices of healthcare services in the country in order to monitor the associated costs carefully. Singapore has developed a co-financing scheme for its health care system that shares the overall burden and financial risk. Its dynamic regulations over the supply and prices have also made its comprehensive system fairly unique when compared with other countries. For example, people are empowered to seek a suitable service provider from the private sector but required to pay a share of health care service charge regardless of the level of subsidy.

To complement its health care financing approach, Singapore has recognized the importance of reducing information asymmetry between the end users and the health care service providers on quality performance. As advocated by Lim (2005), "*Singapore's regulatory framework should not merely consist of 2 parties, namely the regulator (MOH) and the regulated (public and private providers). It should ideally be tripartite, in which empowered and well-informed consumers play their rightful role in selecting health care providers on the basis of price and quality of care provided. Information asymmetry would not be an insurmountable barrier once the full power of information technology plus the role of the media is brought to bear.*" Such an advocated regulatory framework by Lim (2005) is provided in Figure 2.

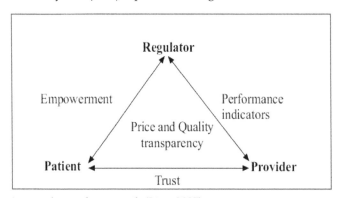

Fig. 2. A tripartite regulatory framework (Lim, 2005)

4. Concluding remarks

As revealed in prior studies, slack could be created when there is rigid budgetary control system and there are certain consequences on the performance delivered by an organization (Bourgeois, 1981; Miller and Adam, 1995; Van der Stede, 2000). A transparent performance measurement system is critical for the stakeholders to monitor quality performance. As a government funded organization, HA of Hong Kong operates under a rather rigid budgetary control culture which reinforces accountability for its cost efficiency and quality of services. However, its mega organizational structure makes monitoring quality performance of its numerous health care entities a challenge and quality transparency with the end-users a difficulty.

Subsequent to HA's incorporation, the organization has been under pressure to strengthen cost efficiency as a publicly funded operation. While cost containment as an important objective that HA has strived to achieve, there is no indication that quality performance expected by the end users has been met. In fact, HA has voluntarily disclosed more cost-related performance indicators than those concerning quality-related, non-financial information. Similar experience is reflected by Daniel et al. (2007) that, lacking an effective performance measurement and control to deal with concerns of the stakeholders, a healthcare service provider could create moral hazard in dealing with slack resources. As a consequence, a phenomenon of "average hospital" that focuses on the cost control might emerge within HA as reflected in a prior study by Llewellyn and Northcott (2005). Hong Kong SAR appears to retain an embedded cost optimization system that operates to maintain acceptable service levels. However, quality performance remains a key concern while there is continuous emphasis on cost containment as the population expands. While prior literatures suggest that not all additional resources could improve performance, an organization needs incentives to better utilize its slack resources towards performance improvement. HA's recently introduced "Pay-for-Performance" incentives with increasing measurement of performance would enable its system to induce optimal use of resources towards pre-determined quality performance targets.

In the case of Singapore, the country proceeds with an increasingly transparent performance measurement system that not only monitors cost efficiency but also quality performance as a key concern among the stakeholders. Performance measurement system plays a critical role in enhancing stakeholders' decision for purchasing services as well as in facilitating the development of a public-private partnership for health care financing that makes the overall health system a relatively more self-sustainable one. Table 1 provides a brief comparison

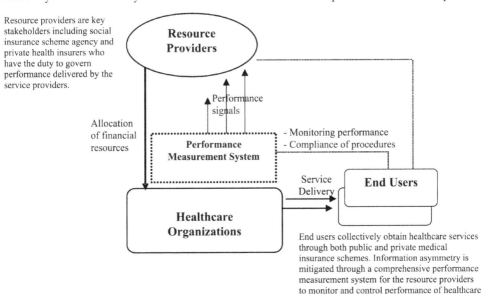

Fig. 3. Enhanced resource allocation mechanism through a balanced performance measurement system (Lee et al. 2007)

	Health care financing	Performance measurement system	Quality improvement initiatives
Hong Kong SAR	- Jointly but separately by public and private sectors - Reliance on a subvention budgetary system to monitor cost efficiency - Advocating self-insured schemes	- Subvention budgetary control measures with disclosures at the corporate level - Emphasis on cost efficiency with selected qualitative data through a high-level corporate disclosures - limited linkage to corporate governance	- Introducing performance-based incentives - External accreditation on hospitals[4]
Singapore	- Well-designed public-private partnership - Multiple sources of funding - Complementary roles and specializations of participants, with active regulatory measures by government	- Extensive disclosures and performance indicators on a range of quality performance by cluster companies[5] - Focusing on both cost efficiency and quality performance - Commitments through corporate governance	- Further focus on quality performance and pertinent indicators - Positioned as the regional hub for health care services

Table 1. Comparison between HKSAR and Singapore in Health Care Financing and Performance Measurement System

between HKSAR and Singapore with respect to health care financing and performance measurement system. It also remarks their initiatives on quality improvement.

In conclusions, this article explores the interplay between resource management for health care service and a balanced performance measurement system within a health care system. Two outstanding health care systems in Asia are reviewed briefly. It argues that an effective health care financing system that empowers the end users to allow financial resources could be enhanced by a transparent performance measurement system that provides relevant information about quality performance of a health care service provider and thereby

---

[4] HA, with the support and collaboration from the Department of Health and Private Hospitals Association in Hong Kong, launched the "Pilot Scheme of Hospital Accreditation" in May 2009 with the following objectives: (i) Establish infrastructure of accreditation, including Standards and Surveyors, (ii) Assess the feasibility of implementing accreditation program, (iii) Enhance public-private collaboration and; (iv) Evaluate and recommend on future model of accreditation in Hong Kong.
[5] For instance, SingHealth discloses clinical outcomes on various measures to track the quality of clinical services provided at its institutions.

reduces information symmetry among the stakeholders (see Figure 3). Second, Singapore has developed a relatively smaller but apparently more optimal corporate structure for her clusters of health care service providers. Such an optimal size facilitates an effective corporate governance function of monitoring performance and accountability for quality when integrated with a balanced performance measurement system.[6] This experience is relevant to other public health care systems that aim to become more effective and responsive to deliver quality health care services.

5. References

Bourgeois, L. (1981) "On the measurement of organizational slack", Academy of Management Review, Vol.6, pp.29-39.

Ballentine, J., Brignall, S. and Modell, S. (1998). "Performance measurement and management in public health services: a comparison of U.K. and Swedish practice", Management Accounting Research, Vol. 9, pp.71-94.

Caulfield, J., and Liu, A. (2006). "Shifting concepts of autonomy in the Hong Kong Hospital Authority." Public Organizational Review, 6, 203-219

Chan, I., and Benitez, M.A. (2006). "Changing Patient Expectations." In G.M. Leung & J. Bacon Shone (eds), Hong Kong's Health System – Reflections, Perspective and Visions, 81-93

Cheng, J.L.C. and Kesner, I.F. (1997) "Organizational slack and response to environmental shifts: the impact of resource allocation patterns", Journal of Management, Vol.23, No.1, 1-18.

Cheung, A.B.L. (2002). "Modernizing public healthcare governance in Hong Kong – A case study of professional power in the New Public Management." Public Management Review, 4, 343-365.

Courty, P. and Marschke, G. (2003) "Dynamics of performance-measurement systems", Oxford Review of Economic Policy, Vol.19, No.2, pp.268-284.

Daniel, F., Lohrke, F.T. and Fornaciari, C.J. (2004) "Slack resources and firm performance: a meta-analysis", Journal of Business Research, Vol.57, pp.565-574.

Goddard, M., Mannion, R. and Smith, P. (2000). "Enhancing performance in health care: a theoretical perspective on agency and the role of information", Health Economics, Vol.9, pp.95-107.

Hurst, J. and Siciliani, L. (2003). Tackling excessive waiting times for elective surgery: A comparison of policies in twelve OECD countries. Retrieved May 18, 2008, from http://www.oecd.org/dataoecd/24/32/5162353.pdf

Lee, S.H., Ng, A.W. and Zhang, K. (2007). "The quest to improve Chinese healthcare: some fundamental issues", International Journal of Health Care Quality Assurance, Vol.20, No.5, pp.416-428.

Lim, M.K. (2005) "Transforming Singapore health care: public private partnership", Annals Academy of Medicine, Vol.34 No.7, pp.461-467.

Llewellyn, S. and Northcott, D. (2005). "The average hospital", Accounting, Organizations and Society, Vol. 30, pp.555-583.

---

[6] For instance, SingHealth - the largest health care cluster in Singapore is incorporated with its own corporate governance structure and oversees only two major public hospitals among other specialty centres and polyclinics. On the other hand, Hong Kong's HA maintains a single board of directors while overseeing seven regional clusters; some of the largest clusters alone contain seven public hospitals.

Miller, J.L. and Adam, E.E. (1996) "Slack and performance in health care delivery", International Journal of Quality and Reliability Management, Vol.13, No.8, pp.63-74.

Moullin, M. (2004), "Eight essentials of performance measurement", International Journal of Health Care Quality Assurance, Vol. 17 No. 3, pp. 1101-12.

Ng, Y.H. (2009), "Complacency led to blunders", South China Morning Post, 24 March.

Radnor Z. and Lovell B. (2003). "Success factor for implementation of the balanced scorecard in a NHS multi-agency setting", International Journal of Health Care Quality Assurance, Vol.16, No.2, pp.99-108.

Solomon, S. (2006). Organizing and managing health Care. Presented at the Medical and Health Research Network International Symposium: Hong Kong's Health System - Reflections, Perspectives and Visions, Hong Kong. Retrieved May 18 2009, from http://www.hku.hk/facmed/mhrn/event/16-17jun2006-prog.html

Tan, J. and Peng, M.W. (2003) "Organizational slack and firm performance during economic transitions: two studies from an emerging economy", Strategic Management Review, Vol.24, pp.1249-1263.

Van der Stede, W.A. (2000) "The relationship between two consequences of budgetary, controls: budgetary slack creation and managerial short-term orientation", Accounting Organizations and Society, Vol.23 No.5, pp.609-622.

Yip W.C. and Hsiao, W.C. (2003). "Autonomizing a Hospital System: Corporate Control by Central Authorities in Hong Kong. In A.S. Preker & A. Harding (eds). Innovations in Health Service Delivery: The Corporatization of Public Hospitals, 391-424. Washington DC: World Bank.

Yuen, P. (1991). "The Implications of the Corporatization of Health Care Delivery in Hong Kong". The Asian Journal of Public Administration, 13, 23-38.

Yuen, P. (1994). "The Corporatization of Public Hospital Services in Hong Kong: A Possible Public Choice Explanation" The Asian Journal of Public Administration, 16, 165-182.

Yuen, P.P. (1999) "Health care financing in Hong Kong: a case for tax-based financing", International Journal of Health Planning and Management, Vol.14, pp.3-18.

Yuen, P. (2004)."The consequence of health care reform impasse. Lessons from Hong Kong." Retrieved May 18, 2009 from
http://swat.sw.ccu.edu.tw/index.php?option=com_jombib&task=showbib &id=738&return=index.php%3Foption%3Dcom_jombib%26amp%3Bcatid%3D117

Yuen P. P. and Gould, D. B. (2006). Priority setting of hospital services: A demonstration project involving clinicians and citizens in Hong Kong. Asian Pacific Journal of Health Management, 1, 30-37.

Yuen P. P. and Lieu, G. (2004). Healthcare reform and the public-private imbalance in Hong Kong: The victim of success. Paper presented in the International Conference on Comparative Health Policy and Reforms in East Asia, Singapore. Retrieved May 18, 2009 from
www.ari.nus.edu.sg/showfile.asp?eventfileid=183_September2004Conf.pdf.

Yuen, P.P. and Ng, A.W. Diagnostic use of performance measurement system after corporatization: case study of the Hospital Authority. Paper presented at Public Policy Research Institute Forum III, The Hong Kong Polytechnic University, Hong Kong, June, 2009.

WHO (2010). The World Health Report: Financing for Universal Coverage.

Permissions

The contributors of this book come from diverse backgrounds, making this book a truly international effort. This book will bring forth new frontiers with its revolutionizing research information and detailed analysis of the nascent developments around the world.

We would like to thank Oreste Capelli, for lending his expertise to make the book truly unique. He has played a crucial role in the development of this book. Without his invaluable contribution this book wouldn't have been possible. He has made vital efforts to compile up to date information on the varied aspects of this subject to make this book a valuable addition to the collection of many professionals and students.

This book was conceptualized with the vision of imparting up-to-date information and advanced data in this field. To ensure the same, a matchless editorial board was set up. Every individual on the board went through rigorous rounds of assessment to prove their worth. After which they invested a large part of their time researching and compiling the most relevant data for our readers. Conferences and sessions were held from time to time between the editorial board and the contributing authors to present the data in the most comprehensible form. The editorial team has worked tirelessly to provide valuable and valid information to help people across the globe.

Every chapter published in this book has been scrutinized by our experts. Their significance has been extensively debated. The topics covered herein carry significant findings which will fuel the growth of the discipline. They may even be implemented as practical applications or may be referred to as a beginning point for another development. Chapters in this book were first published by InTech; hereby published with permission under the Creative Commons Attribution License or equivalent.

The editorial board has been involved in producing this book since its inception. They have spent rigorous hours researching and exploring the diverse topics which have resulted in the successful publishing of this book. They have passed on their knowledge of decades through this book. To expedite this challenging task, the publisher supported the team at every step. A small team of assistant editors was also appointed to further simplify the editing procedure and attain best results for the readers.

Our editorial team has been hand-picked from every corner of the world. Their multi-ethnicity adds dynamic inputs to the discussions which result in innovative outcomes. These outcomes are then further discussed with the researchers and contributors who give their valuable feedback and opinion regarding the same. The feedback is then collaborated with the researches and they are edited in a comprehensive manner to aid the understanding of the subject.

Apart from the editorial board, the designing team has also invested a significant amount of their time in understanding the subject and creating the most relevant covers. They scrutinized every image to scout for the most suitable representation of the subject and create an appropriate cover for the book.

The publishing team has been involved in this book since its early stages. They were actively engaged in every process, be it collecting the data, connecting with the contributors or procuring relevant information. The team has been an ardent support to the editorial, designing and production team. Their endless efforts to recruit the best for this project, has resulted in the accomplishment of this book. They are a veteran in the field of academics and their pool of knowledge is as vast as their experience in printing. Their expertise and guidance has proved useful at every step. Their uncompromising quality standards have made this book an exceptional effort. Their encouragement from time to time has been an inspiration for everyone.

The publisher and the editorial board hope that this book will prove to be a valuable piece of knowledge for researchers, students, practitioners and scholars across the globe.

List of Contributors

Catherine Ogilvie and Edward Fitzsimons
Department of Haematology, Gartnavel General Hospital, Glasgow, UK

Josephine Emole
University of Texas Health Center at Houston, Houston, Texas, USA

Elisabetta Rovatti
Dept. of Pneumology – University Hospital – University of Modena and Reggio Emilia, Italy

Oreste Capelli and Antonio Brambilla
The District Primary Care, Emilia-Romagna Region, Bologna, Italy

Maria Isabella Bonacini
Pharmacy Department, Derriford Hospital, Plymouth NHS Trust, UK

Imma Cacciapuoti
Dpt. of Mental Health, Modena, Italy

Peter Montnemey and Sölve Elmståhl
Lund University, Sweden

Andrew P. Coveney
Department of Vascular Surgery, Cork University Hospital, Cork, Ireland

Kirtan Ganda and Markus J. Seibel
Bone Research Program, ANZAC Research Institute, The University of Sydney at Concord Campus, Sydney, Australia

Susan Kirsh, Renée Lawrence, Lauren Stevenson, Sharon Watts, Kimberley Schaub, David Aron, Kristina Pascuzzi, Gerald Strauss and Mary Ellen O'Day
Louis Stokes Cleveland Veterans Affairs Medical Center, USA

Heike S. Englert
University of Applied Sciences Muenster, Department of Nutritional Sciences, Germany

Hans A. Dieh
Lifestyle Medicine Institute, Loma Linda, CA, USA

Roger L. Greenlaw
Center for Complementary Medicine, SwedishAmerican Health System, Rockford, IL, USA

Steve Aldana
Lifestyle Research Group, Mapleton, UT, USA

Imma Cacciapuoti
Dpt. of Mental Health, Modena, Italy

Laura Signorotti
Dpt. of Prevention, Novara, Italy

Maria Isabella Bonacini
Pharmacy Department, Derriford Hospital, Plymouth NHS Trust, UK

Oreste Capelli, Maria Rolfini and Antonio Brambilla
The District Primary Care, Emilia-Romagna Region, Bologna, Italy

Alex Müller
University of Cape Town, South Africa

Russell H. Searight
Department of Psychology, Lake Superior State University, USA

Artie W. Ng
College of Professional & Continuing Education, The Hong Kong Polytechnic University, Hong Kong, China

Artie W. Ng and Peter P. Yuen
Department of Management and Marketing, Hong Kong, China

Printed in the USA
CPSIA information can be obtained
at www.ICGtesting.com
JSHW011442221024
72173JS00004B/911